ITI Treatment Guide
Volume 15

Stefan Wolfart
Bilal Al-Nawas

International Team
for Implantology

Managing Fully Edentulous Patients

EDITORS
Daniel Wismeijer
Stephen Barter
Nikolaos Donos

QUINTESSENCE PUBLISHING

Berlin | Chicago | Tokyo
Barcelona | London | Milan | Paris | Prague | Seoul | Warsaw
Beijing | Istanbul | Sao Paulo | Sydney | Zagreb

The German National Library has listed this publication in the German National Bibliography. Detailed bibliographical data are available at https://dnb.ddb.de.

A CIP record for this book is available from the British Library.
ISBN 978-1-78698-132-5

QUINTESSENCE PUBLISHING DEUTSCHLAND

Ifenpfad 2–4
12107 Berlin
Germany
www.quintessence-publishing.com

Quintessence Publishing Co Ltd
Grafton Road, New Malden
Surrey KT3 3AB
United Kingdom
www.quintessence-publishing.com

Illustrations: Ute Drewes, Basel (CH), www.drewes.ch
Copyediting: Triacom Dental, Barendorf (DE), www.triacom.com
Layout | Production: Janina Kuhn, Berlin (DE)
Printer: Grafički zavod Hrvatske
Mičevečka ulica 7
HR-10000 Zagreb, Croatia
www.gzh.hr

Printed in Croatia
ISBN 978-1-78698-132-5

The tooth identification system used in this ITI Treatment Guide is that of the FDI World Dental Federation.

The ITI Mission is …

"… to empower dental professionals globally through a collaborative network, cutting-edge education, innovative research, and to cultivate leaders committed to evidence-based practices."

Acknowledgement

The authors would like to express their gratitude to Dr. Kati Benthaus for her excellent support in the preparation and coordination of this Treatment Guide. We would also like to thank Ms. Ute Drewes for the professional illustrations, Ms. Janina Kuhn (Quintessence Publishing) for the typesetting and Ms. Änne Kappeler (Quintessence Publishing) for the coordination of the production workflow and Mr. Per N. Döhler (Triacom Dental) for the language editing.

Preface

The use of dental implants to provide edentulous patients with better function, comfort, and appearance, can also result in considerable improvements in the confidence and self-esteem of this patient group. When such treatment is carefully planned and executed, the resulting psychosocial benefit could be truly life changing. This makes the successful treatment of the edentulous patient one of the most satisfying treatment options for both patient and clinician.

The possibilities for treatment range from the simplest to highly complex. Since the McGill Consensus Conference 2002, the implant-supported overdenture has been accepted as the basic treatment of choice for edentulous patients. As both experience and research have shown us, we are not limited to standard implants; short, narrow, tilted/angled, or even zygoma implants can all be used when treating the edentulous patient to provide complete fixed reconstructions.

The challenges in all such treatments are often substantial; the changes in volume and morphology of both hard and soft tissues, as well as facial appearance, present with a number of factors to be considered. Treatment planning is as important as ever, but equally important is the need to explain to and decide with the patient how best their needs and expectations can be fulfilled.

To help the clinician in the decision-making process, this Volume 15 of the ITI Treatment Guide series introduces the "Patient Profile": a tool that can be used in finding the best option for each individual patient.

In addition, as we move further into an increasingly digital therapeutic environment, technologies that can be used to improve the quality of treatment, with potential reductions in complexity, risk, cost, and morbidity, are also discussed.

Successful treatment is not produced at the delivery of the final prosthesis; the benefits described, together with potential overall health benefits from improved function and a better diet, are measured over years and decades. How the outcomes of treatment will endure as the patient ages and becomes less able to manage the essential home-performed maintenance, will be key considerations if we are to prevent dental disability later in life.

Based on the clinical recommendations of the 6th and 7th ITI Consensus Conferences in Amsterdam (2018) and Lisbon (2023), in this Volume 15 of the ITI Treatment Guide series the reader will find step-by-step clinical cases based on the available evidence, performed by experts in the field, focussing on the various up-to-date treatment options in order to successfully treat edentulous patients.

D. Wismeijer   S. Barter   N. Donos

Editors and Authors

EDITORS

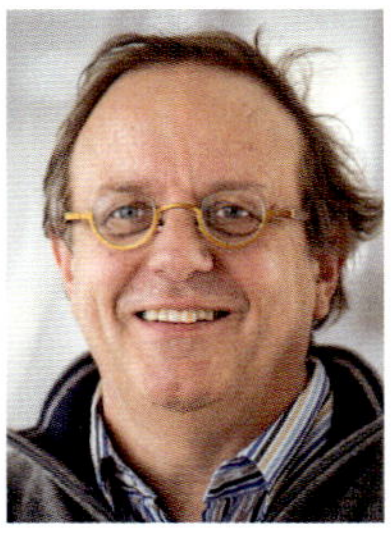

Daniel Wismeijer, Prof, DMD, PhD
Referral Practice for Oral Implantology and Prosthetic Dentistry
De Veluwezoom
p/a Zutphensestraatweg 26
6955 AH Ellecom
The Netherlands
danwismeijer@gmail.com

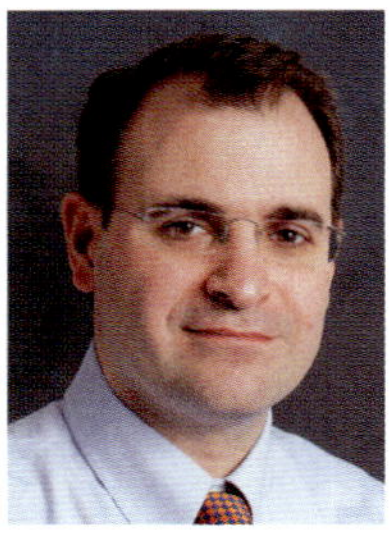

Nikolaos Donos, DDS, MS, FHEA, FDSRCSEngl, PhD
Director of Research
Professor and Chair of Periodontology and Implant Dentistry
Head of Clinical Research
Centre for Oral Clinical Research
Institute of Dentistry
Faculty of Medicine and Dentistry
Turner Street
London E1 2AD
United Kingdom
n.donos@qmul.ac.uk

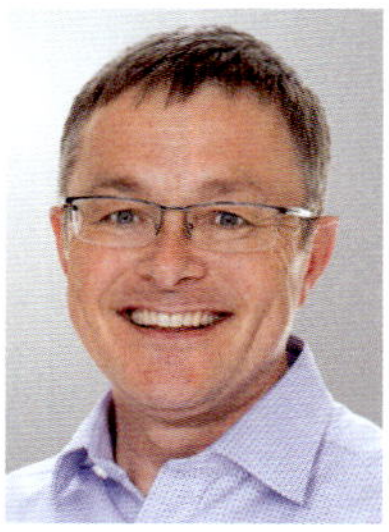

Stephen Barter, BDS, MSurgDent, RCS
Specialist in Oral Surgery
Honorary Senior Clinical Lecturer / Consultant Oral Surgeon
Centre for Oral Clinical Research
Institute of Dentistry
Faculty of Medicine and Dentistry
Turner Street
London E1 2AD
United Kingdom
s.barter@gmx.com

AUTHORS

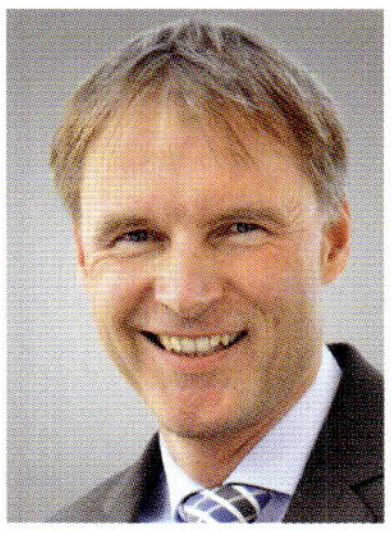

Stefan Wolfart, Univ-Prof, Dr med dent
Head and Chair of the Clinic of Prosthodontics and Biomaterials
Center for Implantology
University Hospital Aachen
Pauwelsstrasse 30
52074 Aachen
Germany
swolfart@ukaachen.de

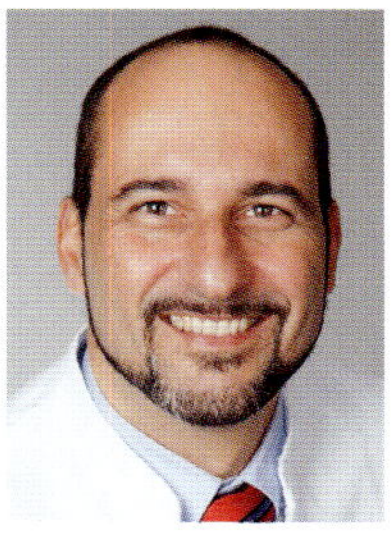

Bilal Al-Nawas, Univ-Prof, Dr med, Dr med dent
Medical Director, Department of Oral, Maxillofacial and Plastic Surgery
University Medical Center of Johannes Gutenberg University
Augustusplatz 2
55131 Mainz
Germany
al-nawas@uni-mainz.de

Contributors

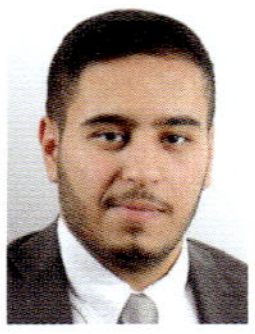

Abdullah Ali A. Alehaideb, DMD, MS, FRCDC
Department of Prosthodontics
Security Forces Hospital
Riyadh
Saudi Arabia
abdullah.alehaideb@gmail.com

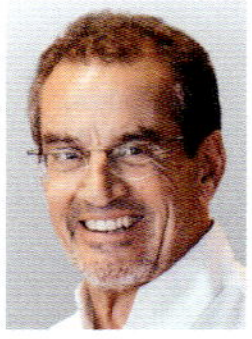

Carlos Aparicio, MD, DDS, MSc, MSc, DLT, PhD
Visiting Research Professor
Indiana University School of Dentistry
Indianapolis, IN 46202
USA

Director of the Zygomatic Unit at Hepler
Bone Clinic, ZAGA Center Barcelona
Roman Macaya 22-24
08022 Barcelona
Spain
carlos.aparicio@zygomaticimplants.org

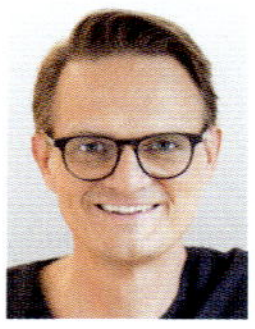

Arne F. Boeckler, Prof Dr med dent habil, DMD, PhD
Zahnzentrum Halle
Lafontainestraße 20
06114 Halle (Saale)
Germany
arne.boeckler@zahnzentrum-halle.de

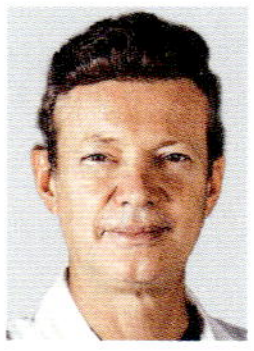

João Caramês, DMD, PhD
Full Professor
Dean of the Faculty of Dental Medicine
Lisbon University
1649-003 Lisbon
Portugal
carames@campus.ul.pt

Implantology Institute
Av. Columbano Bordalo Pinheiro, n° 50
1070-064 Lisbon
Portugal

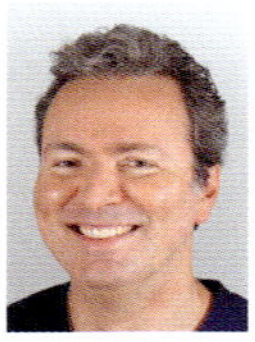

Paolo Casentini, DDS, Dr med dent
Private practice
Studio Dr Paolo Casentini
(Implantology, Oral Surgery, Periodontology, Esthetic Dentistry)
Via Anco Marzio 2
20123 Milan
Italy
paolocasentini@fastwebnet.it

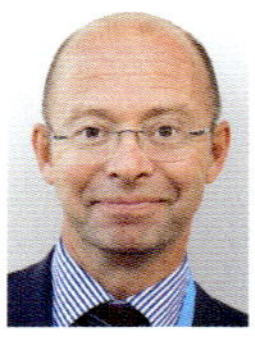

Matteo Chiapasco, MD
Professor, Unit of Oral Surgery
Department of Biomedical, Surgical and Dental Sciences
University of Milan
Via della Commenda 10
20122 Milan
Italy
matteo.chiapasco@unimi.it

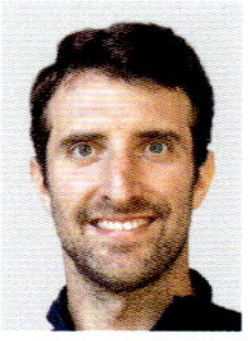

Tommaso Ghedini, DDS, MClinDent Oral Surgery
Adjunct Professor MED School — Humanitas University
Department of Oral Surgery
Humanitas Dental Center
via Rita Levi Montalcini 4
20072 Pieve Emanuele (Milan)
Italy
tommaso.ghedini@hunimed.eu

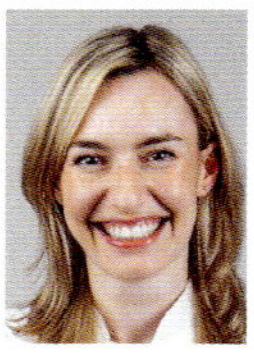

Pauline Gutmann, Dr med dent
Associate Professor
Department of Prosthodontics
Center for Oral Medicine (Carolinum)
Faculty of Medicine at Goethe-University
Theodor-Stern-Kai 7, building # 29
60596 Frankfurt am Main
Germany
gutmann@med.uni-frankfurt.de

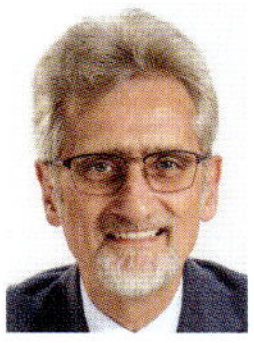

Matthias Kern†,
Prof Dr med dent habil, FADM

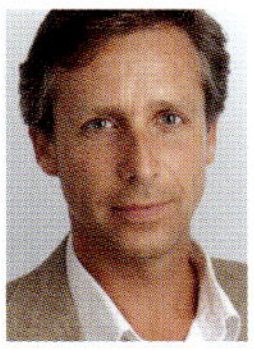

Henny J.A. Meijer, Prof Dr
Department of Oral and Maxillofacial Surgery
and Department of Restorative Dentistry
University Medical Center Groningen
University of Groningen
Hanzeplein 1
9713 GZ Groningen
The Netherlands
h.j.a.meijer@umcg.nl

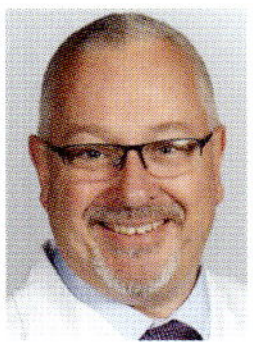

Dean Morton, BDS, MS, FACP
Indiana Dental Association Endowed
Professor, Department of Prosthodontics
Director, Center for Implant, Esthetic and
Innovative Dentistry
Indiana University School of Dentistry
1121 W Michigan Street, DS-S408
Indianapolis, IN 46202
USA
deamorto@iu.edu

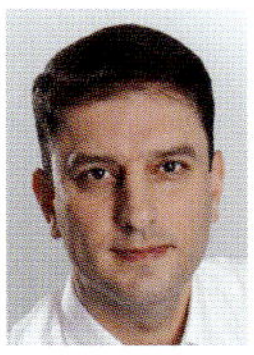

Puria Parvini, Prof Dr med dent habil,
MSc, MSc
Assistant Director
Department of Oral Surgery & Implantology
Center for Oral Medicine (Carolinum)
Faculty of Medicine at Goethe-University
Theodor-Stern-Kai 7, building # 29
60596 Frankfurt am Main
Germany
parvini@med.uni-frankfurt.de

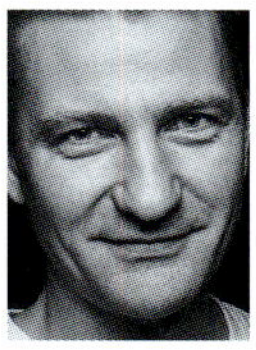

Thorsten Peter, MSc of Dental Technology,
MDT
Head of Department of Dental Technology
Center for Oral Medicine (Carolinum)
Faculty of Medicine at Goethe-University
Theodor-Stern-Kai 7, building # 29
60596 Frankfurt am Main
Germany
t.peter@med.uni-frankfurt.de

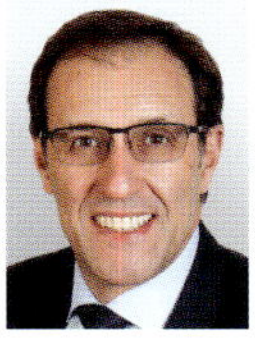

Waldemar D. Polido, DDS, MS, PhD
Clinical Professor, Department of Oral and
Maxillofacial Surgery and Hospital Dentistry
Co-Director, Center for Implant, Esthetic and
Innovative Dentistry
Indiana University School of Dentistry
1121 W Michigan Street, DS 109
Indianapolis, IN 46202
USA
wdpolido@iu.edu

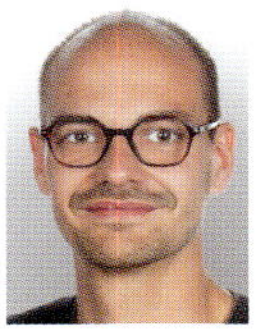

Clemens Raabe, Dr med dent, MAS
Senior Oral Surgeon and Lecturer
Department of Oral Surgery and Stomatology
School of Dental Medicine
University of Bern
Freiburgstrasse 7
3010 Bern
Switzerland
clemens.raabe@unibe.ch

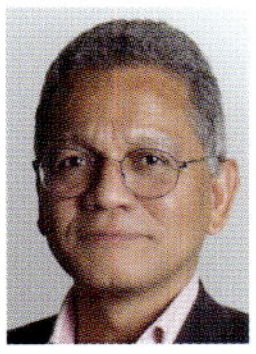

Gerry M. Raghoebar, DMD, MD, PhD
Department of Oral and Maxillofacial Surgery
University of Groningen
University Medical Center Groningen
Hanzeplein 1
9713 GZ Groningen
The Netherlands
g.m.raghoebar@umcg.nl

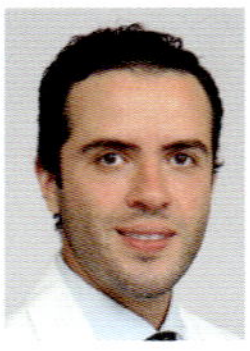

Said Arturo Sánchez, DDS
Specialty in Prosthodontics and Implant Surgery
Private Practice, ProstoPerio Grupo Dental
37130 León
Mexico

Clinical Professor and lecturer
La Salle Bajío University
3602 Juan Alonso de Torres
37458 León
Mexico
said.arturo.sz@gmail.com

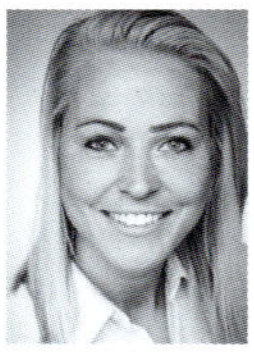

Nicole Schenk, Dr med dent, MAS
Department of Reconstructive Dentistry and Gerodontology
School of Dental Medicine
University of Bern
Freiburgstrasse 7
3010 Bern
Switzerland
nicole.schenk@unibe.ch

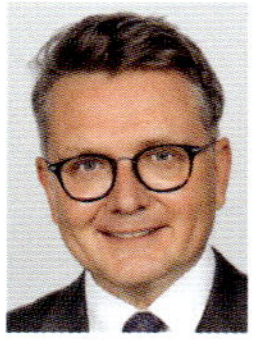

Martin Schimmel, Prof Dr med dent, MAS Oral Biol
Chairman, Department of Reconstructive Dentistry and Gerodontology
School of Dental Medicine
University of Bern
Freiburgstrasse 7
3010 Bern
Switzerland
martin.schimmel@unibe.ch

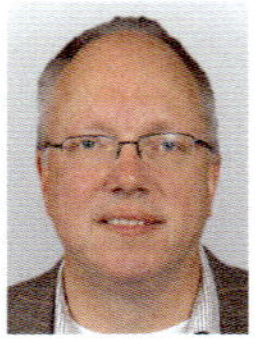

Wim Slot, DMD, PhD
University Medical Center Groningen
Oral Surgery and Implantology
Center for Dentistry and Oral Hygiene
Antonius Deusinglaan 1
9713 AV Groningen
The Netherlands
j.w.a.slot@umcg.nl

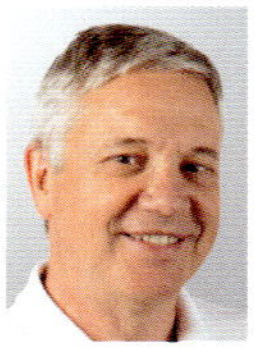

Paul Weigl, Dr med dent, PhD
Head of Department of Postgraduate Education
Head of Department of Medical Technology Research
Center for Oral Medicine (Carolinum)
Faculty of Medicine at Goethe-University
Theodor-Stern-Kai 7, building # 29
60596 Frankfurt am Main
Germany
weigl@em.uni-frankfurt.de

Table of Contents

1 Introduction

S. Wolfart, B. Al-Nawas

The dental health of the population has improved continuously over the past decades. Global disparities in dental health are shaped by access to care, socioeconomic status, public health policies, and cultural factors. While high-income countries have made considerable progress in reducing dental diseases and improving care, many low- and middle-income countries still face serious challenges. In Germany, for example, the proportion of completely edentulous patients in the 65–74 age group decreased from 23% in 2005 to 12% in 2014 and to 5% in 2025 (Micheelis and Schiffner 2006; Jordan and Micheelis 2016; Jordan and coworkers 2025).

In contrast to this, in middle and low-income countries the disease burden of edentulism is high. The World Health Organization (WHO) has estimated that the global prevalence of edentulous adults aged ≥ 60 is 23% (WHO 2023). Many of the factors that contribute to edentulism are preventable and unequally distributed. Globally, patient demand for dental restorations and a good oral health-related quality of life has increased significantly.

Implant treatment options for the edentulous jaw range from implant-supported overdentures to implant-supported fixed restorations. The surgical, prosthetic, and laboratory effort required to place an implant-supported prosthesis varies considerably, depending on the initial clinical/anatomical situation. Extensive augmentation techniques in conjunction with standard implants can be as justified today as the conscious avoidance of augmentation. Short or narrow implants, tilted/angled implants, or zygomatic implants can all be used.

The current surgical and prosthetic treatment options are supported by scientific evidence, resulting in a wide "corridor" for the treatment of the edentulous jaw. Therefore, it is clearly inadequate to consider only the long-term performance and complication rates of different treatment modalities. Instead, patient-related parameters such as the patient's oral health-related quality of life, desires, abilities, and resources must be considered to determine the most appropriate treatment for the individual patient. In high-income countries, the desire for a certain "comfort level" for the patient, i.e., a specific treatment approach, is associated with different levels of invasiveness, treatment time, and cost. The patient's manual dexterity and ability to maintain adequate oral hygiene and care must also be considered. This complex decision-making process is supported in this Treatment Guide by the "patient profile" concept. The decision tree is visually structured by assigning "patient types" to appropriate surgical and prosthetic treatment concepts.

Modern digital technologies, such as CBCT combined with superimposed STL surface data from intraoral scanners, improve the planning accuracy and predictability of surgical and prosthetic treatments. Many contemporary treatment concepts, such as the combination of immediate implant placement and immediate loading, are made more predictable by these technologies. In addition, statically guided implant placement typically reduces surgical time significantly, which can have a positive impact on postoperative discomfort. Three-dimensional planning of the surgical procedure can also make patient education more effective. Last but not least, digital technologies open up new possibilities in dental technology, which can improve the quality of the treatment.

The follow-up and maintenance period begins with the delivery of the implant-supported restoration. Follow-up is often restoration-specific. The clinician should become familiar with the respective maintenance regimen early and communicate it to the patient. In this way, the patient will know what to expect after treatment, and the time and cost involved.

This ITI Treatment Guide aims to systematically discuss the surgical and prosthetic rehabilitation of edentulous patients with dental implants on the basis of currently available scientific evidence, with a consistent focus on patient-related outcomes. The necessary differential diagnoses, implant prosthetic planning, and treatment procedures are presented in detail by internationally renowned clinicians as exemplified by actual cases.

The clinical recommendations of the 6th and 7th ITI Consensus Conferences in Amsterdam (2018) and Lisbon (2023) on the edentulous patient have also been incorporated into this Treatment Guide and play a key role in shaping the structure and recommendations of this book.

2 Basic Principles

S. Wolfart, B. Al-Nawas

2.1 Patient Selection

S. Wolfart

2.1.1 Incidence of Edentulism

The global prevalence of edentulism has decreased over the past few decades due to improvements in dental care and preventive measures. However, it is still estimated that approximately 7–20% of the world's adult population is edentulous, with much higher rates among older adults (GBD 2017). At the same time, patient demand for dental restorations and good oral health-related quality of life has increased significantly. Today, complete dentures are associated with unsatisfactory chewing ability, speech problems, psychological distress, and social impairment (Albaker 2013).

There are large regional differences. In wealthier countries, such as the United States, Canada, and Western Europe, the prevalence of edentulism has declined significantly in recent decades. Improved access to preventive dental care, public health initiatives such as fluoridation, and advances in dental treatments have contributed to this decline. For example, in the United States, the prevalence of complete tooth loss among adults aged 65 and older declined from 50% in the early 1960s to approximately 13–15% by the 2010s (CDC 2015). Similar trends have been observed in Australia and New Zealand, where public health interventions, improved oral hygiene, and access to dental services have led to reductions in edentulism rates (AIHW 2016). Norway, Sweden, and Denmark have some of the lowest edentulism rates in the world, due to strong public health systems and access to high-quality dental care. In these countries, edentulism among older adults has declined to 5–10% in recent decades (Pitts and coworkers 2011).

However, in many low-income regions, such as sub-Saharan Africa and parts of South Asia, edentulism is still a significant problem due to limited access to dental care and preventive services. Rural areas and low-income populations are particularly vulnerable, with edentulism rates often exceeding 20–40% among older adults. Countries such as Brazil, despite significant advances in public health and dental care, still report relatively high rates of edentulism among older adults, with rates as high as 20–30% in certain regions.

In Southeast Asian countries such as India, Indonesia, and the Philippines, edentulism remains prevalent, particularly among older adults and low-income populations. Limited access to dental care as well as high rates of dental caries and periodontal disease contribute to higher rates of tooth loss.

The global prevalence of edentulism is steadily declining in high-income countries due to improved access to dental care, preventive measures, and public health interventions. However, edentulism remains a significant problem in low- and middle-income countries, particularly among older adults, rural populations, and low-income groups. Efforts to improve access to dental care, oral-health education, and preventive public-health measures will be critical in reducing global disparities in edentulism.

2.1.2 Patient-Related Metrics and Patient-Related Outcomes

INTRODUCTORY REMARKS

Given the wide range of clinical options, from complete dentures to implant-supported overdentures and implant-supported fixed dental prostheses, it is essential to consider patient-related factors such as quality of life and comfort. In addition, the degree of invasiveness, cost, and time required for each treatment option must be taken into account. Only by considering these aspects can clinical decisions be effectively tailored to meet the unique needs of each individual patient.

Patient-reported outcomes (PROs) are commonly used for such patient-centered outcome analyses. In the medical field, PROs describe health outcomes that come directly from patients without interpretation by another person. These PROs are collected using various patient-reported outcome measures (PROMs), which are the tools used to collect PROs. In dentistry, specific dental patient-reported outcome measures (dPROMs) are used to measure the patient-reported outcomes of dental care (dPROs). However, the terms "dPROs" and "dPROMs" are often used interchangeably (Schimmel and coworkers 2023).

These patient-related measures include satisfaction with oral health or treatment status as well as other non-clinical assessments, such as satisfaction with treatment esthetics, speech, and masticatory function (Lang and Zitzmann 2012; McGrath and coworkers 2012),

METRICS REPORTED IN CLINICAL TRIALS

Messias and coworkers (2022) used the example of the edentulous jaw with removable or fixed restorations to examine how often these metrics have been used in clinical trials since the definition of dPROMs. Implant failure or survival was the most frequently reported outcome (270 studies). Marginal bone levels, technical complications, and clinical parameters (e.g., assessment of peri-implant soft-tissue and implant stability) were also frequently reported. By contrast, patient-related data were evaluated in only 145 studies and function-based assessments in only 40 studies. While quality of life was assessed using validated instruments, patient satisfaction was assessed using a "common-sense" concept of satisfaction. Economic outcomes were least frequently reported (13 studies) (Messias and coworkers 2022).

To gain a better understanding of the impact of different treatment options on patients, the currently available scientific evidence is presented here, organized by treatment options. Due to the anatomical differences, the maxilla and mandible will be considered separately.

COMPLETE DENTURE

In terms of oral health-related quality of life, patients with complete dentures in both jaws are generally less satisfied than patients with only one complete denture in the maxilla or mandible. Difficulty in biting or chewing food was reported by 79% of study participants, a large proportion of whom were embarrassed to eat in front of others. 45% of study participants reported difficulty speaking with the denture (Albaker 2013).

Most studies on the edentulous mandible show significantly better patient satisfaction and better oral health-related quality of life with implant overdentures compared with complete dentures (Assunção and coworkers 2010). In contrast, complete dentures in the maxilla tend to be well accepted by patients (Thomason and coworkers 2007). A systematic review showed that in patients who are generally comfortable with their complete dentures and have a suitable alveolar ridge, an implant overdenture does not significantly improve function, stability, or patient comfort (Andreiotelli and coworkers 2010). This is contradicted by the findings of Zembic and Wismeijer (2014), who demonstrated an improvement in oral health-related quality of life between newly fabricated complete dentures when these were retained via two Locators in the maxilla. In addition, overall satisfaction with the restoration, chewing function, speech, and denture stability improved (Zembic and Wismeijer 2014).

In summary, a complete denture can be considered a reasonable option in the maxilla when anatomic conditions are favorable, but it is usually not an adequate solution in the mandible. Ultimately, financial aspects and resilience factors also influence a patient's decision for or against an implant-supported overdenture as an alternative to a complete denture (Sharka and coworkers 2019).

MANDIBULAR IMPLANT OVERDENTURE

Already in the 1990s, Wismeijer and co-workers (1995, 1997 and 1999) demonstrated that implants improve the support, retention, and stability of mandibular dentures in edentulous patients and improve patient satisfaction. There is now ample evidence that mandibular implant-supported overdentures can result in higher satisfaction, improved quality of life, or other improved dPROs compared to conventional complete dentures (De Bruyn and coworkers 2015). Specifically, an overdenture supported by two interforaminal implants shows improvements regarding comfort, speech, stability, and masticatory function. In terms of esthetic appearance, there was no improvement over the complete denture. There was even a subjective deterioration in oral hygiene (Egido Moreno and coworkers 2021).

Based on existing studies, an overdenture on two implants is considered the first choice for the treatment of the completely edentulous mandible (Feine and coworkers 2002).

To evaluate the appropriate number of implants to support the overdenture in the edentulous mandible, several studies have investigated overdentures supported by no, one, two, or three implants, assessing masticatory function and oral health-related quality of life. Masticatory performance and oral health-related quality of life improved regardless of the number of implants (one, two, three, or four) (Wismeijer 1996). The best masticatory performance was achieved with two implants (Passia and coworkers 2022). A multicenter study with more than 150 patients also showed a significant improvement in both prosthetic satisfaction and masticatory function for the mandible with a single midline implant and a ball attachment (Passia and coworkers 2017a; Passia and coworkers 2017b).

These results are supported by a recent meta-analysis. Support by a single implant results in better oral health-related quality of life and satisfaction compared with a complete denture. Mandibular prostheses supported by either one or two implants showed no significant differences in terms of satisfaction with speech, comfort, esthetics, and social life. However, prostheses supported by two implants showed better masticatory performance (Fu and coworkers 2021).

In an early crossover clinical trial first reported in 2000, 18 edentulous subjects with complaints about their mandibular dentures received two implants and a new denture with magnet, ball, or bar/clip attachments that were placed in random order. At the end of the study, the attachment type of their choice was placed in the overdenture. After 10 years, 7 subjects with a ball and 7 subjects with a bar/clip attachment were available for evaluation. Four subjects were lost to follow up. There was no significant difference in satisfaction between subjects with ball-attachment and bar/clip-retained mandibular overdentures at initial evaluation and after 10 years of function. Patient appreciation of implant-supported dentures was high and remained high over time (Cune and coworkers 2010).

In another crossover study, 30 patients received three different overdentures for 1 year each. Support was provided by either four implants splinted with a bar, two implants splinted with a bar, or two ball attachments. Restorations with two ball attachments were rated equal to or better than bar restorations for most metrics, with the bar on four implants showing the highest retention. After wearing all options, patients reported the highest satisfaction with ball attachments (Burns and coworkers 2011).

MANDIBULAR IMPLANT-SUPPORTED FIXED DENTAL PROSTHESIS

Fixed mandibular restorations were rated better than overdentures in three quality-of-life subscales: functional limitations, physical disability, and physical pain. Fixed restorations also improved satisfaction in terms of comfort, mastication, retention, and stability compared to overdentures. The same was true for overall oral health-related quality of life and patient satisfaction. Only satisfaction with cleanability was better for overdentures (Borges and coworkers 2022). In clinical cases where both options are considered, patient expectations and cost should be the determining factors in deciding which treatment option to choose (Tsigarida and coworkers 2021).

MAXILLARY IMPLANT OVERDENTURE

Removable restorations in the maxilla can be supported on implants using either ball attachments, bar attachments, or telescopic crowns. In situations where only two Locators are used for support, good oral health-related quality of life scores were achieved, but functional limitations can be expected. This may be due to the linear axis of rotation around the two fixtures, which has a detrimental impact on function (Zembic and coworkers 2019). This linear axis primarily causes the denture to tilt during biting with the anterior teeth, which are typically positioned anterior to the alveolar ridge. The more the denture tilts, the more likely it is that the attachments will loosen at the same time.

However, even with an overdenture supported on four implants with Locators, inconsistent results were seen. Within a 5-year observation period, a significant number of implant losses (19%), prosthetic complications (44%), and refabrications (15%) occurred. After 5 years, oral health-related quality of life deteriorated as a result and returned to the baseline levels achieved with complete dentures (Bouhy and coworkers 2023).

Other studies collected dPROs using only unvalidated patient satisfaction questionnaires. For example, Zou and coworkers (2013) tested different anchorage systems (telescopes, bars, and Locators) supported by four implants each in the maxilla over a 3-year observation period. Patients reported being “completely satisfied” with their restorations in terms of comfort, speech, and function.

Patients treated with bar-supported overdentures on four or six implants reported a significant improvement in terms of prosthetic satisfaction and chewing ability compared with complete dentures (Boven and coworkers 2017; Slot and coworkers 2016; Slot and coworkers 2019).

Anchoring maxillary overdentures on six implants with implant-supported telescopic crowns also resulted in a significant improvement in patient satisfaction compared to baseline with a complete denture. This high level of satisfaction remained stable over the 5-year observation period (Eerdekens and coworkers 2014).

MAXILLARY IMPLANT-SUPPORTED FIXED DENTAL PROSTHESIS

The data for the edentulous maxilla are not as conclusive as for the edentulous mandible. However, there are isolated studies that do not measure oral health-related quality of life but measure patient satisfaction through questionnaires. For example, patients with fixed restorations on six to eight implants for more than 8 years in function reported high overall satisfaction with function, esthetics, speech, and restorations (Mertens and Steveling 2011). Zhang and coworkers (2016) also found excellent patient satisfaction with multi-unit FDPs, 10 years after loading, in terms of esthetics, comfort, masticatory ability, and overall satisfaction.

In the field of immediate restorations, a recent systematic review analyzed the treatment of edentulous patients using the all-on-four concept. The 693 patients included in the review demonstrated high levels of oral health-related quality of life and patient satisfaction (Gonçalves and coworkers 2022).

PALATE-FREE DESIGN FOR REMOVABLE PROSTHESIS

When a patient receives a removable prosthesis, the question arises as to whether the prosthesis should be designed to cover the palate or leave the palate exposed. A covered palate has advantages in terms of inherent and positional stability of the prosthesis. In contrast, a palate-free design supports improved patient articulation, especially for “S”-type sounds

(Fonteyne and coworkers 2019). Taste perception is also rated better by patients (Zembic and coworkers 2015). The clinical implementation of the palate-free design has been successfully implemented with four to six implants and a supporting polygonal framework in some clinical studies (Sadowsky and Zitzmann 2016).

In terms of improved speech function (articulation) and taste perception, a palate-free design is recommended, based on scientific evidence, when four to six well-distributed implants are available to support a removable prosthesis.

REMOVABLE VS. FIXED RESTORATIONS

A recent systematic review compared dPROs regarding implant-supported overdentures and implant-supported fixed restorations from 8 prospective and 5 retrospective studies. In general, the two types of restorations showed no significant differences when comparing dPROs, with a slight trend toward the superiority for fixed restorations. However, conflicting results were observed for aspects such as chewing function, speech function, overall satisfaction, and esthetics (Yao and coworkers 2018). For example, most patients preferred the maxillary removable overdenture to the fixed restoration. This was due to was better speech function and ease of cleaning (Heydecke and coworkers 2003).

In summary, the absolute advantage of fixed or removable implant-supported restorations is not evident from patient-reported metrics, especially since factors such as patient preferences and expectations play a key role (Yao and coworkers 2018).

PATIENT FACTORS AND TREATMENT DECISIONS

The attitude of the edentulous patient is important in the decision for or against an implant-supported restoration. Patients are more likely to choose implant-supported restorations if they explicitly request implant therapy or are unable to adapt to or tolerate a complete denture. Financial aspects and adaptability also influence patient tolerance of both treatment modalities (Sharka and coworkers 2019). Education, income, and patient-perceived quality of life are potential predictors of edentulous patients' preferences for implant rehabilitation. These factors may be important for clinicians to consider when planning treatment for edentulous patients (Leles and coworkers 2019).

LEVEL OF INVASIVENESS TOLERATED BY EDENTULOUS PATIENTS

Particularly in the implant treatment of the edentulous jaw, more invasive augmentation techniques should be weighed against minimally invasive placement techniques, depending on the patient type. In this context, a review article included 37 studies reporting on minimally invasive implant treatment. Patient satisfaction averaged 91% with flapless implant placement, 89% with short implants, 87% with narrow-diameter implants, 90% with a reduced number of implants, 94% with tilted implant placement, and 83% with zygomatic fixtures.

An indirect comparison showed that patients tended to prefer tilted implant placement to a reduced number of implants or to zygomatic implants. Although this comparison did not provide direct evidence of patient preference for minimally invasive treatment alternatives over surgical bone augmentation, it can be concluded that patient satisfaction with non-graft solutions is generally high (Pommer and coworkers 2014).

This underscores the need to balance the use of less invasive treatment approaches with more complex augmentation procedures, often involving extraoral grafts. Three-dimensional radiographs, combined with a prosthesis-oriented set-up, can be valuable in this complex decision-making process (see Chapter 3.1 for details).

CLINICAL RECOMMENDATIONS BASED ON DPROS

In summary, the current data on dPROs in edentulous patients are good, allowing important clinical recommendations to be derived, which were formulated at the 7th ITI Consensus Conference (2023) as follows:

Clinical recommendation 1

In fully edentulous patients, based on dPROs, both complete implant-supported fixed dental prostheses and implant overdentures result in an improvement in stability and comfort compared to complete dentures. For the highest levels of stability, retention, and comfort, complete implant-supported fixed dental prostheses may be recommended over implant overdentures whenever clinically indicated. Clinical decisions should also consider other relevant factors including speech, esthetic concerns, prosthetic space requirements, costs, stability, retention, maintenance requirements, and manual dexterity. Continuous assessment of the patient's ability to manage the prosthesis and maintain plaque control should be performed (Schimmel and coworkers 2023).

Clinical recommendation 2

In fully edentulous patients, both splinted and unsplinted attachments are equally effective from a patient's perspective and can be recommended (Schimmel and coworkers 2023).

Clinical recommendation 3

In fully edentulous patients, mandibular implant overdentures retained by one or two implants show positive effects on dPROs compared to a mandibular complete denture, with two implants being the optimal number. Additional implants do not offer further improvements in dPROs. Based on expert opinion, if the opposing maxilla is dentate or restored with a fully implant-supported prosthesis, more than two standard-diameter implants in strategic positions are recommended to support mandibular implant overdentures to avoid complications and fractures of the implants and prosthetic components. More than two implants are also recommended to enable implant support over mucosal support in compromised anatomical situations (e.g., highly resorbed posterior mandible) and/or compromised mucosal conditions (e.g., hyposalivation) (Schimmel and coworkers 2023).

Clinical recommendation 4

Oral function significantly improves in completely edentulous patients when the mandible is restored using a complete implant-supported fixed dental prosthesis or implant overdenture compared to complete dentures. Therefore, these can be recommended as the best treatment options. The availability of these treatment modalities should be actively promoted in all edentulous communities, including those with limited means or limited access to medical care (Schimmel and coworkers 2023).

Use this code to download the Proceedings of the 7th ITI Consensus Conference (2023)

2.1.3 Patient Profiles

INTRODUCTORY REMARKS

The decision of whether to rehabilitate a patient with fixed or removable implant prostheses cannot be based solely on dPROMs (see Chapter 2.1.2). Such decisions should be guided by the specific anatomy and clinical parameters of the individual case, as well as the patient's needs and wishes. In cases where either treatment is feasible, a proper assessment of the patient's pre-treatment expectations and desires is critical before deciding on a fixed or a removable prosthesis (Feine and coworkers 2018).

To make this assessment, it is necessary to have a comprehensive understanding of the patient, beyond clinical findings and diagnoses. In this context, education, income, and the patient's perceived quality of life are the potential predictors for edentulous patients' preference for implant rehabilitation (Leles and coworkers 2019). In addition, a patient is more likely to choose an implant restoration if he or she explicitly requests implant therapy or cannot adapt to or tolerate a complete denture (Sharka and coworkers 2019).

The sum of these individually weighted patient factors results in the patient profile (Wolfart 2023). It considers the patient's wishes and expectations on the one hand and essential anatomical and general medical factors on the other. The patient profile helps the clinician to guide and moderate this complex decision-making process together with the patient.

The individual components considered in the patient profile are:

Patient wishes and expectations:

1. Resilience (and willingness to undergo invasive procedures, while considering the patient's general health)
2. Function (expectations of the restoration)
3. Retention
4. Esthetics

Patient-related baseline factors:

5. Tissue loss (vertical and horizontal)
6. Financial resources
7. Individual risk of implant loss

When evaluating the patient profile, it is important to also assess the esthetic, surgical, and prosthetic risks using the SAC classification for edentulous patients in implant dentistry (Dawson and coworkers 2022). To fully inform the patient, it is necessary to consider their wishes and options as well as the SAC risk assessment and the level of surgical and prosthetic difficulty. Based on this information, a joint decision can be made regarding the most suitable treatment plan. The SAC classification can help determine whether the clinician can meet the surgical and prosthetic demands or whether specialist intervention may be required. See Table 1 for more information.

MAIN ASPECTS OF THE PATIENT PROFILE

Resilience: Since patients usually have limited knowledge of the surgical procedures involved in oral implantology, they should be provided with a clear description of the duration and invasiveness of the procedure, and of the expected degree and duration of postoperative discomfort. A subjective evaluation of this factor should also include the patient's age, morbidity, and any additional measures associated with the procedure, such as endocarditis prophylaxis or anticoagulant therapy (Wolfart 2023). Measures to reduce exogenous stress, e.g., by providing a quiet surgical environment, good planning, and empathic perioperative care are important, especially since the patients concerned are often elderly. Targeted sedation, the use of anti-inflammatory medications, and preventive pain management have also been shown to be effective in reducing stress. By incorporating flapless implantation techniques, the use of short, narrow, or angled implants, or zygomatic implants, augmentation can be avoided, and patient distress may be reduced. Similarly, the treatment burden can be reduced by providing fewer implants and an implant-supported overdenture.

Function: Functional aspects in edentulous patients mainly relate to the question of whether they can accept a removable implant-supported overdenture or whether they prefer an implant-supported fixed restoration. In the case of removable restorations, the number of implants and the retention element used are important, because both have a direct influence on the stability of the prosthesis and are therefore relevant to the functionality of the prosthesis. In the case of fixed restorations, the question is whether a shortened dental arch up to the second premolar is advisable, or whether the masticatory function must be maintained up to the first molar.

Retention: A distinction must be made here between supportive function and fixed support without mobility, which in part determines the type of retention element(s) used. Bar attachments and telescopic crowns can achieve very rigid anchorage, giving the patient the feeling of having "fixed teeth again." Stud attachments such as ball, Locator or Novaloc attachments, on the other hand, usually exhibit a certain amount of movement, which gives the patient the feeling of a "fixed prosthesis," but not the feeling of having fixed teeth. In addition to this patient preference, the required vertical height of the prosthesis and the parallelism of the implants also influence the choice of the retention element. The smaller the vertical distance to be bridged and the more parallel the implants are placed, the more suitable the stud attachments systems are for the restoration. In the other case, bar attachments or telescopic crowns are more appropriate.

Esthetics: In edentulous patients, esthetic considerations may influence the decision to use a fixed or removable restoration. Three examples are given in the following:

- For example, if a patient insists on maximum dental and (artificial) gingival esthetics, ceramic restorations will be required, but these can only be achieved with fixed full-arch restorations.
- On the other hand, if the vertical tissue loss is extensive, the missing soft and hard tissues can be esthetically reconstructed with pink acrylics using removable overdentures. Improved lip support is also easier to achieve with overdentures.
- Another important aspect is the visibility of the transition between the natural soft tissue and the artificial gingiva. If this transition is visible while laughing, it can reveal the restoration as artificial. This can be concealed with a removable prosthesis that includes a labial pink plastic saddle, for example. Alternatively, during implant placement, reducing the alveolar ridge in an inconspicuous area is a possible approach for fixed restorations; however, this procedure is questionable due to its high invasiveness.

Tissue loss: The extent of the vertical tissue loss determines whether vertical bone augmentation is necessary or whether the existing tissue loss can be prosthetically compensated (see Chapter 3.5). The latter may be a strong indication for an implant overdenture, which can compensate for any tissue loss much more easily than a fixed prosthesis.

Financial aspects: The financial aspects depend on the patient's social situation, insurance coverage, and specific choices. Especially in the case of edentulous patients, planning implant overdentures rather than complete implant-supported fixed dental prostheses provides a wide margin of maneuver in terms of treatment costs.

Risk: To assess the individual risk of implant loss, it is necessary to analyze the patient's medical history regarding certain concomitant general medical factors (see Chapter 2.2). In addition, factors such as smoking, a history of periodontitis, and patient resilience (oral hygiene) are considered here.

PRESENTATION OF THE PATIENT PROFILE

The seven factors of the patient profile are each presented as a scale with a low and high endpoint (see Fig 3). Each of the seven scales has four levels (low, moderate, moderately high and high). This effectively consolidates all the data for parameters important for treatment planning, making them easily assessable and readable at a glance.

PATIENT PROFILE AND PROSTHETIC APPROACH

An individual patient profile can be created for each patient. This profile can be used to make different recommendations regarding surgical procedures and the number of implants. Most importantly the profile largely determines the most appropriate prosthetic approach (see Table 3, Chapter 3.6). It thus supports the clinical recommendation of the 6th ITI Consensus Conference (2018) that the planned final prosthesis should be considered when determining the surgical treatment of the edentulous jaw (Morton and coworkers 2018).

At the same time, the concept of the patient profile makes it clear in principle that as soon as individual parameters in the evaluated profile change significantly, the most suitable dental prosthesis for this patient will also change (see Table 3, Chapter 3.6).

THE SAC CLASSIFICATION IN THE EDENTULOUS JAW

The patient profile provides an initial assessment of the individual prosthetic restoration concept (see Chapter 3.6). The degree of esthetic, surgical, and prosthetic difficulty associated with the clinical situation should be recorded in parallel (see Chapters 5.3, 5.7, and 5.9 for detailed patient examples).

Table 1 Edentulous esthetic risk assessment (EERA) (The SAC Classification in Implant Dentistry; Dawson and coworkers 2022).

Esthetic risk factors - Edentulous	**Level of risk**		
	Low	**Medium**	**High**
Arch	Mandible		Maxilla
Facial support (fixed)	Alveolar process provides adequate facial support	Minimal changes tolerated by the patient	Flange required for adequate facial support
Facial support (removable)	Flange provides adequate facial support	Minimal changes tolerated by the patient	Insufficient space for a flange
Labial support	Designed tooth position provides satisfactory labial support	Minimal changes tolerated by the patient	Designed tooth position causes unsatisfactory labial support
Upper lip length	Long upper lip (> 20 mm)		Short upper lip (< 20 mm)
Buccal corridor* (atrophic ridge)	Removable prosthesis		Fixed prosthesis
Smile line	No display of the ridge(s) at full smile (maxilla or mandible)		Display of the ridge(s) at full smile (maxilla or mandible)
Maxillomandibular relationship	Class I	Class II	Class III

*Desired narrow corridor in definitive prosthesis.

The introduction of the SAC classification for edentulous patients in implant dentistry (Dawson and coworkers 2022) has provided a valuable tool for this purpose. It encompasses both a general risk assessment and a specific esthetic risk assessment. As an illustration of the intricacy of the assessment, the individual decision criteria and categorization of esthetic risk levels in edentulous patients are presented in Table 1.

Furthermore, the case is classified as straightforward (S), advanced (A), or complex (C) based on anatomical and specific surgical and prosthetic factors. This classification is made separately for surgery and prosthetics. The use of the SAC classification is exemplified in the case presentation in Chapter 5.9. In general, the risk for each clinical case can be assessed using the ITI's online SAC Assessment Tool.

Use this code to access the online SAC Assessment Tool.
The online SAC Assessment Tool takes you through each step necessary to identify the degree of complexity and potential risk involved in individual clinical cases.

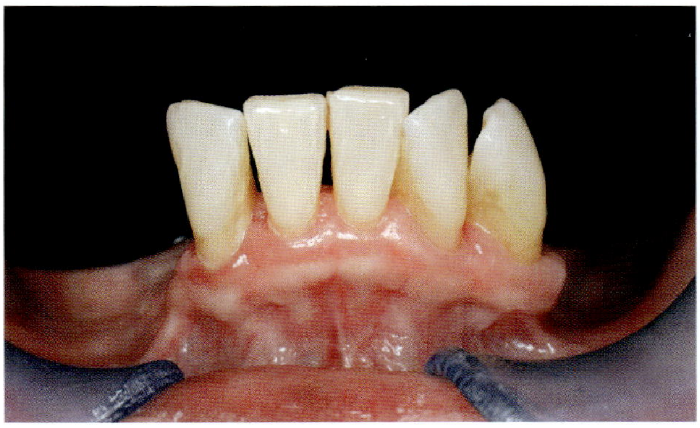

Fig 1 Initial situation: Residual mandibular dentition.

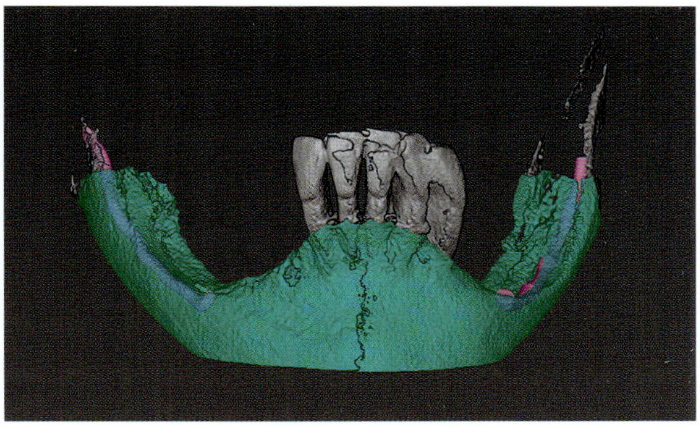

Fig 2 Initial situation: CBCT analysis of the mandible. The CBCT showed a significant difference in bone height between the highly atrophic posterior region and the mandibular residual dentition.

CLINICAL EXAMPLE: PRACTICAL APPLICATION OF A PATIENT PROFILE

A 67-year-old female patient had no teeth left in the maxilla and was wearing a complete denture, which she tolerated very well. A few periodontally compromised residual teeth were present in the anterior mandible. The difference in the vertical dimension between this region and the very severely atrophied posterior region was considerable (Figs 1 and 2). Due to this difficult anatomical situation, the patient was very dissatisfied with her current mandibular prosthesis with its cast-metal framework. The prosthesis was unstable during chewing. The patient complained of "stabbing nerve pain" in the posterior region when chewing. This was immediately attributed to impaction of the mental nerve, as the mental foramina were located almost directly on the severely atrophied alveolar ridge.

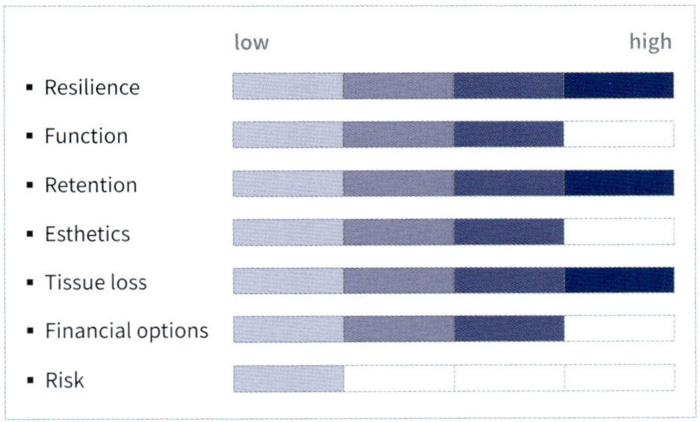

Fig 3 Patient profile of the 67-year-old patient.

The patient was a retiree who reported that she had saved a considerable amount of money in her life: she said that financial considerations "should only play a subordinate role in treatment planning for now." She wanted a restoration that provided a significant functional improvement, was free of phonetic restrictions and was esthetically pleasing and in harmony with her youthful appearance. She stated emphatically that she was willing to go to great lengths to try and improve her quality of life, which had been severely compromised by her difficult oral situation.

There were no general medical conditions that would have increased the risk of implant loss. The patient did not smoke. Her oral hygiene was good. Only the presence of periodontitis indicated an increased risk of implant loss.

The initial consultation provided the clinician with the information needed to establish the patient profile (Fig 3).

Resilience: Based on her very good general health, the patient's athletic appearance, her assertion that she was ready to make a great effort to achieve her goal, and her unremarkable general medical history, her resilience was rated as high (level 4).

Function: Based on the patient's comments and the fact that she was satisfied with the function of her maxillary complete denture and did not want any other type of restoration, it was clear that the patient would be satisfied with a significant improvement in the function and esthetics of her mandibular prosthesis. Her functional expectations were rated as moderately high (level 3).

Retention: The patient had been dissatisfied with the retention of the mandibular partial denture for years. She wanted a significant improvement in this area. At the same time, the new prosthesis should not exert any pressure on the severely atrophied posterior region in order to prevent the associated nerve pain. Since a secure anchorage of the mandibular prosthesis was therefore an essential wish of the patient, her expectations regarding the retention of the prosthesis were rated as high (level 4).

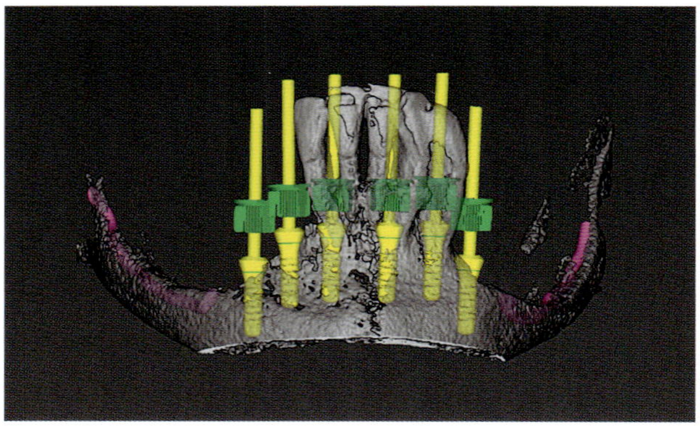

Fig 4 Implant planning, taking into account the narrow alveolar ridge and reducing the large height difference between the anterior and posterior alveolar bone.

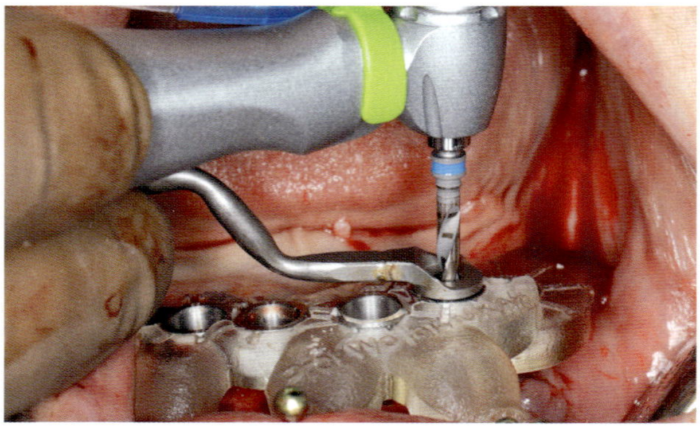

Fig 5 Surgical guide in place. Execution of the drilling protocol with appropriate drill keys and shaping drills.

Esthetics: The patient wanted an esthetic improvement but was not really dissatisfied with her current appearance. In relation to the current situation, the patient's esthetic expectations for her prosthetic restoration were rated as moderately high (level 3).

Tissue loss: The CBCT confirmed a very severe loss of vertical dimension in the posterior mandible (level 4).

Financial aspects: Based on the patient's statement that financial considerations "should only play a subordinate role in treatment planning" and the fact that she had private dental insurance, no major limitations were expected (level 3).

TREATMENT PLAN AS DERIVED FROM THE PATIENT PROFILE

The patient profile shown in Figure 3 was derived from these considerations. Based on this profile, the complete maxillary denture was replaced and a mandibular overdenture supported by six interforaminal implants was fabricated (Figs 4 to 14). In this case, six implants were planned instead of four because the patient wanted absolute assurance that no pressure would be exerted on the posterior region during mastication and that this would be ensured even in the event of implant loss.

In addition to the severe periodontal destruction, the narrow alveolar process in the anterior mandible was unfavorable for the planned implant restoration. The buccal and lingual bone plates were extremely thin, especially in the root area. The vertical bone level needed to be adjusted to ensure a favorable implant distribution while maintaining a clinically acceptable height difference between the implants. For this purpose, the implants were ideally positioned in the CBCT dataset (Fig 4).

After extraction of the remaining mandibular teeth and adjustment of the vertical height of the alveolar ridge, immediate implant placement was performed using a surgical guide (Figs 5 and 6).

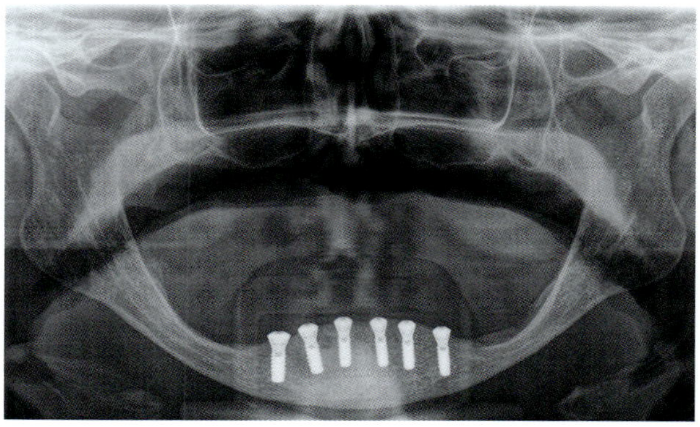

Fig 6 Postoperative panoramic radiograph.

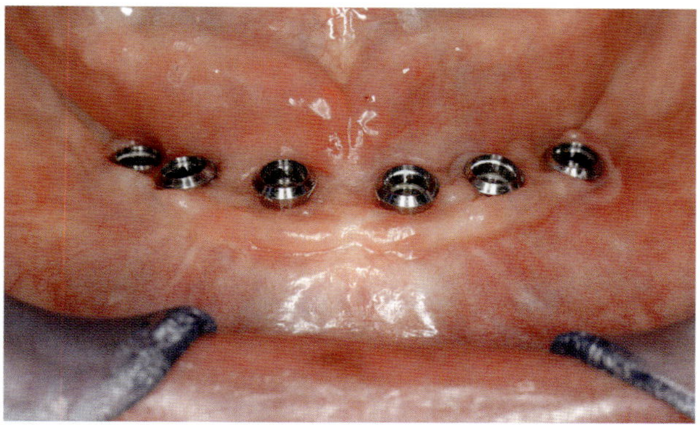

Fig 7 Reentry 3 months after implant placement.

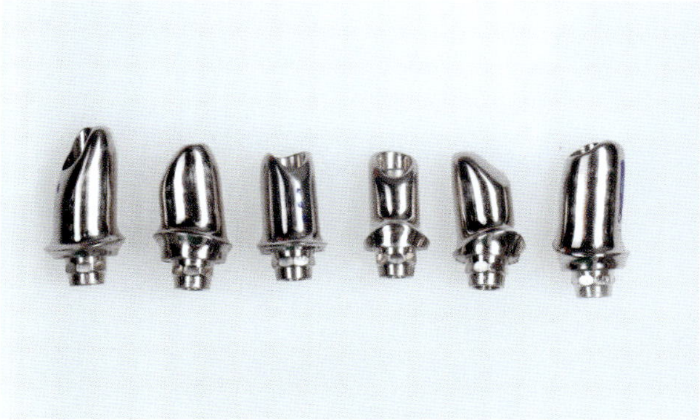

Fig 8 CAD/CAM titanium abutments (milled primary telescopes) before placement.

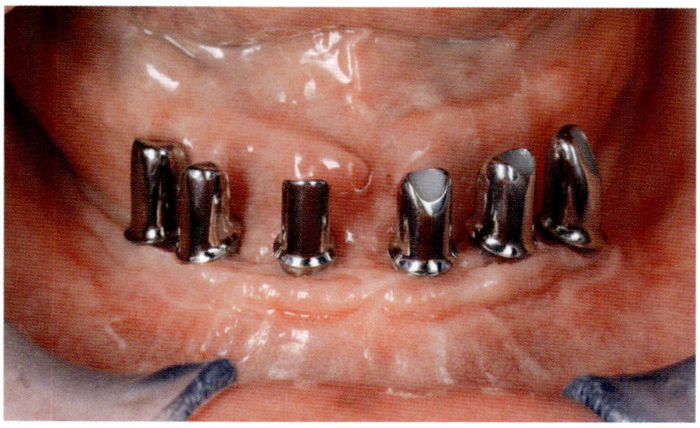

Fig 9 Primary telescopes in place with sealed screw access channels.

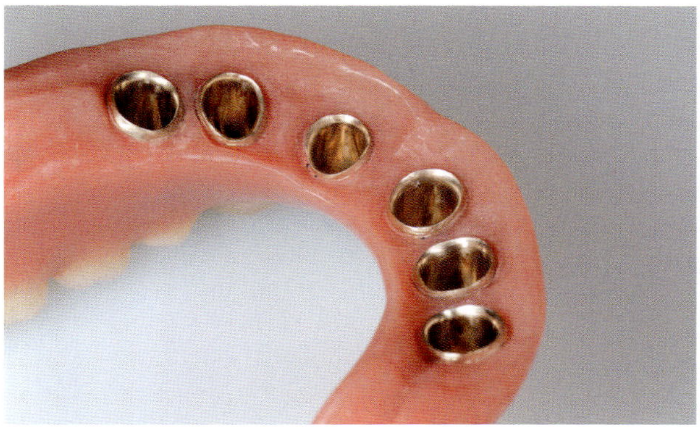

Fig 10 Basal view of the overdenture.

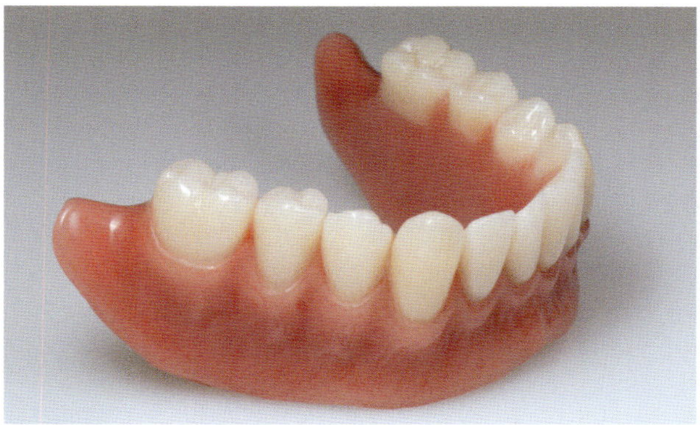

Fig 11 Lateral view of the overdenture.

Re-entry surgery was performed 3 months after implant placement (Fig 7). The implants were restored with a removable overdenture on telescopic crowns (Figs 8 to 12). This restorative concept ensured that the severe vertical tissue loss was compensated in an anatomically appropriate manner. The implants were easy to clean, and the restoration would remain functional even in the event of implant loss, without the need to modify the overdenture.

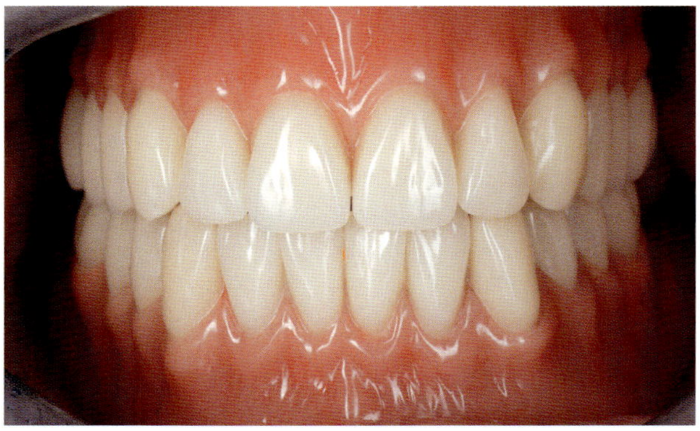

Fig 12 Treatment outcome 3 months after delivery. The maxillary complete denture was also new.

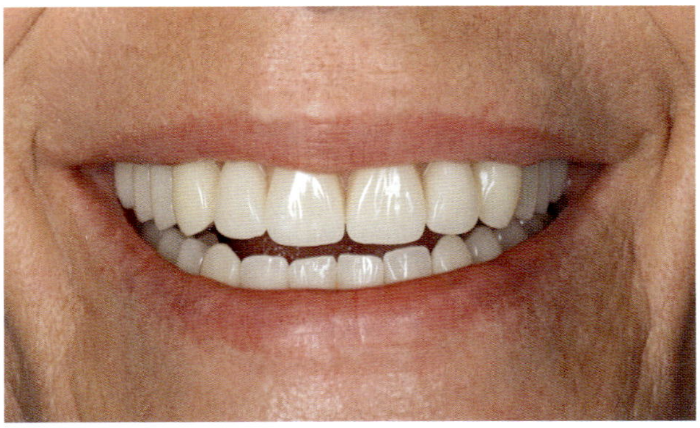

Fig 13 The patient's smile.

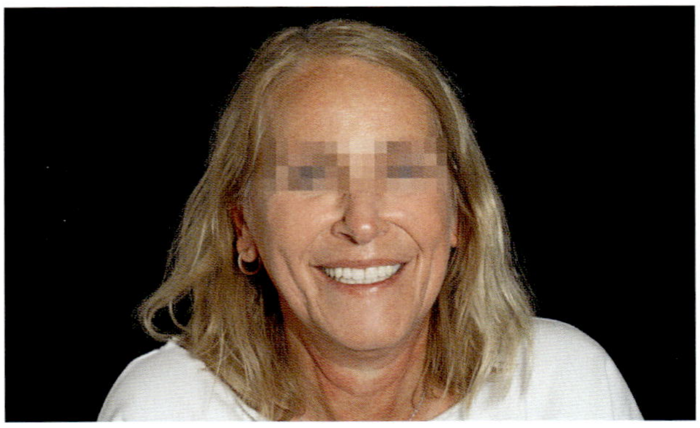

Fig 14 Portrait of a satisfied patient at the 1-year follow up.

At 1 year after delivery, the patient was still very satisfied with the restoration, both with the function of the prostheses and their esthetic appearance (Fig 14).

2.2 Edentulous Patients and Restorative Risks

B. Al-Nawas

The numerical age of a patient does not necessarily correlate with the perioperative risks associated with a given procedure. Similarly, the process of osseointegration is not affected by age (Boboeva and coworkers 2021). Conversely, the number of risk factors increases with age. For example, patients with a mean age of 40 years and older often have more than one risk factor, and patients 70 years and above often have more than two and a half risk factors (Turrentine and coworkers 2006; Barnett and coworkers 2012) (Fig 15).

The most significant risk factor is cardiovascular risk. It is of the utmost importance to objectively assess and document the patient's physical status, in particular his or her exercise capacity, and the ASA classification or metabolic equivalent is an appropriate and practical way to do this. These are validated scores that assess perioperative risk (Table 2) (Abouleish and coworkers 2020). Such a score allows the dentist to objectively assess the patient's physical resilience, facilitating the identification of the most appropriate level of invasiveness for a given dental treatment.

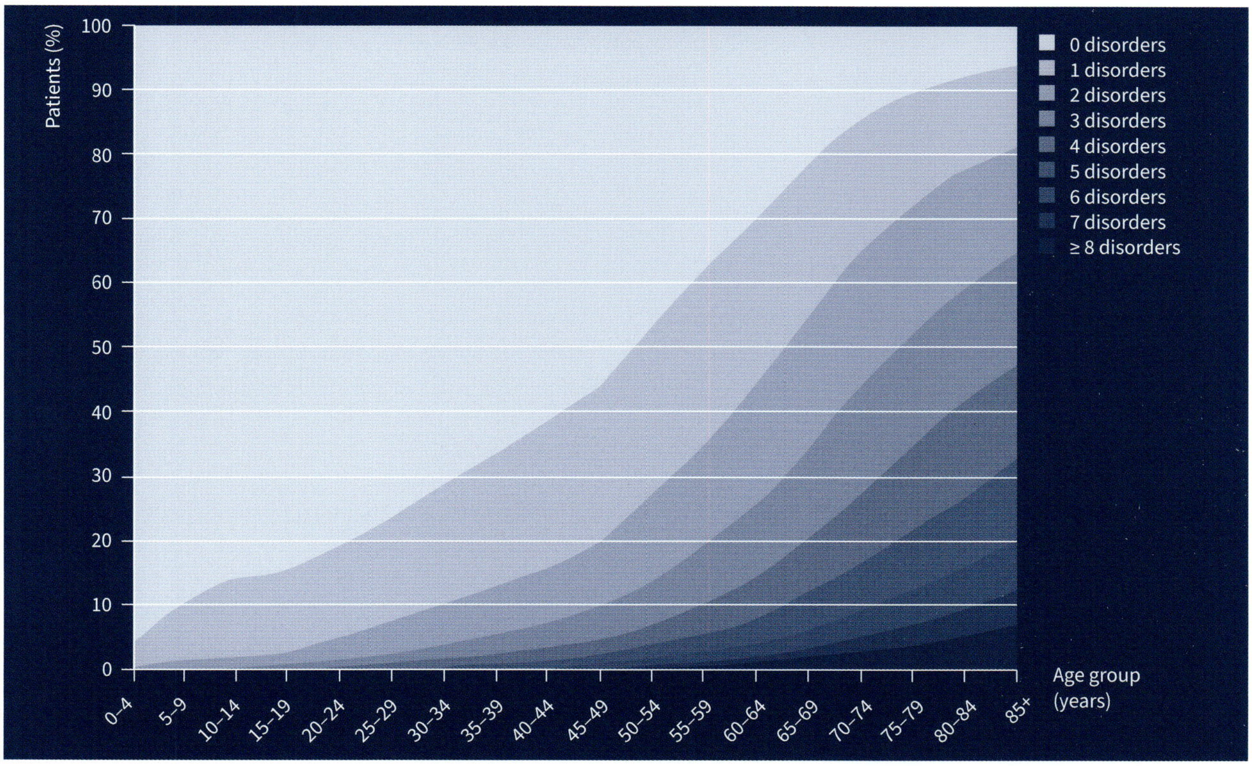

Fig 15 Average number of risk factors as a function of patient age (Barnett and coworkers 2012. In: ITI Treatment Guide, Vol. 9. Implant Therapy in the Geriatric Patient. Müller and Barter 2016).

Table 2 Surgical risk classification for outpatient surgery according to the American Society for Anesthesiology, including patient examples (Abouleish and coworkers 2020).

ASA Classification	Definition	Adult examples, including, but not limited to
ASA I	A normal healthy patient	Healthy, non-smoking, no or minimal alcohol use.
ASA II	A patient with mild systemic disease	Mild diseases only without substantive functional limitations. Current smoker, social alcohol drinker, pregnancy, obesity (Body Mass Index BMI 30–40), well-controlled diabetes, mild lung disease.
ASA III	A patient with severe systemic disease	Substantive functional limitations: One or more moderate to severe diseases. Poorly controlled diabetes, COPD, morbid obesity (BMI ≥ 40), active hepatitis, alcohol dependence or abuse, implanted pacemakers, moderate reduction of ejection fraction, history (> 3 months) of myocardial infarction, TIA, or stents.
ASA IV	A patient with severe systemic disease that is a constant threat to life	Recent (< 3 months) myocardial infarction, TIA, or stents, ongoing cardiac ischemia or severe valve dysfunction, severe reduction of ejection fraction.

Table 3 Overview of medical risk factors and their relevance to the risk of implant surgery.

	Low risk	Intermediate risk	High risk
Anticoagulants	Aspirin	Coumarins, direct oral anticoagulants	New stent (last 12 months) Cardiac infarction
Immunosuppression	Healthy or well controlled diabetes HIV under treatment	Diabetes uncontrolled or with inadequate control	Immunosuppression (chronic polyarthritis, organ graft)
Radiation therapy	None or < 50 Gy	Radiation > 50 Gy	Radiation (last 12 months)
Bone physiology	Osteoporosis	Antiresorptives in osteoporosis (low dose) Low vitamin D level	Antiresorptives in oncology (high dose)

Another aspect related to cardiovascular risks is the frequently used medical anticoagulation or antiplatelet therapy. It is rarely possible to interrupt or modify the procedure without additional risks. It may be advisable to contact to the prescribing physician, but this does not absolve the dentist of the responsibility for the procedure.

This assessment of the medical background results in subjective risk categories that are not always related to the chronological age of the patient. Table 3 helps facilitate decision-making. For instance, recent myocardial infarction (within the previous 12 months) is a relative contraindication for elective interventions (red category). However, the commonly prescribed aspirin is usually not restricted, even for extensive augmentative procedures (green category). Patients taking on coumarins or direct oral anticoagulants can often discontinue them for short periods. This makes them suitable for simple local bone procedures and circumscribed augmentation. There are more frequent indications for dimensionally reduced implants (yellow category) (Römer and coworkers 2022).

A similar system, which is subjective but practical, can be used for patients under immunosuppression with disturbances in bone physiology, or with similar effects after radiotherapy. In patients with high doses of antiresorptive drugs, e.g., in oncological indications, the decision for an implant-supported restoration or even augmentation must be made with great caution (red category). In contrast, in low-dose therapy, in osteoporosis, implant-supported measures and circumscribed augmentation can be planned successfully (yellow category) (Al-Nawas and coworkers 2023) (Fig 16).

There is limited scientific information on patients with compromised mucosa, such as those with oral lichen planus or those with post-irradiation xerostomia. In these cases, there may be a clear relative contraindication to tissue-supported dentures. The question must therefore be raised to what extent purely tissue-supported full dentures can still be considered as a therapeutic option for certain patient groups, e.g., after radiotherapy in the head and neck region or difficult mechanical or immunological soft-tissue conditions (e.g., oral lichen planus) (Pawlowski and coworkers 2023).

The general medical situation must be taken into account when deciding how to restore the edentulous jaw, as it can affect the load-bearing capacity of the soft tissue and bone. This refers not only to the reduced physical resilience and perioperative risks, but also to the bone and soft-tissue physiology.

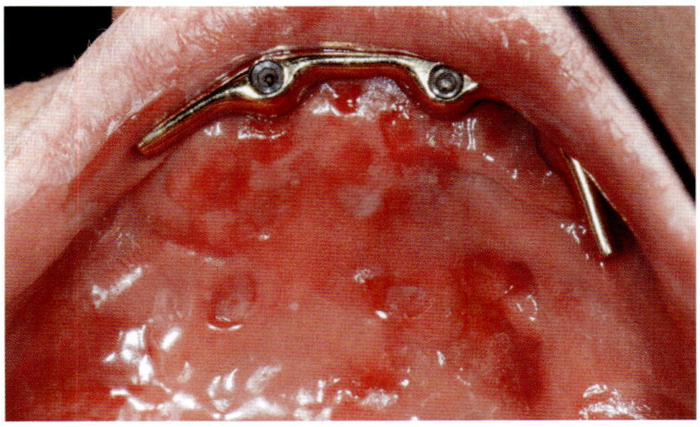

Fig 16 Patient with "lichen-like" mucosal inflammation due to graft-versus-host disease. Implant-supported prostheses may reduce mechanical irritation to the mucosa.

2.3 Anatomical Conditions and Changes over Time

B. Al-Nawas

2.3.1 Morphology and Atrophy

The anatomy of the edentulous jaw is well-described, with special attention to the peculiarities of its morphology.

One aggravating factor is the physiological loss of the alveolar process after tooth extraction. Another factor is the wearing of tissue-supported dentures for many years (Tallgren 1975; Cawood and Howell 1988) (Fig 17). The different trajectory of atrophy in the maxilla compared to the mandible leads to typical incongruence of the upper and lower tooth positions relative to the available bone (Fig 18). It is therefore essential to consider the relative position of the jaws when planning fixed or removable restorations (Figs 19 to 21).

The maxillary sinuses also become increasingly pneumatized. Elevation of the maxillary sinus floor is a common requirement for implant placement. This is a form of “internal atrophy” (Figs 22a-b). Typical horizontal and vertical bone loss is expected to occur in the maxillary anterior and premolar regions after tooth extraction. This makes single-stage implant placement difficult and results in typical loss of facial soft-tissue support.

A history of periodontitis will also exacerbate the vertical loss of alveolar bone. A number of clinical classifications can assist in accurate pre-implant analysis (Cawood and Howell 1988) (Fig 18). The complexity of the anatomical situation and the challenges of the prosthetic restoration require the analysis of 3D image data in many cases, especially for fixed restorations.

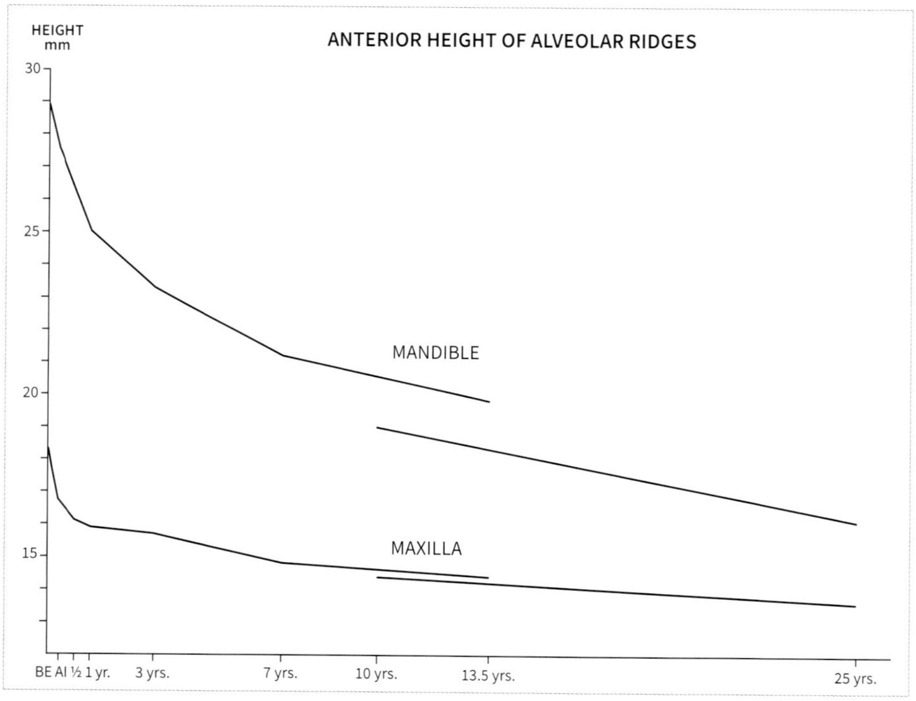

Fig 17 Continuous reduction of the residual alveolar ridges in complete-denture wearers over 25 years (based on Tallgren 1972).

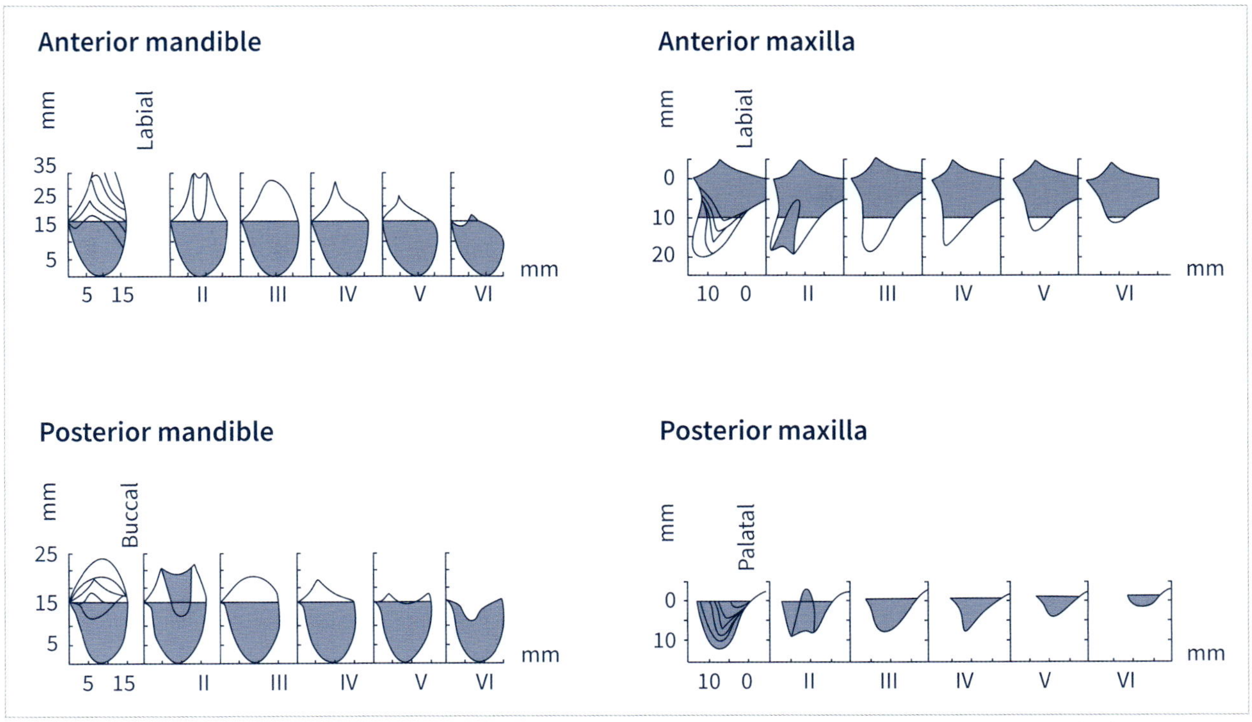

Fig 18 Classification of alveolar ridge morphology according to Cawood and Howell (1988). Class I: Dentate ridge. Class II: Ridge immediately after extraction. Class III: Broad and rounded ridge with adequate height and width. Class IV: Knife-edge ridge with sufficient height but inadequate width. Class V: Flat ridge with insufficient height and width. Class VI: Depressed ridge with a cup-shaped surface. (Blue: Basal bone. White: Alveolar bone.)

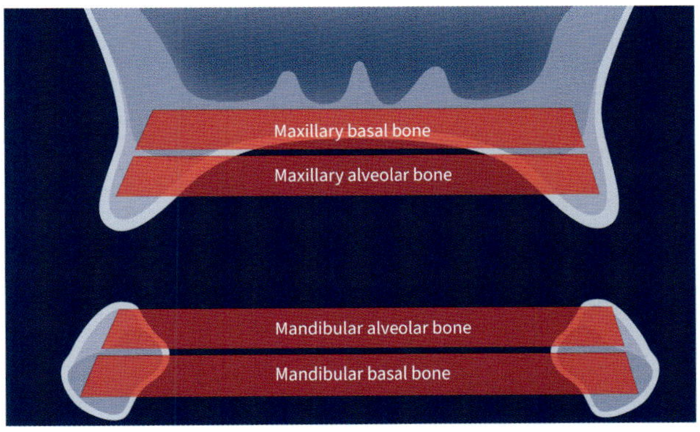

Fig 19 Atrophy developing in different directions in the maxilla and mandible (ITI Treatment Guide, Vol. 7. Ridge Augmentation Procedures in Implant Patients: A Staged Approach. Cordaro and Terheyden 2014).

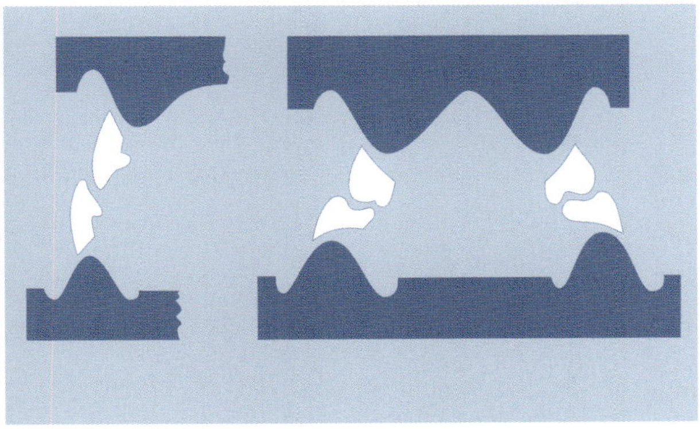

Fig 20 Crossbite in relation to different directions of atrophy in the mandible and maxilla.

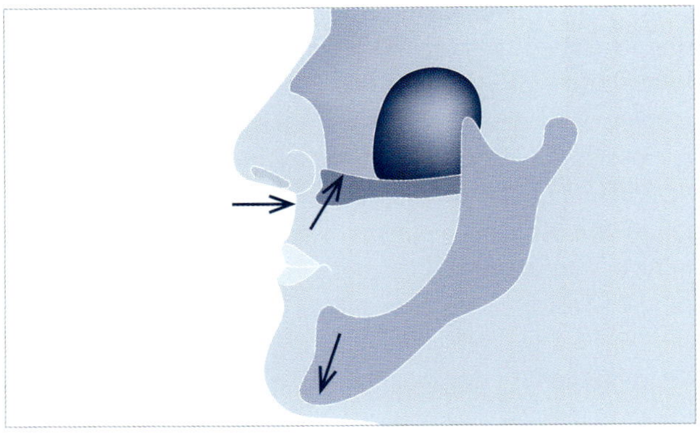

Fig 21 Loss of lip support and establishment of a class III jaw relationship in relation to different directions atrophy in the mandible and maxilla.

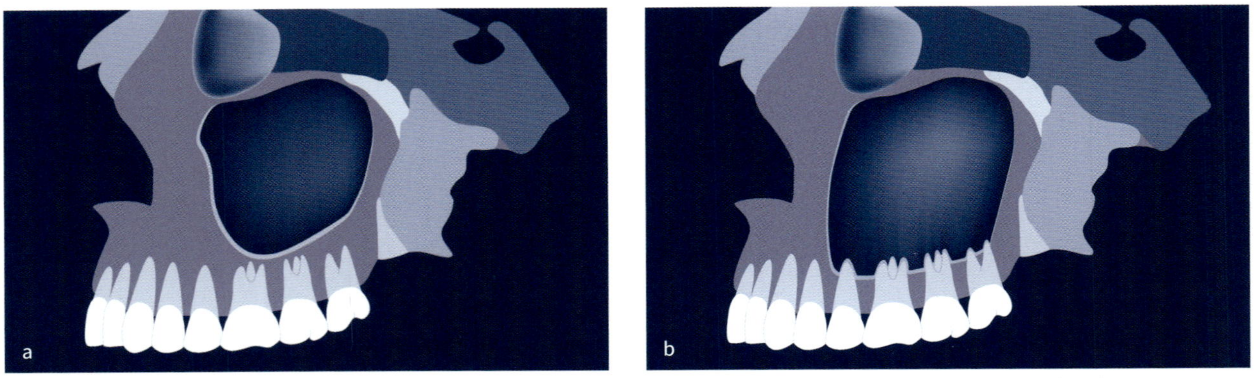

Figs 22a-b "Internal atrophy" of the maxilla due to pneumatization of the sinus floor with indication for elevation of the maxillary sinus floor (ITI Treatment Guide, Vol. 5. Sinus Floor Elevation Procedures. Katsuyama and Storgård Jensen 2011).

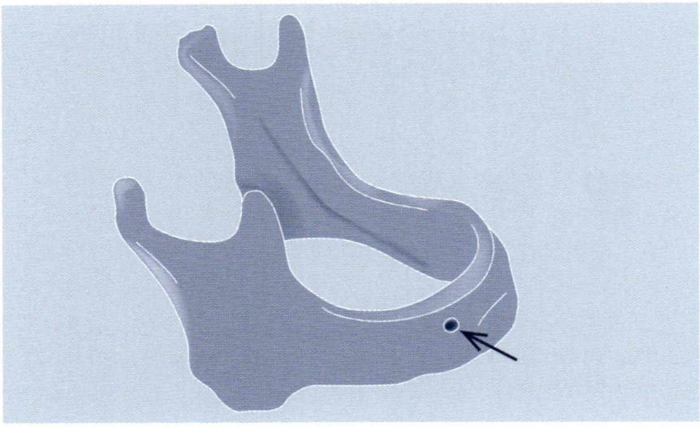

Fig 23a Typical lateral position of the mental foramen.

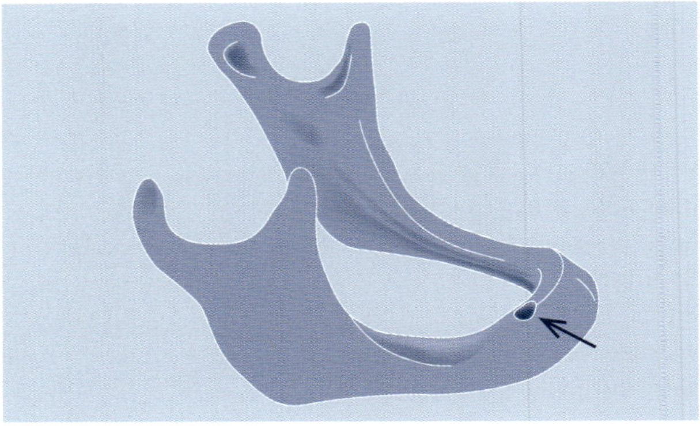

Fig 23b Crestal position of the mental foramen in severe mandibular atrophy.

In the mandible, the inferior alveolar nerve is a typical limitation. From an implant surgical perspective, the position of the so-called anterior loop is of particular interest, as this site is crucial for interforaminal implant placement. The combination of physiological loss of the alveolar process after tooth extraction and pressure atrophy due to tissue-supported dentures worn for many years also plays a role.

Sharp knife-edge ridges are a significant clinical challenge. They often require the use of reduced-diameter implants or bone augmentation. In cases of extreme atrophy, the loss of crestal bone ultimately places the nerve exit point on the alveolar ridge. This can cause chronic pain and is a clear indication for ridge augmentation or implant-supported dentures. In the posterior region, on the other hand, the vertical dimension will undoubtedly be a challenge, often requiring the use of short implants or complex augmentation procedures. Typical undercuts below the mylohyoid line (submandibular fossa) or in the lingual region of the chin (sublingual space) must be considered. Perforations into the floor of the mouth can be a critical complication (Figs 23a-b).

Severe atrophy of the mandible can even lead to pathological fractures (Fig 24).

2.3.2 Bone Physiology: Osteoporosis and Osteoimmunology

Bone physiology has received limited attention in recent years. Implants heal successfully, even in the "oldest old" patients. However, there is a clear need for more research into the success of complex augmentation procedures (such as vertical augmentations) in older patients. The role of long-term inflammation in bone and the possible consequences, such as the impact on osteoimmunology and in the risk of osteonecrosis, are also controversial topics. In the mandible, for example, histological signs of osteomyelitis and osteonecrosis can still be seen 1 year after tooth extraction (Kassolis and coworkers 2010).

Reduced cortical plate thickness and increased trabeculation are often observed in the maxilla compared to the mandible. Therefore, the development of osteoporosis is particularly relevant in the maxilla. In some cases, it might be difficult to achieve sufficient primary stability of dental implants in this situation, which is particularly relevant for immediate loading. Modern implant systems with high primary (mechanical) stability are currently popular solutions to this problem. This is particularly relevant for immediate loading concepts. And

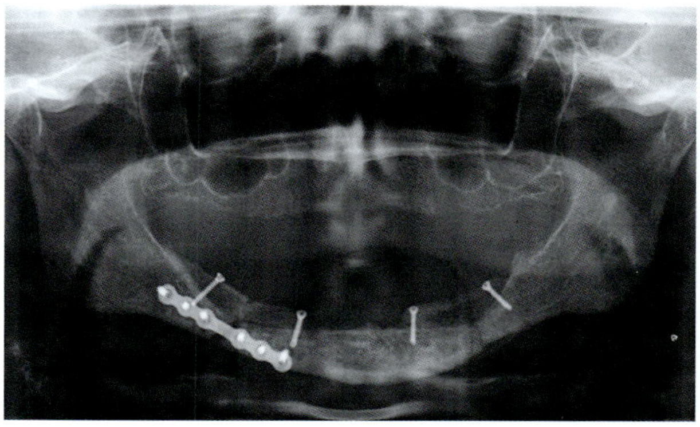

Fig 24 Pathological fracture due to atrophy treated with a mini-plate and iliac crest grafting.

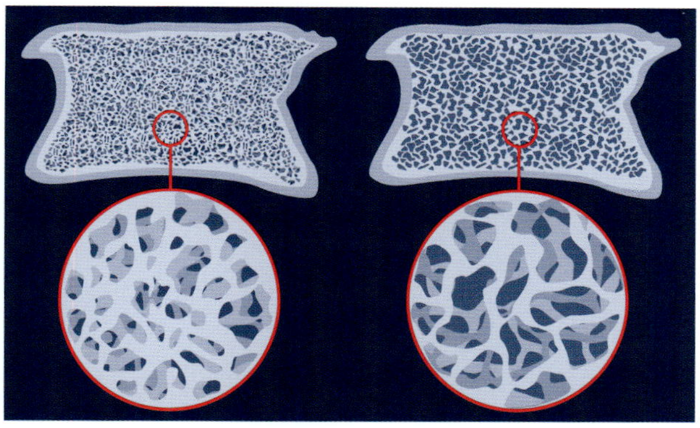

Fig 25 Bone density changes in osteoporosis in men (left) and women (right) (here: vertebral bone) (ITI Treatment Guide, Vol. 9. Implant Therapy in the Geriatric Patient. Müller and Barter 2016).

while bone density values (Hounsfield units) can provide an indication of bone density on a CT, a CBCT is much less reliable for such an analysis (Flanagan and coworkers 2021). Drilling protocols must be adapted to the clinical situation. It is therefore likely that difficulties with distal implants in bone with reduced cortical thickness are underreported, especially with immediate loading.

In the mandible, however, the very dense cortical bone can also be a significant challenge requiring precise and sensitive preparation of the implant cavity.

In addition, it is critical to evaluate medications and their effects on bone physiology. Low-dose antiresorptive agents, such as those used in osteoporosis (Fig 25), decrease the rate of bone remodeling and may even cause implant-associated bone necrosis. Immediate loading is not recommended here under any circumstances (Al-Nawas and coworkers 2023). However, other drugs such as steroids also slow down bone healing and lead to osteoporosis. These must be taken into account when designing the treatment concept.

2.3.3 Mechanical Aspects: Mandibular Torsion

While the maxilla allows rigid splinting of multiple implants, mandibular torsion during opening and closing of the mouth is a well-known problem. Clinical work has demonstrated a change in the distance and angle between the mandibular posterior teeth during jaw movement (Richter 1999; Thongpuong and coworkers 2022; Raymond and coworkers 2016) (Fig 26). There is considerable individual variation. However, the relevance for prosthetic restorations is still controversial. Historically, the interforaminal implant position in the mandible has been proven for fixed restorations. Most clinicians avoid splinting into the molar region and prefer to employ modular restorations rather than a single cross-arch mandibular restoration.

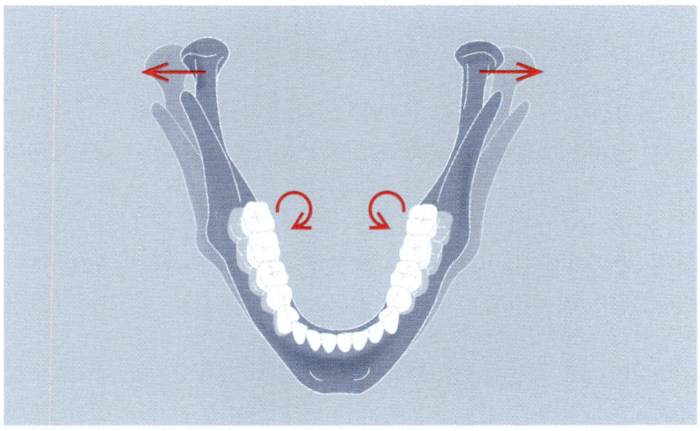

Fig 26 Mandibular deformity during mouth opening and chewing.

2.4 Implant Designs and the Edentulous Patient

B. Al-Nawas, C. Aparicio

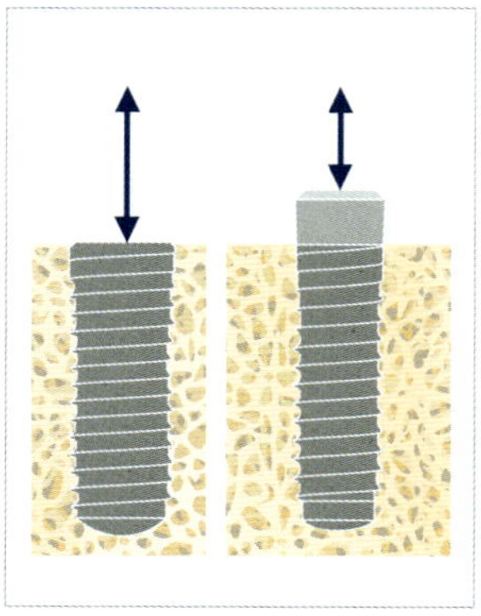

Fig 27a Reduced vertical bone dimension with long crown: soft-tissue level implants offer shorter technical crown lengths.

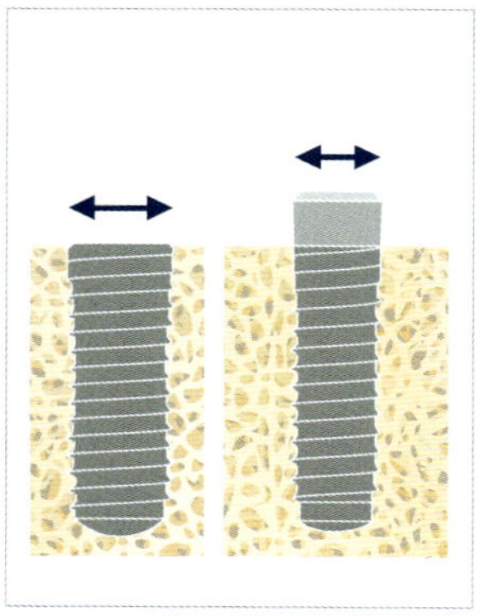

Fig 27b Reduced horizontal bone dimension with narrow-diameter implant: soft-tissue level implants offer wider and stronger neck designs.

The rapid development of implant designs in recent years has also led to clinical changes and indication expansion. The scientific rationale for short implants is well established in randomized studies, compared to vertical ridge augmentation and longer implants (Jung and coworkers 2018). Even 4-mm implants have been documented in studies. Today, 8-mm implants are no longer considered short. In the future, 6- and 7-mm implants will be in the focus of clinical and scientific work.

In contrast to implant length, reduced-diameter implants have rarely been the subject of comparative studies. Fractures of these implants have been documented, particularly in the molar region. The incidence is unclear, and the importance of splinting has not been sufficiently investigated. Current implant designs feature highly stable crestal structures, and it is clear that reduced-diameter implants are increasingly being used in the edentulous jaw. One-piece mini-implants are a special variant that has been scientifically established in larger study cohorts.

Biomechanical forces and cantilever play a limiting role, especially with short implants, but also in the case of reduced-diameter implants. The renaissance of the soft-tissue level concept has also allowed for a more stable neck design and shorter vertical cantilever arms (Figs 27a-b). Overall, the reduction in implant dimensions allows for less insertion morbidity and a reduced need for bone augmentation.

Almost all modern implant systems are designed with the explicit goal of increasing primary stability (Heimes and coworkers 2023; Jokstad and coworkers 2018) (Figs 28 and 29). This is achieved in part by slightly tapered implant shapes, but more importantly by cutting rather than compressing thread geometries. This not only provides stability even in less dense osteoporotic bone, but also frequently allows for immediate loading.

Implants are now available that can be placed in the atrophic maxilla without the need for major bone augmentation. For example, zygomatic implants have been on the market for over 20 years and are scientifically well documented. Implants placed at the junction of the maxillary tuberosity and the pterygoid process have also been documented in case series and are helpful in truly exceptional situations (Figs 30a-b).

Recently, additively manufactured subperiosteal implants (Fig 31) that are placed over a large area of the bone and fixed with screws ("osseofixation") have also been used. This is an understudied technique that needs to be rigorously evaluated (Van den Borre and coworkers 2022). It is important to evaluate explantation morbidity and bone loss in the event of inflammation/infection following the use of bulky implants. Taken together, these specific implant designs may allow for augmentation-free restorations even in difficult situations.

Implant design strategies (Table 4) follow a clear trend toward fewer augmentations. Digital planning allows the use of the available bone volume; smaller implant dimensions or angulated implants may also allow the use of a limited bone bed. Together with the focus on primary stability, this explains the trend toward more immediate restorations.

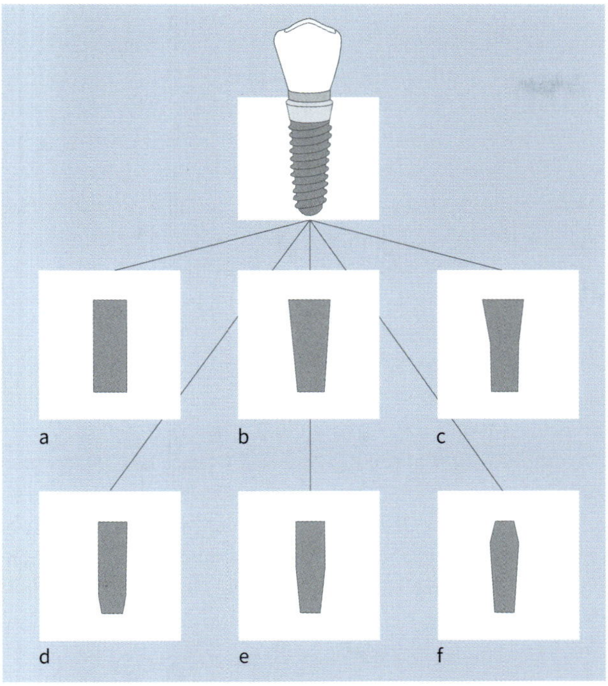

Fig 28 Implant body designs. Cylindrical design (a). Conical design (b). Hybrid design (apically cylindrical and crestally conical) (c). Cylindrical design with apical taper (d). Hybrid design (apically conical and crestally cylindrical) (e). Conical design with crestal back taper (f).

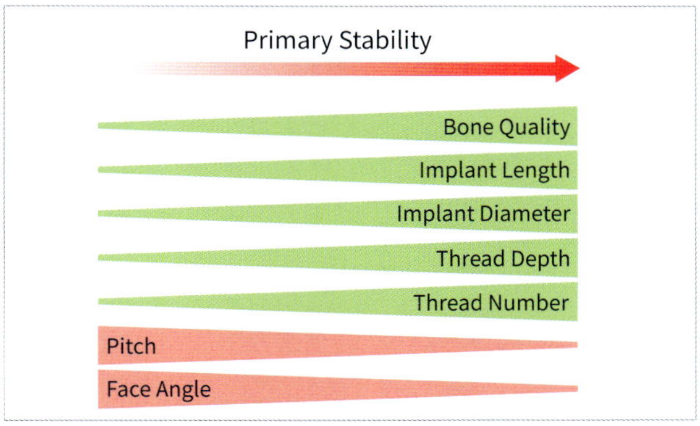

Fig 29 Characteristics of the implant macro design. Thread helix angle: angle between the horizontal of the thread helix to the longitudinal axis of the implant. Apical face angle: angle between the horizontal of the thread face to the longitudinal axis of the implant. Pitch: distance between the center of a thread to the next thread in the longitudinal axis of the implant or implant length divided by the number of threads. Thread depth: distance between the outer contour of the thread and the implant base body. Thread width: distance between the most coronal and the most apical portion of the same thread.

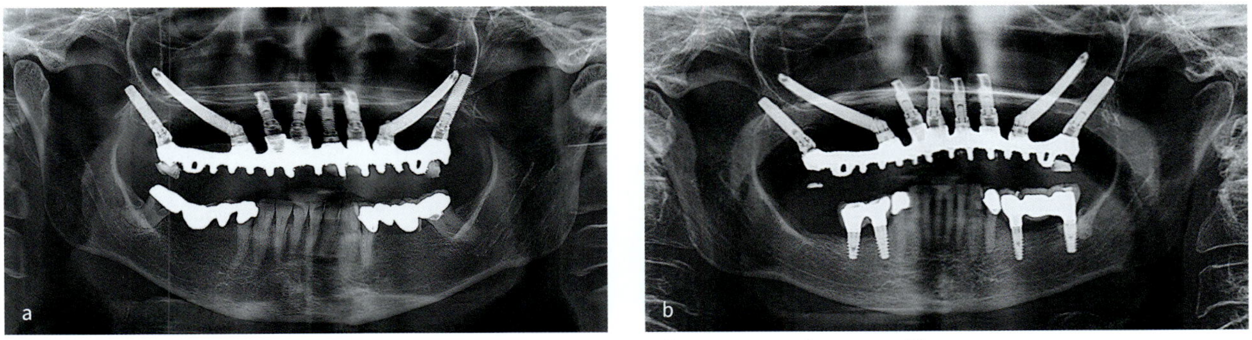

Figs 30a-b Pterygoid, zygomatic, and regular implants 10 years after placement (a). The same patient after 20 years (b).

Table 4 Implant design strategies that allow augmentation-free restorations and therefore immediate restorations.

Short implants
Reduced-diameter implants
Tilted implants
Zygomatic implants
Pterygoid implants (Fig 30)
Subperiostal implants (Fig 31)

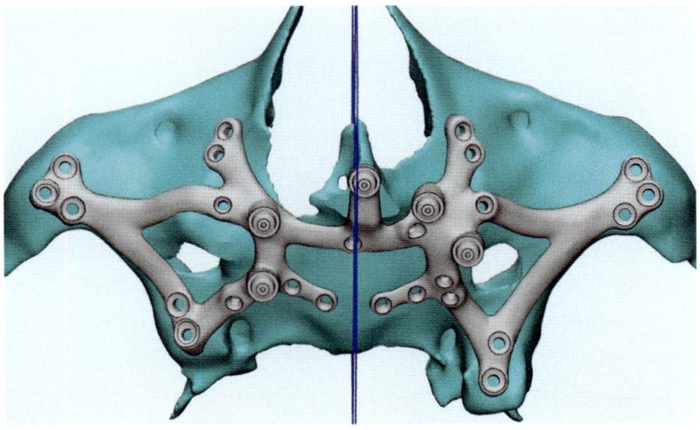

Fig 31 Subperiostal implant planned for a discontinuous maxillary bone by Dr9 Taras Yurov, ZAGA Center Saint Petersburg.

2.4.1 Zygomatic Implants

Zygomatic implants were originally developed to rehabilitate patients with severe mid facial alveolar bone defects. They play a critical role in the prosthetic rehabilitation of severely resorbed maxillae, whether the patient is fully or partially edentulous. While we often assume that non-specialist clinicians have a basic understanding of “what zygomatic implants are and what they are used for,” the reality is quite different. Due to limited usage and restrictive indications, most clinicians remain unfamiliar with the various placement techniques, the differences in implant design, and the impact these factors can have on long-term outcomes and the development of complications.

The placement of zygomatic implants should be regarded as a major surgical intervention—complex in nature and, in many cases, representing the final opportunity to restore fixed dentition in patients with extreme maxillary atrophy. Adequate and specialized training is, therefore, essential. These implants are indicated only in cases of severe maxillary bone loss, with the “king indication” being the complete absence of both anterior and posterior maxillary bone. As a result, the number of suitable cases in an average dental practice will be very limited, leading to a steep and prolonged learning curve for clinicians.

Moreover, in recent decades, a range of placement protocols and implant designs have been introduced—many without long-term clinical validation. This situation is further complicated by the aggressive marketing strategies of some companies, which often promote the technique as simple and accessible following just a short weekend course. Such oversimplification risks clinicians adopting unproven techniques or using implants designed without sufficient consideration for biological principles, potentially leading to suboptimal outcomes and an increased incidence of complications.

This introductory chapter aims to encourage the responsible and evidence-based use of zygomatic implants. We also wish to highlight the value of employing a well-documented and protocol-driven approach tailored to the specific anatomy of each patient and physiology based: the zygoma anatomy-guided approach (ZAGA).

When planning the osteotomy for a zygomatic implant, it is important to understand that a zygomatic implant may follow different trajectories depending on the anatomical situation. Consequently, adapting the treatment strategy to each patient’s situation is a key factor in the evolution of zygomatic treatment concepts. From this critical perspective, a site-specific implant design that can adapt to the patient-specific anatomy appears to be crucial.

The original Brånemark protocol, known as the original surgical technique (OST), included one implant in each zygoma, traversing the sinus, combined with two to four conventional anterior implants (Parel and coworkers 2001; Brånemark and coworkers 2004). In subsequent years, the original technique has been refined with respect to sinus position and crestal emergence to allow for better individual anatomical and prosthetic adaptations. The sinus-slot technique (Stella and Warner 2000) reduces the size of the first osteotomy, decreases inflammation by elevating a less extensive flap and after a second osteotomy achieves a prosthetically guided crestal position of the implant platform. To avoid bulky prostheses and at the same time respect the integrity of the sinus membrane, Aparicio and coworkers (2008), Ouazzani and coworkers (2006), and Miglioranza and coworkers (2006) proposed the exteriorized technique for the placement of zygomatic implants in patients with extreme buccal concavities in the anterior maxillary wall. Later, an extra-maxillary approach was advocated by Malo and coworkers (2008) eliminating the alveolar bone to anchor the implant exclusively in the zygomatic bone.

In 2010, the ZAGA concept was described by Aparicio based on a cross-sectional study of 200 human clinical and radiographic sites (Aparicio 2011). This approach was organically introduced as a refinement of his exteriorized technique for different anatomical situations from the flat maxillary wall to the concave or atrophic maxilla. By following specific prosthetic, biomechanical, and anatomical factors, the determination of the entry point and final implant path depends on the vertical and horizontal resorption of the alveolar/basal process and the anterior maxillary wall curvature. The differences between OST and the ZAGA concept when it comes to placing implants in an atrophic maxilla are shown in Fig 32. This figure illustrates, in a two-dimensional view, the length of the implant’s contact areas with the bone. L-1 is the length of the implant-bone contact in its dorsal area. We can see that when we apply OST to an atrophic maxilla (Fig 32, left), contact L-1 occurs in a narrow area, limited only to the neck of the implant with the thin bone of the palatal area. When the ZAGA concept is applied to an atrophic maxilla, such as the one shown in Fig 32, right, no early “window” osteotomy is made in the maxillary wall. Instead, a channel is carved into the maxillary wall and the implant pathway is externalized using both the remaining alveolar bone and the maxillary wall as support. This lengthens the L-1 segment, which also occupies a large part of the maxillary wall. L-2 and L-3 represent the implant contact areas at the level of the zygomatic bone. The intrasinus path of the original procedure (OST) forces the entry of the implant through the palatal area. When a functional force is applied to the implant, a concentration of forces occurs on the palatal alveolar segment L-1 which, over time, can lead to bone destruction, micromovements of the implant under load, and end up in orosinusal communication. When we analyze the right-hand side of Fig 32, we

Fig 32 The left-hand side of this figure shows an image of the OST being used on a patient with posterior atrophy of the ZAGA 4, which represents approximately 60% of cases. Due to its intrasinus path, the functional force represented by the white arrow is concentrated in the L-1 alveolar segment, which can cause its destruction, micromovements, and OAC. On the right-hand side, the ZAGA concept is illustrated in the same situation. Here, a single minimally invasive osteotomy is applied, externalizing the implant and significantly increasing the L-1 segment for the same masticatory force. The total BICA, represented by the sum of the L-1, L-2, and L-3 segments, in the ZAGA protocol is clearly superior. The possibility of sinus infection is reduced in the ZAGA protocol, and the implant platform is located on the bone crest.

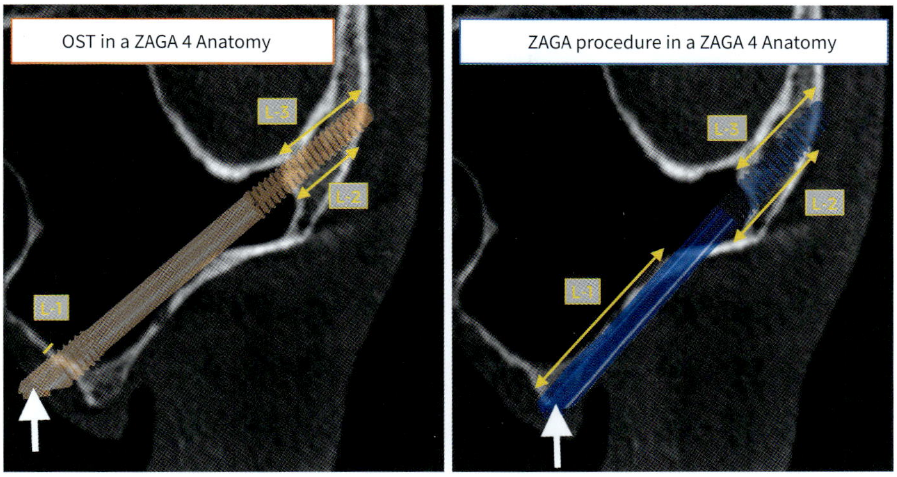

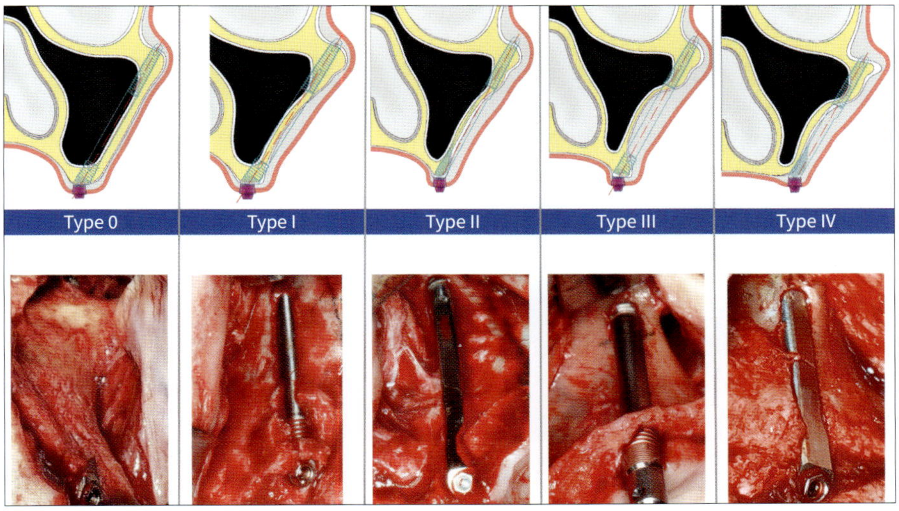

Fig 33 The simulation at the top represents the ZAGA classification, while the simulation at the bottom represents the different paths that the implant can take depending on the residual anatomy. Within the ZAGA concept, the trajectories can be intrasinus, parasinus, or externalized. In addition, the design of the implant will also be chosen according to the nature of the osteotomy used.

understand that under the ZAGA protocol, the functional load is distributed performed over a much longer L-1 segment, and therefore the distribution is much improved. The ZAGA concept has been used for years in teaching and clinical decision making (Aparicio and coworkers 2021). Fig 33 shows the ZAGA classification for posterior areas. The most frequent anatomies are ZAGA types 4 and 3, with 57.4% and 18.7%, respectively (Aparicio and coworkers 2021). The reader can observe in the same figure that the implant design is chosen according to the residual anatomy. According to the ZAGA protocol, the oral rehabilitation of extreme maxillary atrophy shown in Figs 34 to 39 illustrates the importance of adapting the planning of the type of osteotomy, implant path, and implant design to the patient's anatomy to obtain a tailored, predictable, long-lasting result similar to the original prosthodontic situation.

A scheme of criteria for evaluating the outcome of zygomatic implants proposed by Aparicio and coworkers (2020) is shown in Table 5.

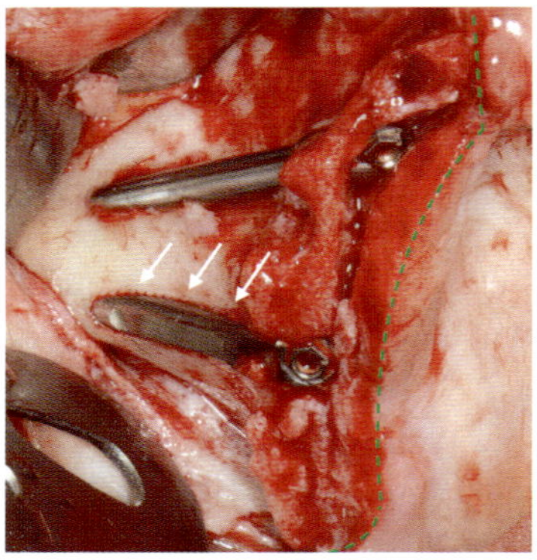

Fig 34 The two zygomatic implants (Institut Straumann AG, Basel, Switzerland) in situ. The anterior one has a mixed path: intraalveolar (ZAGA tunnel osteotomy); then extramaxillary; finally, intrazygomatic. The anterior osteotomy was closed with a ZAGA Round implant. The posterior implant (ZAGA Flat) has an externalized path from the crest (ZAGA channel osteotomy). The white arrows indicate the precision of the osteotomy. No previous window or slot osteotomy was performed prior to implant placement. The dashed green line indicates the edge of the palatal incision which will easily prevent soft-tissue dehiscence by displacing keratinized tissue buccally (ZAGA: zygoma anatomy-guided approach).

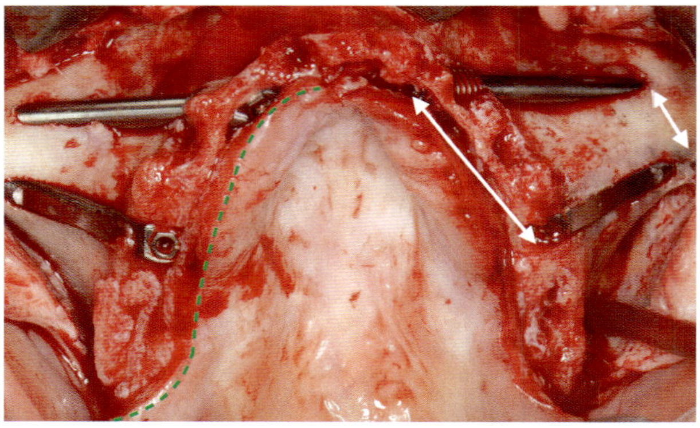

Fig 35 Occlusal view of the four zygomatic implants in their final position. The anterior implants (ZAGA Round) were placed with preservation of the remaining alveolar bone. The two posterior implants (ZAGA Flat) were placed in an externalized position. The green dashed line indicates the perimeter of the incision. The double white arrows show that thanks to the reduced diameter of the implants (3.4 mm diameter in the first 10 mm of their apical part), an excellent anterior-posterior distribution of the masticatory load was achieved.

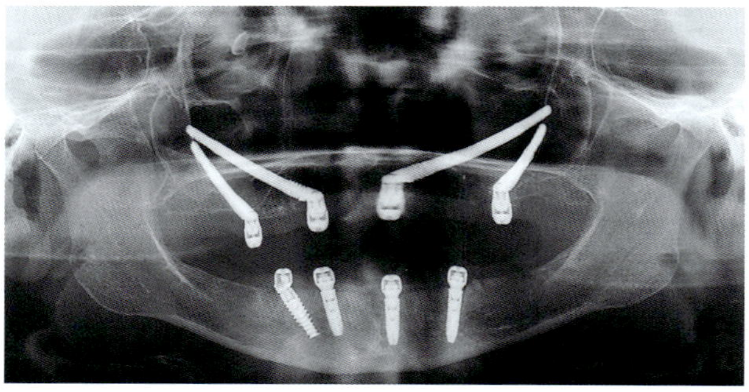

Fig 36 Panoramic radiograph immediately after surgery.

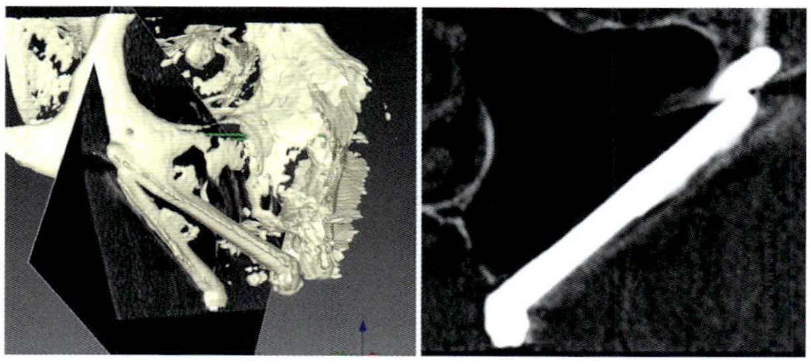

Fig 37 Radiographic situation of the implant at site 15/16 after the first year of loading.

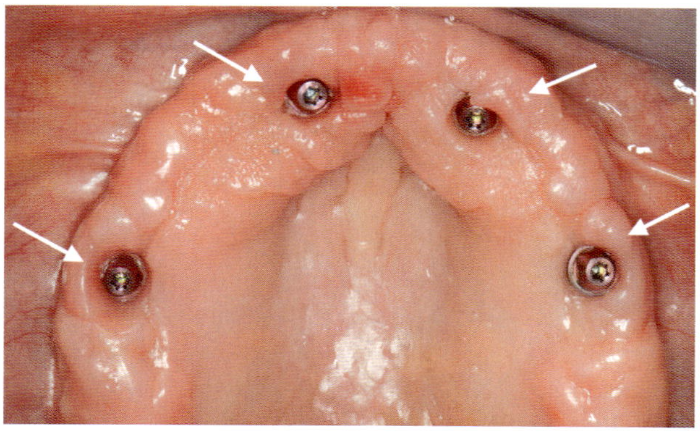

Fig 38 Clinical image taken at the follow-up visit 1 year after immediate loading. The white arrows indicate the quality and quantity of the soft tissue. Thanks to the palatal incision, an additional thickness of keratinized tissue was transported from the palatal area of the alveolar ridge. As a consequence to the ZAGA palatal rolled flap, the keratinized tissue has increased in thickness and will be further strengthened because the connective pedicle has the genetic capacity to transform into keratinized tissue.

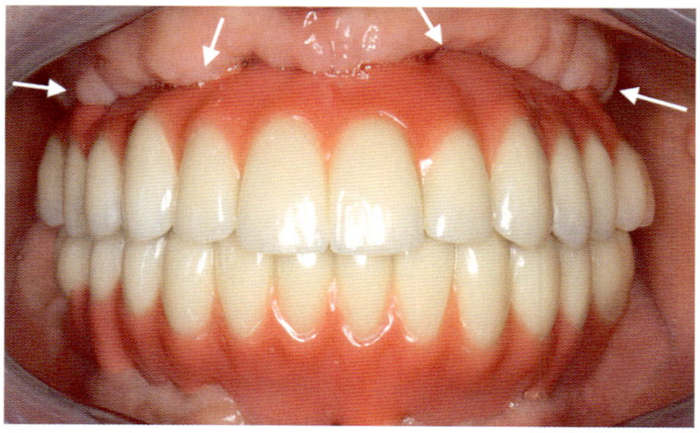

Fig 39 Frontal view of the oral rehabilitation performed by Dr Peter Simon and Dr Madalina Simon (ZAGA Center Stuttgart, Germany). The white arrows indicate how the prosthesis should ideally relate to the soft tissue to facilitate hygiene and good maintenance.

Table 5 Description of the specific criteria (ORIS) that classify zygomatic implants (Aparicio and coworkers 2020) as successful in grades I, II, and III (conditions I to III); survival (condition IV); or failed (condition V). The condition of the four ORIS criteria (i.e., O-1/R-3/I-2 /S-4 would be classified as survival). L-K: Lanza and Kennedy task force on rhinosinusitis criteria for the diagnosis of rhinosinusitis. Prosthetic offset: distance from the center of palate to the center of residual alveolar ridge minus distance from the center of palate to the implant head. Positive values correspond to zygomatic implants placed palatally, while negative values correspond to zygomatic implants placed buccally to the alveolar crest.

Zygomatic implant condition					
	I	**II**	**III**	**IV**	**V**
ORIS* criteria	**Success**			**Survival**	**Failure**
O Prosthetic offset (mm)	0 ≤ d ≤ 6 –3 ≤ d ≤ 0	6 ≤ d ≤ 10 –4 ≤ d ≤ –3	10 ≤ d ≤ 15 –5 ≤ d ≤ –4	Implant not tested following ORIS criteria	d > 15 d < –5
R Rhinosinus-associated pathology	L-K (–) No increased opacity between pretsurgical and post surgical CBCT	L-K (+) or increased opacity between pretsurgical and post surgical CBCT	Occasional rhinosinusitis responding positively to medical or surgical treatment		Persistent or recurrent rhinosinusitis refractory to treatment
I Peri-implant soft-tissue condition	No recession No signs of inflammation or infection	Stable recession No signs of inflammation or infection	Progressive recession Occasional signs of inflammation or infection responding positively to treatment		Recession + Permanent or recurrent signs of soft tissue inflammation or infection refractory to treatment or no esthetic acceptance
S Stability (individually tested)	No mobility No pain No rotation	Light mobility No pain No rotation	Clear mobility (no evidence of disintegration of the apex of the implant) No pain No rotation		Clear mobility (evidence of disintegration of the apex of the implant) Rotation and/or pain

In 2023, the ITI Consensus Workshop on Zygomatic Implants evaluated the current literature to reach consensus and provide evidence-based recommendations for the safe use of zygomatic implants. The Proceedings of the First ITI Consensus Workshop on Zygomatic Implants are available for download below.

Use this code to download the Proceedings of the First ITI Consensus Workshop on Zygomatic Implants (2023).

The clinical recommendations below were derived from the First ITI Consensus Workshop on Zygomatic Implants (2023).

To download the full Proceedings of the First ITI Consensus Workshop on Zygomatic Implants, which also include the consensus statements derived, please scan the code or click on the link on this page.

PLANNING

Clinical recommendation 1
Who should perform zygomatic implant treatment? Zygomatic implants are considered a complex treatment. The success of the treatment is highly dependent on the clinician skill and experience. There is a need for surgical and restorative expertise to address all potential difficulties and complications. This clinical recommendation is based on the systematic review from Polido and coworkers (2023).

Clinical recommendation 2
Who is a candidate for zygomatic implants? Zygomatic implants are an evidence-based alternative to support fixed or removable prostheses to restore partially or completely edentulous maxillae, allowing high survival rates when splinted to other implants. Zygomatic implants are an alternative when the maxillary bone is completely or partially absent, secondary to resection, trauma or congenital defects. Zygomatic implants are an alternative when the maxillary bone is completely or partially absent, secondary to failure of previously placed implants and/or bone grafts. This clinical recommendation is based on the systematic review from Polido and coworkers (2023).

Clinical recommendation 3
What diagnostic tools are recommended to assess the surgical field? A CT/CBCT including the midface, allowing for 3D assessment of the maxillary and zygomatic bone volume and sinus health should be obtained. Preoperative evaluation for a lack of existing sinus pathologies is recommended. The use of specific software for planning, including the image of the planned prostheses and 3D anatomic models is an option. This clinical recommendation is based on the systematic review from Polido and coworkers (2023).

Clinical recommendation 4
What is the degree of maxillary atrophy to consider zygomatic implants? Objective criteria should be utilized to determine the amount of bone atrophy. A 3D assessment of the maxillary and zygomatic bone volume is recommended. The most cited anatomical classification is Cawood and Howell (1988), with class IV, V and VI. Each site should be individually analyzed, and treatment options should be discussed with the patients, considering the risks, benefits, the final prosthetic outcome, total treatment time, long-term outcomes and patients preference and conditions. This clinical recommendation is based on the systematic review from Polido and coworkers (2023).

Clinical recommendation 5
Can I consider zygomatic implants for maxillofacial defects? Zygomatic implants in maxillofacial rehabilitation cases have additional complexity and considerations. Factors such as surveillance of malignant disease, radiation, bone and soft tissues quality and quantity, patient compliance should be considered. This clinical recommendation is based on the systematic review from Polido and coworkers (2023).

SURGERY

Clinical recommendation 6
Can I place zygomatic implant at the same time as dental extractions? Factors such as presence of infection, hard and soft-tissue quality and quantity, clinician experience and patient preference should be considered. Risks may be increased when performing zygomatic implants at the same time as tooth extractions. This clinical recommendation is based on the systematic review from Polido and coworkers (2023).

What is the role of guided surgery or dynamic navigation for inertion of zkygomatic implants? Direct visualization of the surgical field is paramount to avoid disorientation and anatomical complications (e.g.. to the orbital cavity or the infra-temporal fossa). This clinical recommendation is based on expert opinion.

Clinical recommendation 7
Should the sinus membrane be elevated ("preserved") for insertion of zygomatic implants? Neither the literature nor expert consensus on preserving the sinus membrane for zygomatic implant placement exists. This clinical recommendation is based on expert opinion.

RESTORATION

Clinical recommendation 8
Do specific loading protocols have an influence on the long-term outcomes of zygomatic implant therapy? Zygomatic implant survival rates appear to be slightly higher for immediate over delayed loading protocols subject to adequate primary implant stability. Immediate loading also confers benefits to the patient through immediate functional rehabilitation. However, delayed loading techniques are also clinically acceptable. This clinical recommendation is based on the systematic review by Brennand Roper and coworkers (2023).

Clinical recommendation 9
When zygomatic implants are used, what type of prosthesis can be utilized? Once generally accepted restorative concepts for implant-supported-prosthesis are followed, removable or fixed restorations can be considered, provided that all implants are splinted. Factors to be considered include prosthetic material, esthetic factors (e.g., lip support, smile line), condition of the opposing dentition, available space for the prosthesis, planned implant distribution, presence and length of cantilever, space available for hygiene and maintenance, proper abutment selection and timing of implant

platform position, patient preference and compliance. This clinical recommendation is based on the systematic review from Polido and coworkers (2023).

OUTCOMES

Clinical recommendation 10
What are the long-term therapeutic advantages of zygomatic implants? Current survival data support the use of zygomatic implants as a long-term therapeutic option. Zygomatic implants present an opportunity to rehabilitate patients who either lack the desire to undergo extensive augmentation procedures, or lack the anatomical structures required to deliver conventional implant therapy in the maxilla. Zygomatic implants may confer treatment time benefits to patients due to the possibility of immediacy in reconstruction. This clinical recommendation is based on the systematic review by Brennand Roper and coworkers (2023).

Clinical recommendation 11
How does zygomatic implant survival perform long-term when compared to conventional implants? Survival of zygomatic implants appear to be comparable to conventional implants when used for reconstruction of the atrophic maxilla. This includes techniques such as short implants, tilted implants, and implants placed in grafted sinuses. With this in mind, zygomatic implants may be considered as an option to support maxillary reconstructions. This clinical recommendation is based on the systematic review by Brennand Roper and coworkers (2023).

Clinical recommendation 12
What is the long-term performance of zygomatic implant-supported reconstructions? Within the context of long-term data survival analyses, zygomatic implant reconstructions are comparable to, and have similar survival characteristics to reconstructions supported by conventional implants. They are subject to similar mechanical complications. Although no additional technical considerations are required, zygomatic implant reconstruction should be considered as a complex procedure. This clinical recommendation is based on the systematic review by Brennand Roper and coworkers (2023).

Clinical recommendation 13
What are the long-term mechanical complications associated with zygomatic implants? The most common mechanical complications include zygomatic implant prosthesis abutment or screw fracture, abutment or screw loosening, and chipping or loss of the veneering acrylic or ceramic materials. These complications may occur whether the zygomatic implant reconstructions are splinted to conventional implants or supported by zygomatic implants alone, through a Quad Zygomatic implant approach. Zygomatic implant fracture or reconstruction framework fracture have been reported as rare complications. In light of these findings, conventional prosthetic techniques to mitigate such factors are recommended. This clinical recommendation is based on the systematic review by Brennand Roper and coworkers (2023).

Clinical recommendation 14
What are the long-term biological risks associated with zygomatic implants? The most reported long-term biological complication was sinusitis. This may be successfully treated through antibiotic and/or surgical interventions. If these therapies are unsuccessful, the zygomatic implant may be lost. Oro-antral communications, peri-implant infection of the soft tissues, peri-implant mucositis, bleeding on probing and increased probing pocket depths have also been reported. Patient education in oral hygiene maintenance is paramount. This clinical recommendation is based on the systematic review by Brennand Roper and coworkers (2023).

Clinical recommendation 15
How should sinus infections in relation to zygomatic implants be treated? Sinus infections are generally treated with antibiotics with a satisfactory resolution. In the absence of resolution, refractory maxillary sinus infections may need exploration of the patency of the osteo-meatal complex and other paranasal sinuses. This clinical recommendation is based on expert opinion.

PATIENT'S PERSPECTIVE

Clinical recommendation 16
Do patients perceive a long-term benefit from the zygomatic implant treatment experience? Most patients report an increase in oral health-related quality of life and satisfaction with the treatment outcome. This clinical recommendation is based on the systematic review by Brennand Roper and coworkers (2023).

Clinical recommendation 17
Are unique challenges faced by patients receiving zygomatic implants and their reconstructions? Zygomatic implants and their reconstructions may require a higher level of professional maintenance. There are also lim-

itations on the range of acceptable masticatory loads. Patients' expectations need to be managed in line with the biological and technical complexities faced by zygomatic implant therapies. This clinical recommendation is based on the systematic review by Brennand Roper and coworkers (2023).

3 Clinical Aspects

S. Wolfart, B. Al-Nawas

3.1 Radiographic Analysis, Augmentation Requirements, Implant Planning, and Surgical Guide

S. Wolfart

A basic distinction is made between two-dimensional implant planning using a panoramic radiograph and three-dimensional planning using a CBCT scan. In both cases, the radiograph of the edentulous jaw is ideally taken in situ with an individualized radiographic template. Elements of the clinical recommendations from the 6th ITI Consensus Conference 2018 (Wismeijer and coworkers 2018) are a good starting point for a state-of-the-art radiographic analysis, implant planning, and implant placement.

- Static computer-aided implant surgery (s-CAIS) should be considered as an additional tool for comprehensive diagnosis, treatment planning, and surgical procedures (see Chapter 3.1.3).
- s-CAIS should be prosthetically driven (see Chapter 3.1.1).
- Surgical experience and general comprehensive training are desirable to achieve an accurate and favorable outcome for implants placed using s-CAIS.
- While recent studies indicate improved accuracy when using s-CAIS in partially edentulous cases, a safety margin of 2 mm from critical anatomical structures should be maintained.
- The alignment of surface scans, including the prosthetic planning, with 3D volumetric imaging data is recommended to improve the accuracy of the anatomical position of the implant (see Chapter 3.1.3).
- Surgical guides should be digitally designed on surface scan files that have been aligned with DICOM data, which is more accurate than using DICOM data alone (see Chapter 3.1.3).
- Flapless s-CAIS may be beneficial in fully edentulous cases in relation to postoperative pain intensity compared with open-flap procedures.
- Flapless s-CAIS may lead to implant placement outside the zone of keratinized mucosa; therefore, the quality and quantity of the keratinized mucosa must be assessed before planning s-CAIS to avoid this or determine the need for keratinized soft-tissue grafting.

Use this code to download the Proceedings of the 6th ITI Consensus Conference (2018)

3.1.1 Prosthetically Guided Implant Planning

FROM SET-UP TO RADIOGRAPHIC TEMPLATE

Implant planning should be prosthetically guided in all cases. For this purpose, the prospective tooth set-up must be known in all dimensions prior to implant planning and must meet the patient's functional and esthetic requirements. If a suitable complete denture is available, it can be used as the basis for further planning. If there is no appropriate complete denture that reflects the appropriate vertical, horizontal, and sagittal alignment of the future restoration, it is strongly recommended that an adequate final prosthetic set-up be fabricated first and used as a diagnostic try-in. For this purpose, the occlusal plane and the vertical dimension of occlusion (VDO) are determined using maxillary and mandibular bite blocks.

The required radiographic template is then created based on the appropriate prosthesis, or on the clinically tested and approved set-up.

THE RADIOGRAPHIC TEMPLATE AS A MEASURE OF ATROPHY

The radiographic template consists of a clear plastic base with white barium sulfate teeth and should clearly show the cementoenamel junction and the adjacent roots of the teeth on the proposed prosthesis. When the radiographic template is inserted, the alveolar ridge should be visible through the template and the vertical and horizontal degree of atrophy of the soft and hard tissues can be assessed (Fig 1). The

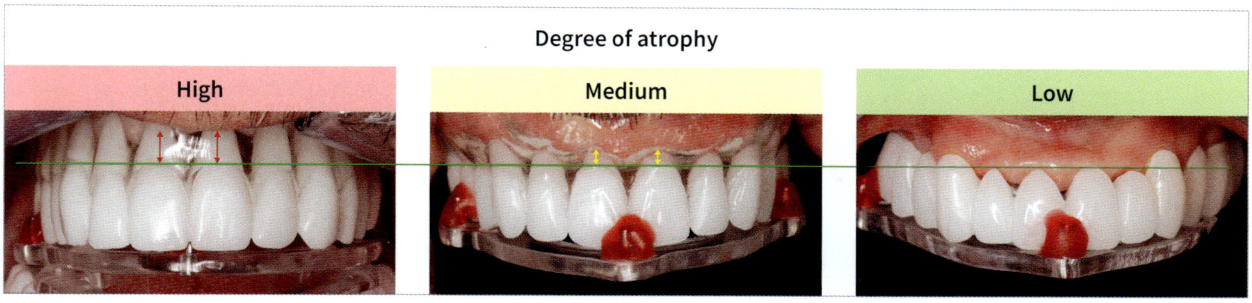

Fig 1 Degree of atrophy: The alveolar ridge can be seen through the radiographic template and the vertical (arrows) and horizontal degrees of soft- and hard-tissue atrophy can be estimated.

degree of atrophy has a direct impact on possible prosthetic treatment approaches and the associated degree of difficulty (see Chapter 3.5). Accordingly, the degree of atrophy present determines whether a clinical case is classified as Advanced or Complex according to the SAC classification for edentulous patients in implant dentistry (Dawson and coworkers 2022).

3.1.2 2D Radiographic Analysis for Orientation-Based Implant Planning

In orientation-based implant planning, metal spheres or sleeves (fiducial markers) are attached to the radiographic template above the regions of the planned implants. These cues broadly represent the planned position of the implants as radiopaque shadows during the radiographic measurements. Another function of the metal spheres is certainly to determine the magnification factor of the plain radiograph to be taken.

Based on the resulting (usually panoramic) radiograph, the template is converted into a surgical guide. There is no direct relationship between the drill hole defined by the template and the radiographic image. In other words, the indicated drilling direction is only a rough guide; the template does not define the drilling depth or implant angulation. However, since any implant rehabilitation of the edentulous jaw must be considered Advanced or Complex according to the SAC classification, static computer-guided implant placement with 3D radiographic analysis is preferable to orientation-based implant planning.

3.1.3 Static Computer-Assisted Implant Surgery (s-CAIS) with 3D Radiographic Analysis

In the edentulous jaw, the fabrication of a guide template is mandatory for static computer-assisted implant surgery (s-CAIS). This requires a CBCT scan with a barium sulfate (radiopaque) template inserted. Axis-centered holes corresponding to the tooth set-up are created to indicate implant positions in the radiographic template (Figs 2a-b).

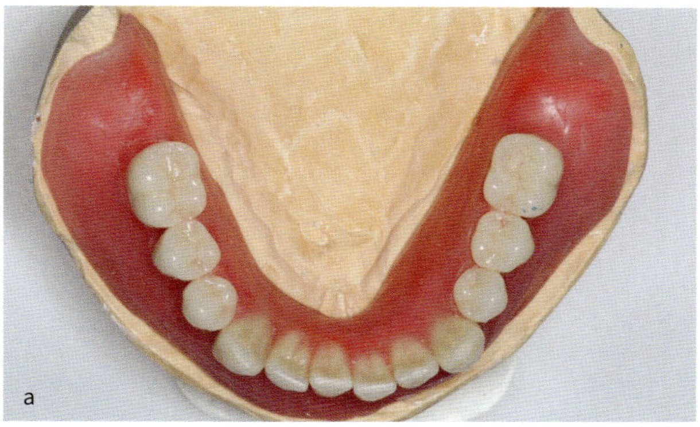

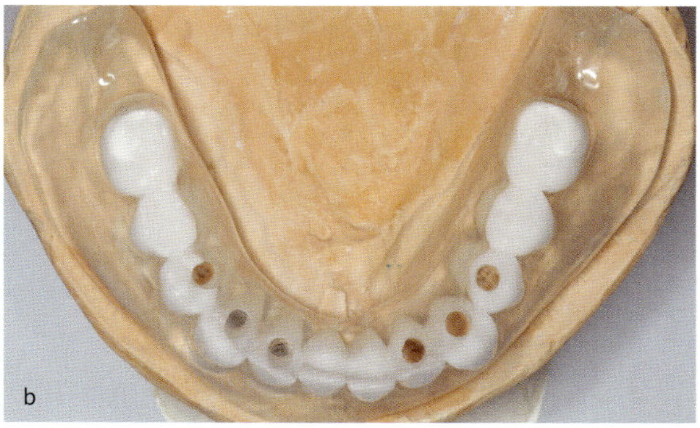

Figs 2a-b Radiographic template (classical method): The set-up as tried on intraorally is transferred to a radiographic template with teeth containing barium sulfate. The reference holes in the teeth reflect the ideal prosthetic implant axis.

A surgical guide is then digitally designed through a complex planning process and manufactured by CAM. The surgical guide allows precise placement of the implants in terms of position, angulation, and insertion depth via integrated guide sleeves using defined drilling sequences. This requires secure anchoring of the surgical guide, which is not possible in an edentulous jaw without the use of specific accessories, provided that the implant is also inserted using the template. Additional retention pins ensure positive fixation of the guide.

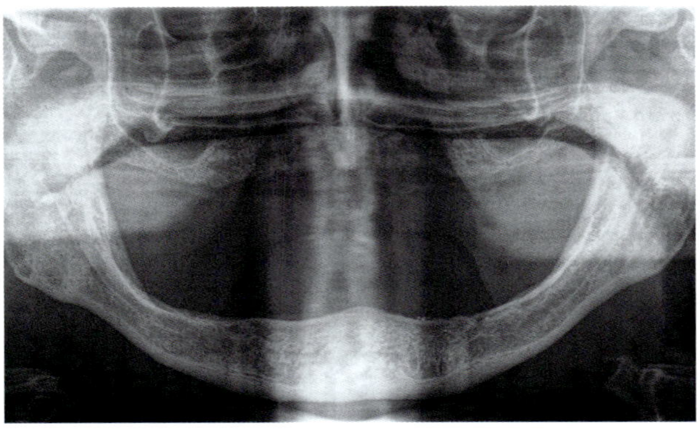

Fig 3 Panoramic radiograph of the edentulous jaw with pronounced mandibular atrophy. The mental foramina are located almost at the level of the alveolar ridges.

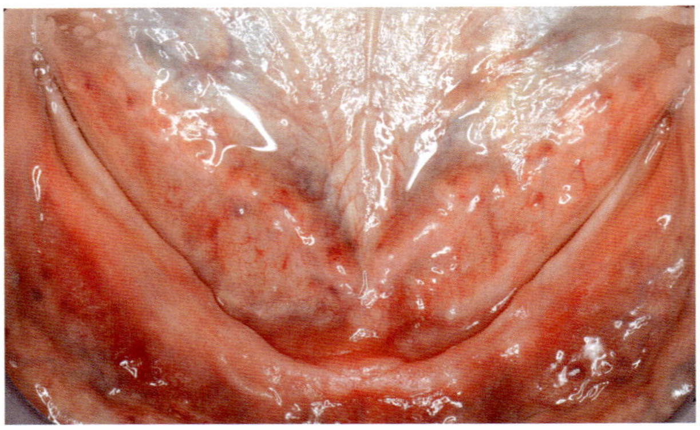

Fig 4 Initial situation: Occlusal view with severely atrophied alveolar ridges.

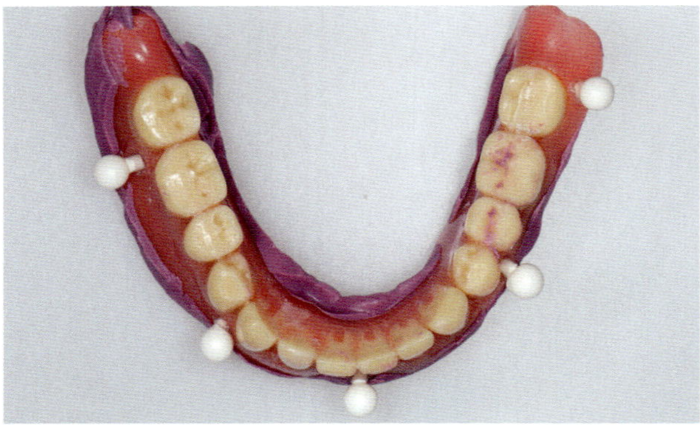

Fig 5 Radiographic template (using the existing complete denture): Relining of the denture for optimal congruency between the denture base and the alveolar ridge. Radiopaque cues (zirconia measuring spheres) are placed on the denture base at regular intervals. Sufficient distance from the denture is required for the spheres to be fully visible in subsequent scans.

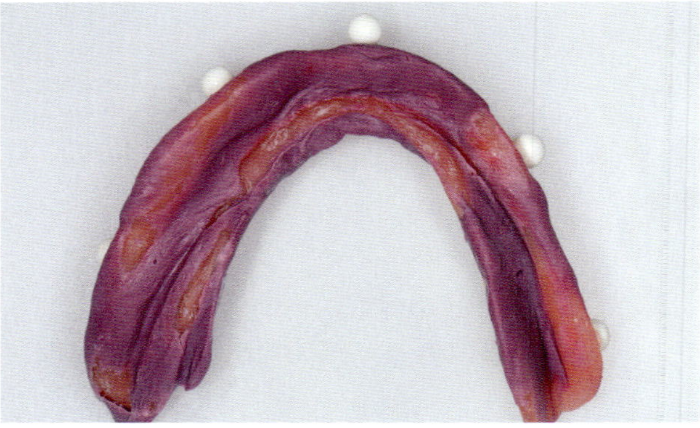

Fig 6 Basal view of the denture after relining.

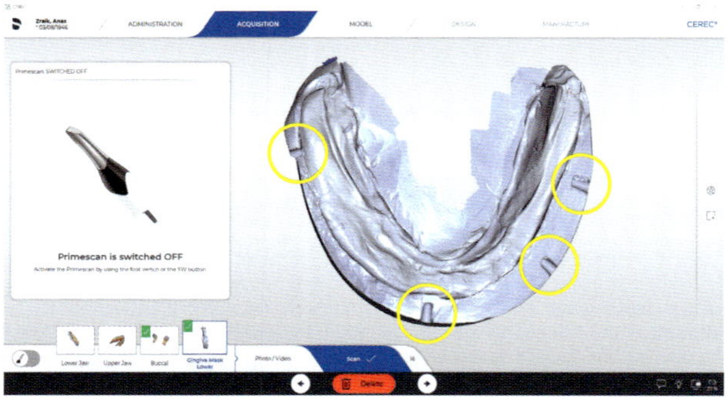

Fig 7 A stone cast of the denture base is made. Reference markers are incorporated (yellow circles) and the cast is scanned with an intraoral scanner.

CAD/CAM SURGICAL GUIDES IN THE EDENTULOUS JAW

In the clinical case presented in this chapter (Figs 3 and 4), a functional and esthetic analysis of the existing complete dentures concluded that it met all the projected requirements and could be used directly as a radiographic template. The radiographic measurements were taken with the existing prosthesis, followed by the CAD/CAM fabrication of the surgical guide. The procedure consists of the following steps (Tuna and coworkers 2024):

1. The denture is relined to ensure maximum congruence between the denture base and the alveolar ridge (Figs 5 and 6).
2. A stone cast of the denture base is made (Fig 7).
3. Since the denture itself has no radiopaque structures, fiducial markers (e.g., zirconia measuring spheres) are regularly spaced and attached to the denture base (Fig 5). These markers must not visually overlap with the prosthesis but should maintain a sufficient distance from the acrylic denture teeth and metallic framework structures within the denture.
4. Reference markers are placed on the outer surfaces of the cast (Fig 7).
5. Four datasets are created:
   a. STL dataset: The cast alone is scanned with an intraoral scanner (*cast-only* scan, Fig 7).
   b. STL dataset: The complete denture with the radiopaque measuring spheres is scanned with an intraoral scanner (*denture-only* scan).
   c. STL dataset: The complete denture with the radiopaque measuring spheres is scanned on the cast with an intraoral scanner (*denture-on-cast* scan, Fig 8).

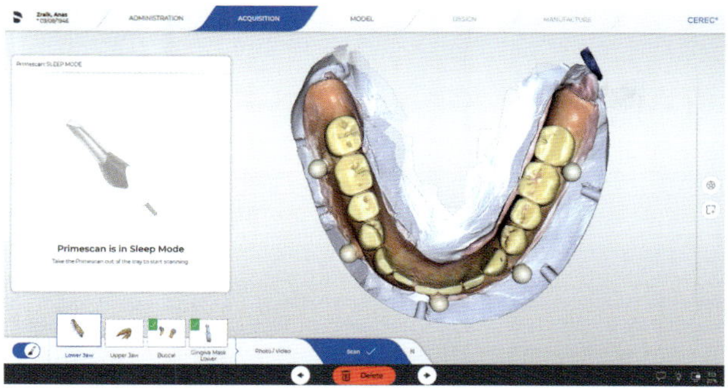

Fig 8 The denture is returned to the cast and scanned with it. Another scan is made of the denture only.

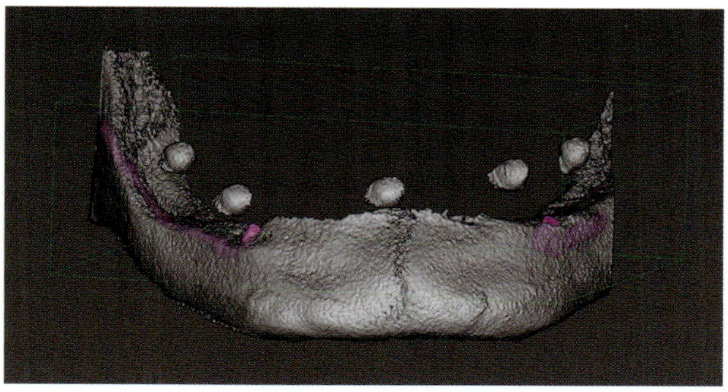

Fig 9 CBCT with the mandibular complete denture inserted. Only the reference bodies are visible.

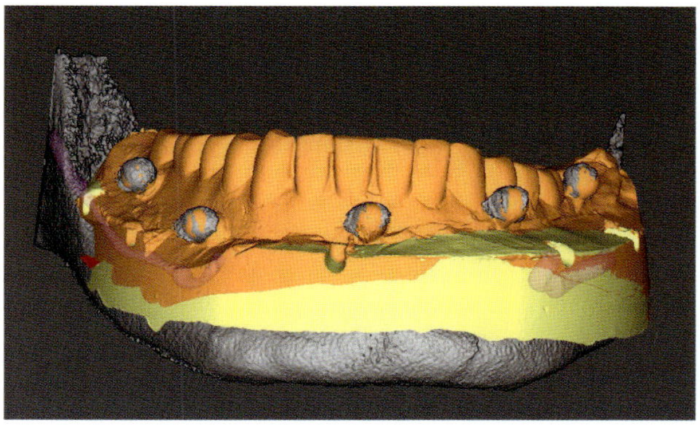

Fig 10 The measuring sphere is used to match the CBCT with the denture-on-cast STL dataset.

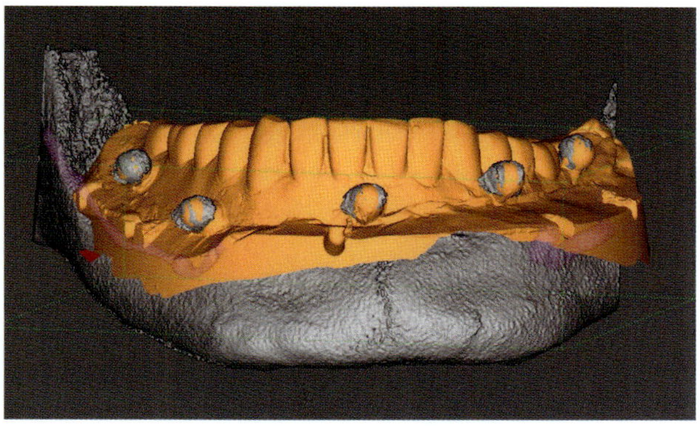

Fig 11 The measuring sphere is used to match the denture-on-cast STL dataset with the denture-only STL dataset.

d. DICOM dataset: A CBCT scan is made with the complete denture (including the measuring spheres) in place (*CBCT-with-denture*, Fig 9).

6. Finally, the measuring spheres and the temporary relining impression are removed from the denture.

The different datasets are superimposed and merged using the different reference structures (measuring spheres and markers in the dental stone):

In the first step, the *CBCT-with-denture* dataset is matched with the *denture-on-cast* dataset using fiducial markers (Fig 10). Next, the *denture-only* dataset is matched with the *denture-on-cast* dataset, again using the **fiducial markers** (Fig 11). Subsequently, the *denture-on-cast* dataset is matched with the *cast-only* dataset using the **reference markers** on the cast (Fig 12). The merged datasets can be individually added or subtracted as needed in the following steps.

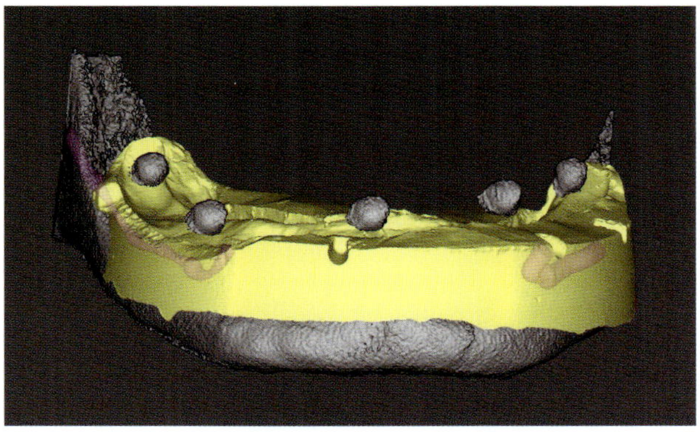

Fig 12 The reference marks on the cast are used to match the denture-on-cast STL dataset with the cast-only STL dataset.

The implants are assigned prosthetic positions in the DICOM dataset (Figs 13 and 14) for the subsequent design of the surgical guide. The guide is supported by the alveolar ridge over as large an area as possible so that it can be clearly positioned in the mouth (Figs 15 and 16). The design of the basal surface of the guide (the surface that contacts the alveolar ridge) is created according to the surface textures of the *cast-only* scan. This results in maximum congruence between the surgical guide and the alveolar ridge (Fig 17).

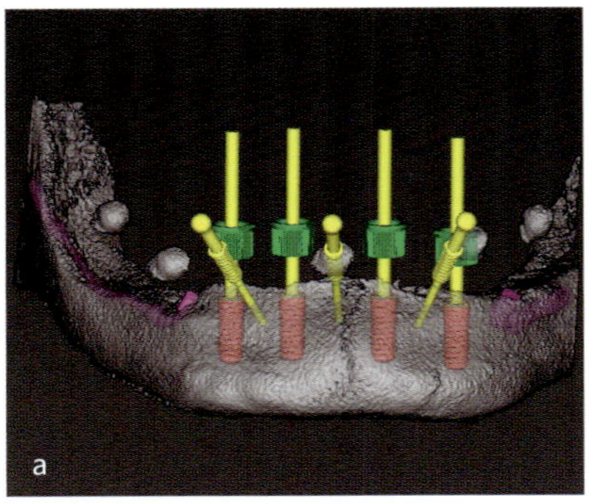

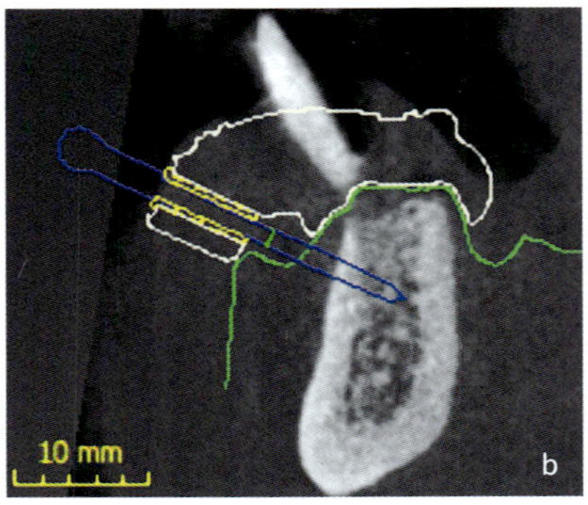

Figs 13a-b Implant planning and design of the three additional pin channels with precision guide inserts (a). The pins are adequately anchored in the jawbone (b).

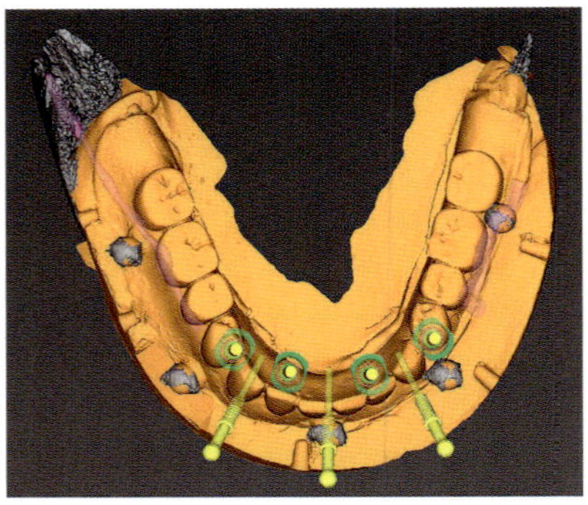

Fig 14 The implants are positioned as prosthetically guided.

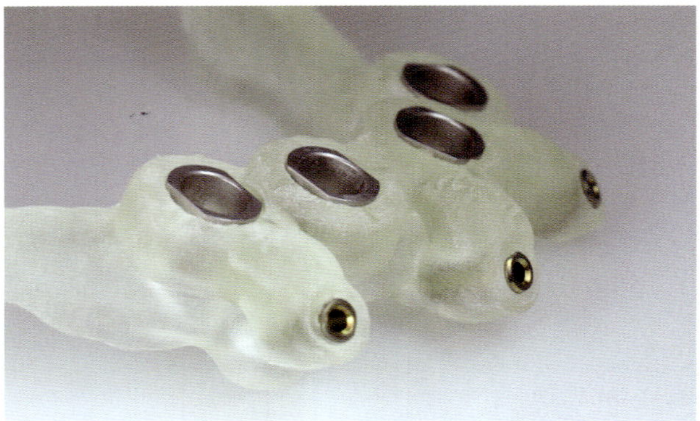

Fig 15 Finished printed surgical guide with bonded guide sleeves for the implants and guide inserts for the retention pins (basal surface constructed from the STL surface structures of the cast-only scan).

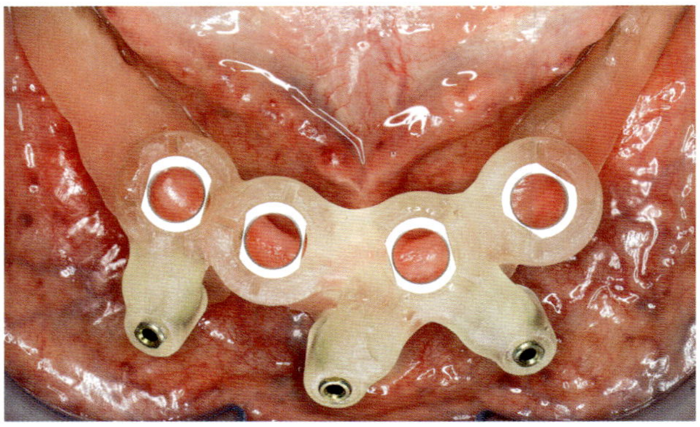

Fig 16 The characteristic saddle areas allow the surgical guide to be clearly positioned on the alveolar ridges.

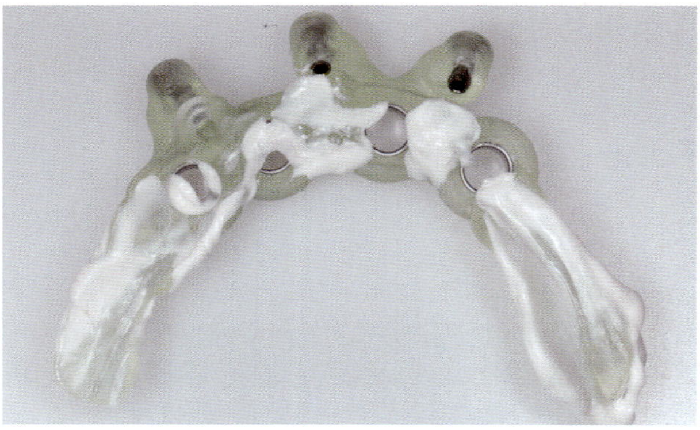

Fig 17 A visible thin line of flow silicone confirms that the surgical guide is fully seated.

3.1.4 Guided Implant Placement with Fixation Pins

To increase the accuracy of guided implant placement in the edentulous jaw, the guide should be attached to the alveolar ridge with additional fixation pins (e.g., Neodent Guided Surgery). For this purpose, the position and penetration depth of the pins are planned at the time the surgical guide is fabricated (Figs 13a-b). In addition to the implant guide sleeves, the finished guide has three pin channels with precision guide inserts (Fig 15). The holes for the retaining pins are drilled through the mucosa. All three retaining pins are then inserted and the guide is secured (Figs 18 to 20). The flap is then reflected. After exposing the alveolar ridge, the guide is reattached with the pins. At this point, it would no longer be possible to use anatomical structures alone for clear positioning (Fig 21).

With the surgical guide in place, the implants are inserted according to the drilling protocol. The drill keys reduce the diameters of the guide sleeves to different internal diameters, so that the pilot drills of different diameters are always precisely guided. A drilling protocol also specifies the drill bit length to be used and the height of the drill keys. The drill keys have a height of either 1 mm or 3 mm. This clearly defines both the drilling axis and the drilling depth (Figs 22 to 24). The implants can also be inserted through the surgical guide to prevent angulation changes during placement (Figs 25 to 29).

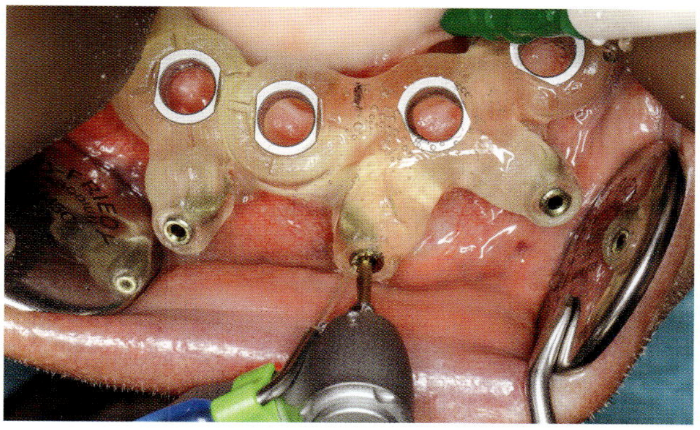

Fig 18 The pre-drills were guided through the pin channels and drilled through the mucosa into the bone with the guide in its optimal position. No flap should be reflected at this time.

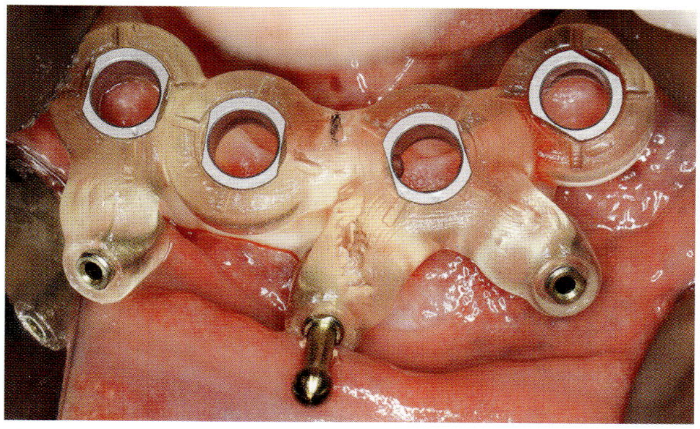

Fig 19 The first pin is inserted through the guide into the bone. The retention of the surgical guide has already improved before drilling the remaining pin channels.

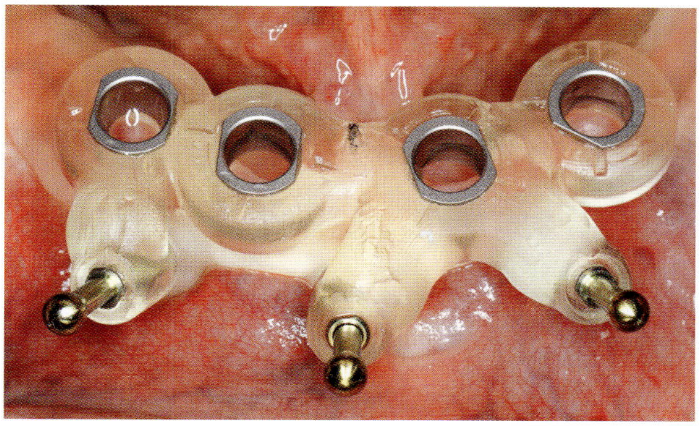

Fig 20 After drilling the remaining pin channels, all three pins are inserted as far as they will go.

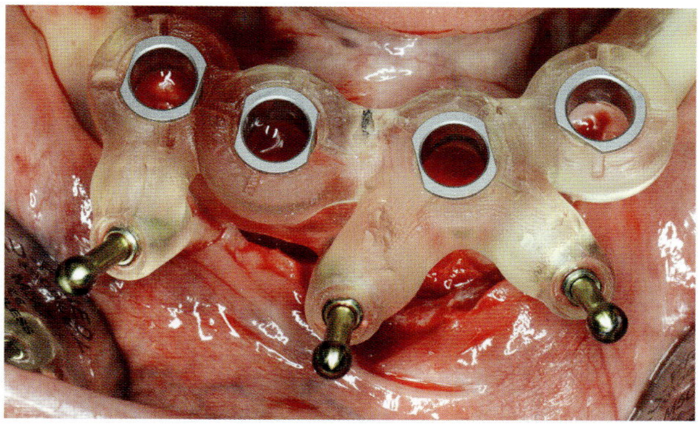

Fig 21 Flap reflection and insertion of the surgical guide with pins. The guide is now firmly anchored and securely fixed by the pins. The pin inserts aid in lip retraction and improve the view of the surgical field.

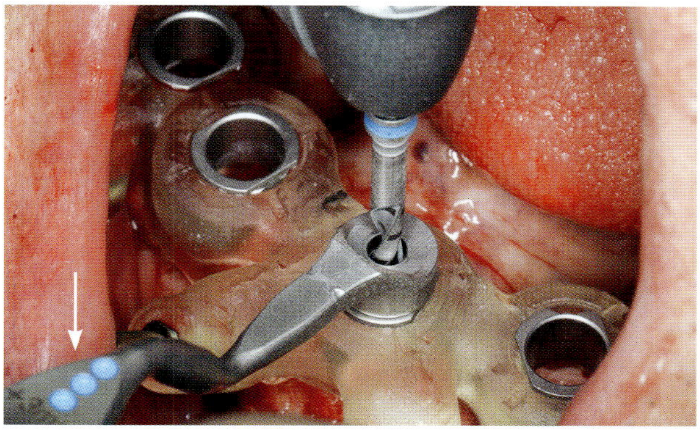

Fig 22 The drill keys reduce the diameters of the guide sleeves to different internal diameters, so that the pilot drills of different diameters are always precisely guided. A drilling protocol also specifies the drill bit length to be used and the height of the drill keys. The drill keys have a height of either 1 mm (one dot) or 3 mm (three dots, see arrow). This clearly defines both the drilling axis and the drilling depth.

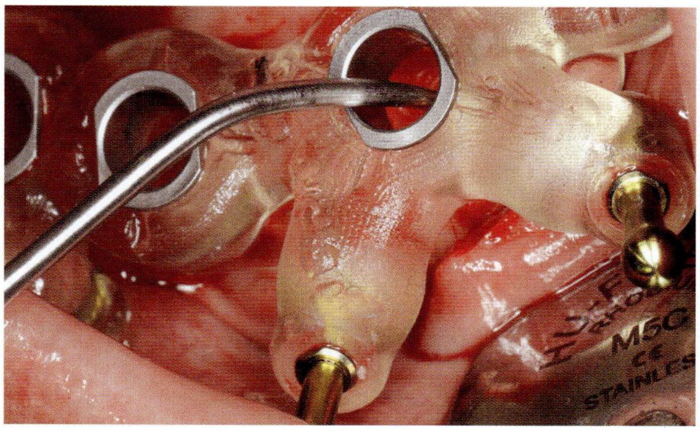

Fig 23 The cloverleaf probe can be used to probe the implant site through the surgical guide.

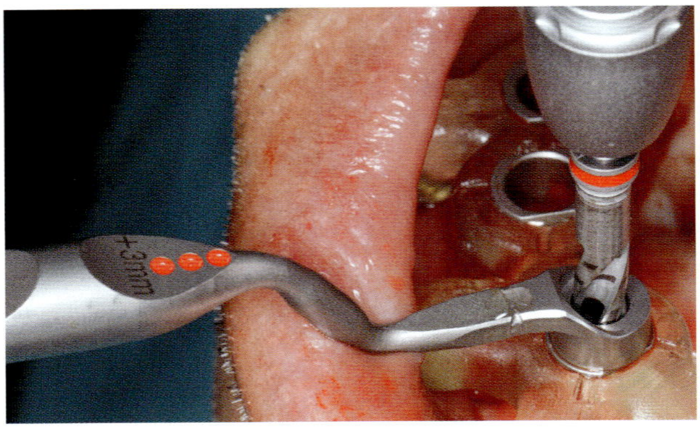

Fig 24 Final shaping drill with corresponding drill key.

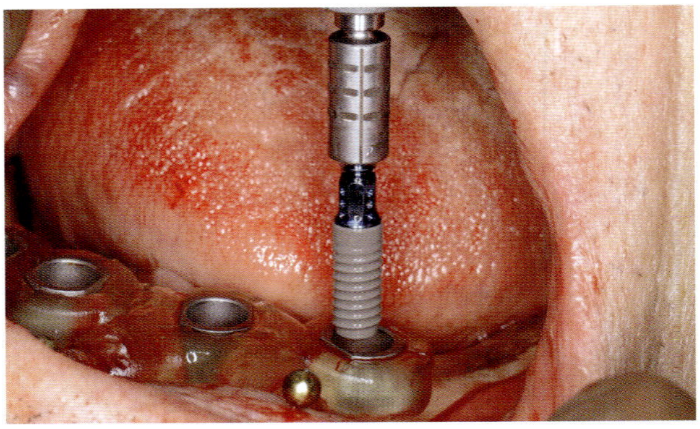

Fig 25 The implants can also be inserted through the surgical guide.

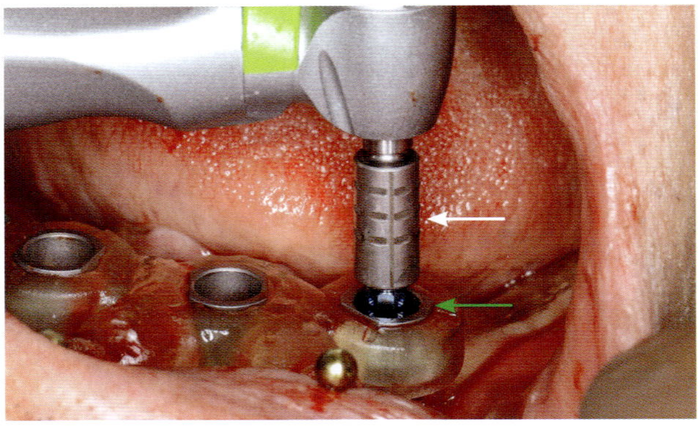

Fig 26 The insertion depth is determined by the horizontal markings on the insertion tool. When finished, the mark (white arrow) specified by the drilling protocol must be flush with the surgical guide (green arrow).

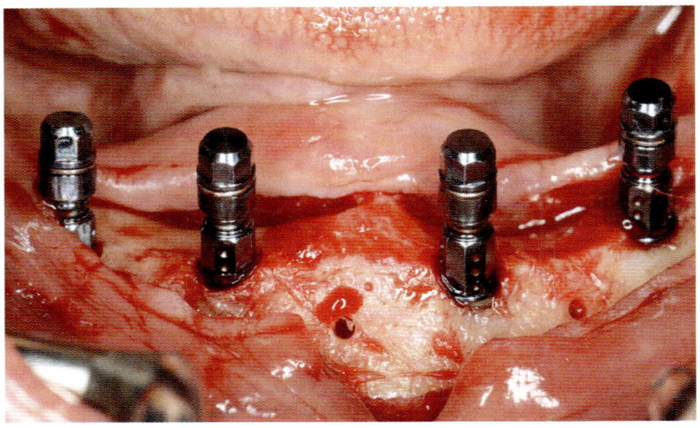

Fig 27 The implants are positioned in parallel with each other.

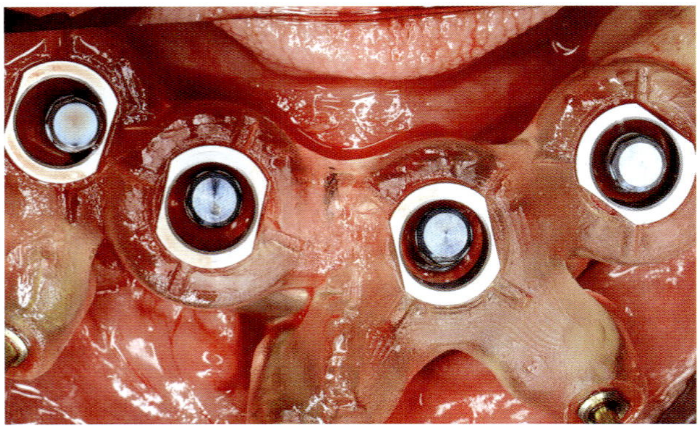

Fig 28 Verification of implant positions (with insertion posts) in relation to the surgical guide.

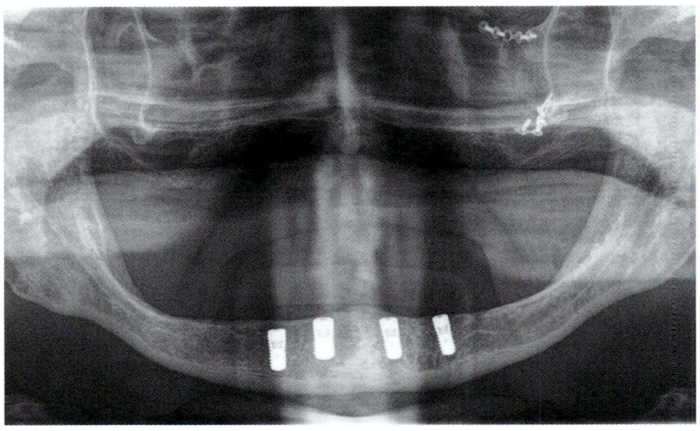

Fig 29 Postoperative panoramic radiograph.

3.1.5 Implant Planning/Placement and dPROs

Patients generally prefer digital technologies for implant planning and placement. However, no difference in intraoperative or postoperative comfort was observed whether implant placement was performed freehand, orientation-based, or with a surgical guide. Only flapless procedures were associated with improved dPROs (Bishti and coworkers 2021).

Three-dimensional planning allows the clinician to predict the course of surgery and the necessary surgical techniques much more accurately (Wismeijer and coworkers 2018; Dawson and coworkers 2022). Based on this accurate planning, it also allows for more sophisticated patient education, which becomes much more vivid and easier to understand when three-dimensional imaging techniques are available. This, better illustrated, patient education suggests an easier understanding of the patient regarding the upcoming surgical procedure. This can further strengthen the dentist-patient relationship (Gross 2012). In addition, the use of a surgical guide typically significantly reduces the surgical time, which in turn can have a positive impact on postoperative (dis)comfort (Wismeijer and coworkers 2018).

3.2 Augmentation Techniques in the Edentulous Jaw

B. Al-Nawas

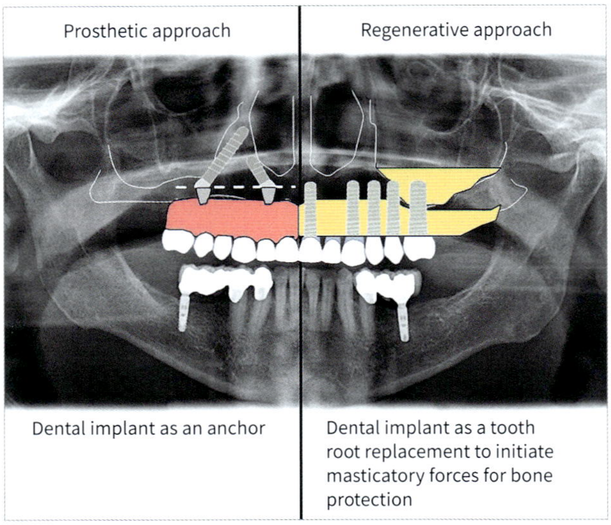

Fig 30 Prosthetic strategy (left) with dental implant serving as anchor vs. regenerative strategy (right) with dental implant serving as dental root replacement for directing the chewing forces in order to protect the bone (Terheyden 2022).

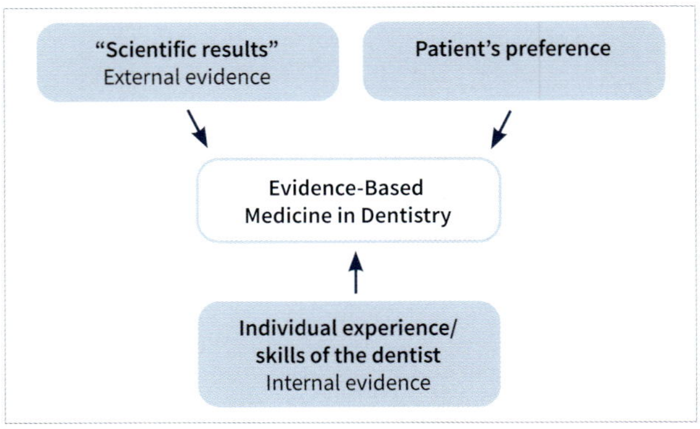

Fig 31 Evidenced-Based Medicine in Dentistry as a basis for individual decision-making processes.

3.2.1 The Decision-Making Process: Avoiding Augmentation

Bone (and soft-tissue) deficiencies are common in the edentulous jaw. Systematically, bone and soft-tissue reconstructive procedures (augmentation) can be contrasted with approaches involving prosthetic reconstruction (Fig 30). The latter often involves the use of implants with reduced dimensions. The number and quality of clinical trials for a given procedure vary, resulting in different levels of external evidence. Guidelines and consensus conferences can help to maintain an overview of evidence-based clinical guidelines.

Individual decision-making includes this external evidence, but also the individual skill and experience of the clinician (internal evidence). For the clinician, open information about treatment alternatives is a must, although of course internal evidence (i.e., the clinician's personal skill and specialty) will also guide the patient's decision.

All clinicians should adopt an evidence-based approach to clinical practice (Fig 31). The key is to recognize and document the constant variation in all three elements of the Evidence-Based Implant Dentistry (EBID) definition, and to maintain the appropriate relative balance between them. To assist clinicians with implementation in practice, the ITI has developed the online 3E Check Tool, whereas the three E's refer to external Evidence, clinician Experience, and patient Engagement (Fig 32).

Use this code to access the ITI's 3E Check Tool

3.2.2 One-Stage vs. Two-Stage Augmentation Techniques

The success of complex extraosseous augmentation is more difficult to predict than for intraosseous defects. Regeneration also depends on the available bony bed and is usually limited to an increase in bone dimensions of 3 to 5 mm, depending on the material used. Therefore, in cases of extensive sinus lifts or complex augmentations, two-stage concepts with secondary implant placement are justified. The long reconstructive phase and the often extremely difficult provisional phase add to the challenges faced by the clinician and patient in this type of treatment. It is not uncommon for the duration of therapy to exceed one year. It is therefore clear that single-stage procedures with implant placement at the time of bone augmentation are also more attractive from the patient's point of view.

In recent years, the topic of immediate restoration has gained new momentum. The paradigm shift behind this topic is complex:

- Shorter, narrower, or angled implants have become established treatment protocols, allowing augmentation-free reconstruction of missing tissue via the prosthetic restoration.
- 3D planning systems allow precise prediction of implant possibilities in the local bone to match the restoration.
- Compared to augmentation, chewing function is achieved earlier with the temporary restoration. The trend is therefore clearly moving away from complex augmentation procedures and toward simpler, single-stage or augmentation-free procedures.

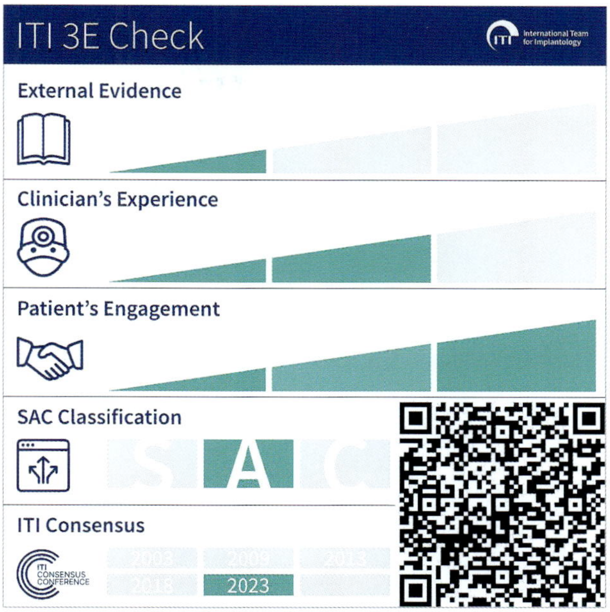

Fig 32 Example of a 3E check created with the ITI 3E Check Tool.

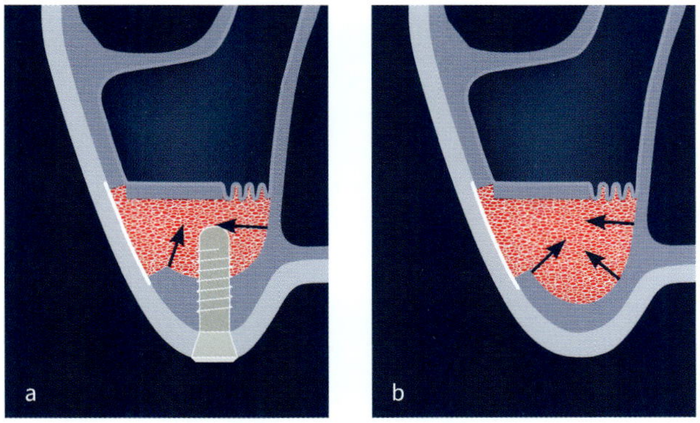

Figs 33a-b Approximately 4 mm of regeneration can be expected from the bony walls. A good regeneration capacity of a "small" sinus floor elevation allowing simultaneous implant insertion (a). Critical regeneration capacity of a large sinus floor elevation requiring staged implant insertion (b) (ITI Treatment Guide, Vol. 5. Sinus Floor Elevation Procedures. Katsuyama and Storgård Jensen 2011).

3.2.3 Sinus Lift

The sinus lift is a special procedure in the field of augmentation. The technique is highly developed, well documented and allows the experienced surgeon a very low patient burden and a high degree of predictability. Residual bone height plays a minor role. With the exception of eggshell-thin bone, modern implant systems can stabilize even in a residual alveolar bone height as little as 2 mm. Recent studies have once again shown the regeneration potential depending on the width of the sinus and the vertical proportions in the sinus. Here, too, approximately 4 mm of regeneration can be expected, starting from the bony walls (Troeltzsch 2016) (Figs 33a-b). This must be taken into account during planning.

In combination with narrow implants in the canine and premolar region, an external sinus floor elevation often allows a favorable implant distribution in a single-stage surgical procedure (Figs 34a-d and 35a-b).

If it is assumed that 8-mm implants also represent a sufficient long-term prognosis, i.e., the implants tend to become shorter overall, the indication for an internal sinus lift also increases compared to the external one. It is important to exclude or evaluate assess sinus mucosal pathology prior to sinus lift surgery. In the case of more extensive mucosal swelling, preoperative evaluation and revision by a specialist may be considered.

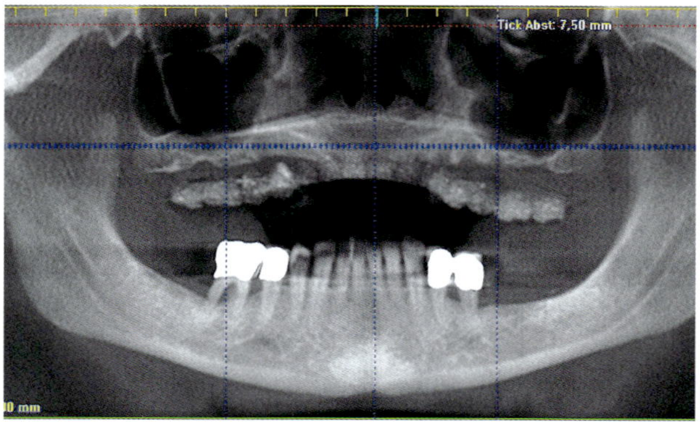

Fig 34a Preoperative CBCT including radiografic templates showing the need for a sinus lift; residual paranasal bone.

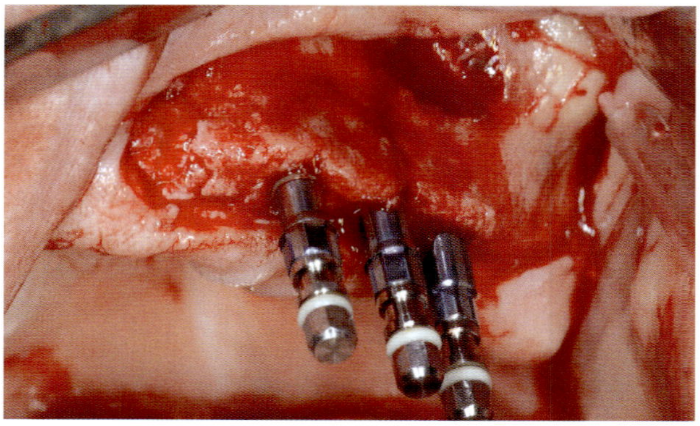

Fig 34b Sinus lift using a bone scraper for access. Narrow-diameter implants in the canine and premolar regions.

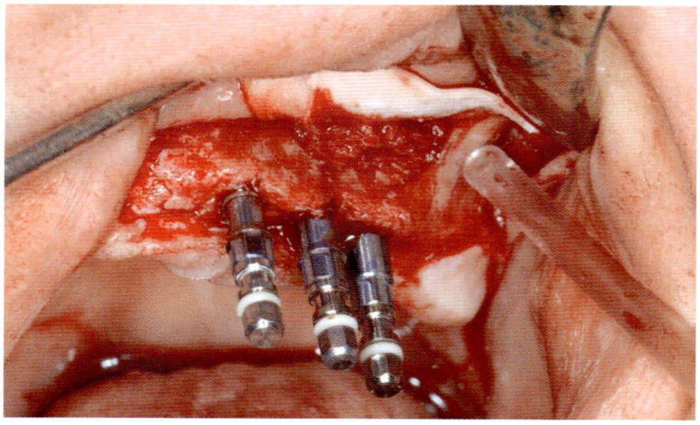

Fig 34c Membrane, autologous scraper bone, and xenogeneic bone substitute in situ.

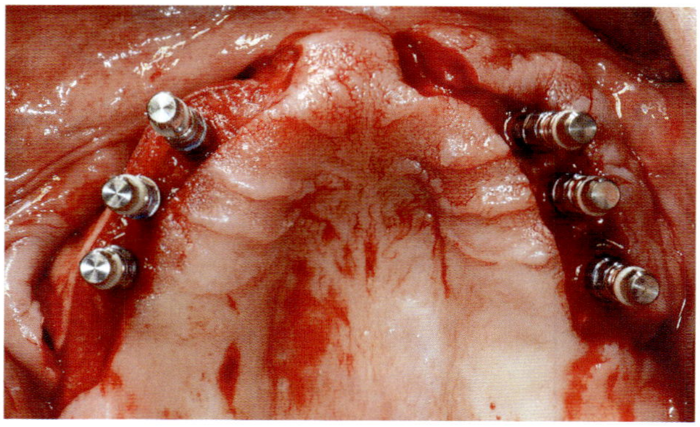

Fig 34d Palatal incision line and implant distribution.

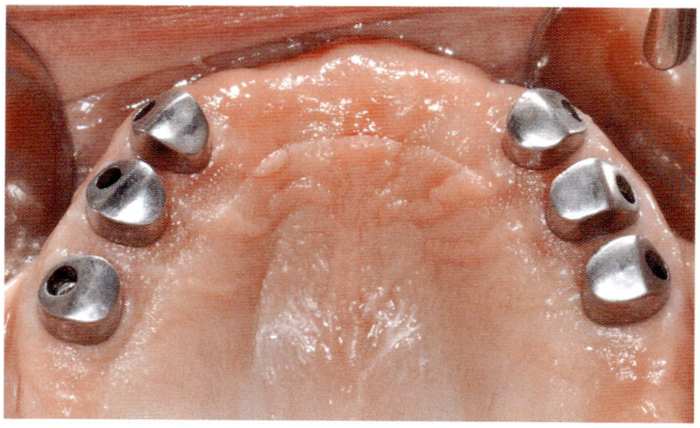

Fig 35a 5-year follow-up of telescoping crowns and removable denture.

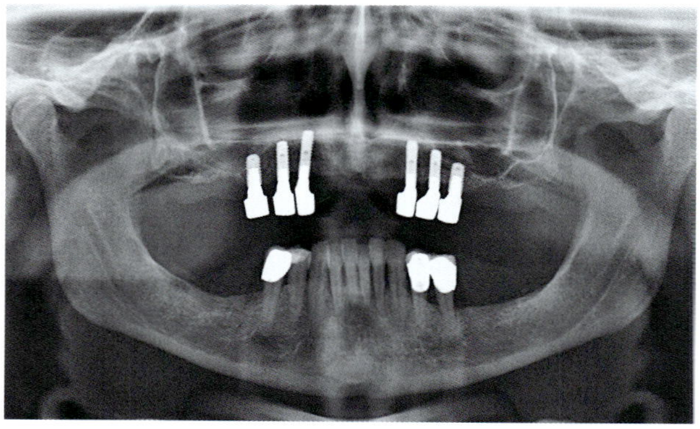

Fig 35b Radiograph at the 5-year follow-up.

Postoperative sinusitis is a not entirely uncommon complication with an incidence of approximately 2–5% (Testori 2023). It is diagnosed clinically and can usually be treated conservatively. In rare cases, especially with the use of alloplastic or xenogeneic materials, chronic sinusitis has been reported, often due to aspergillosis. This usually responds well to surgical intervention without the need for complete implant removal or bone augmentation. The sinus lift thus represents the "workhorse" of maxillary augmentation and is often the only procedure required to provide a sufficient base for implant-supported reconstruction.

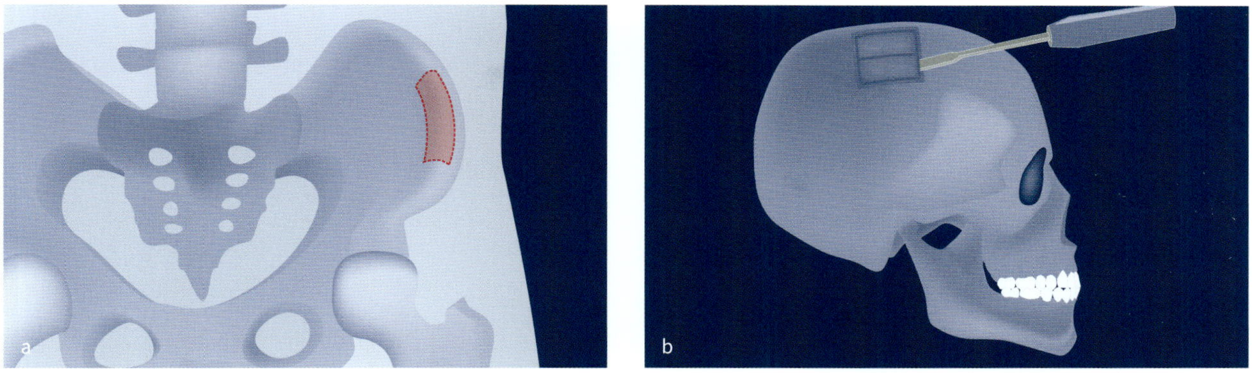

Figs 36a-b Typical extraoral sources of autologous bone. Iliac crest (a). Calvaria (b) (ITI Treatment Guide, Vol. 7. Ridge Augmentation Procedures in Implant Patients: A Staged Approach. Cordaro and Terheyden 2014).

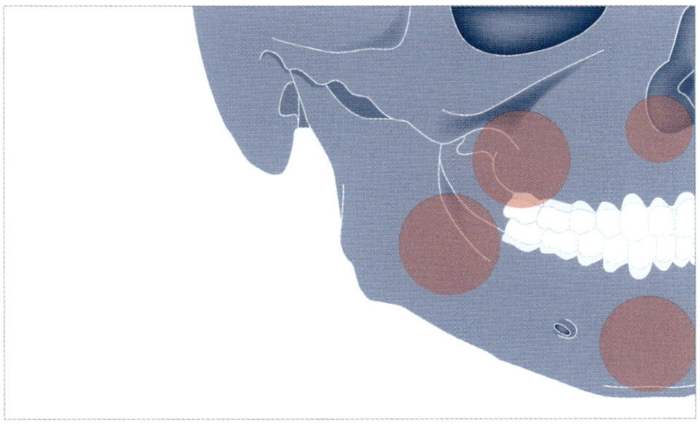

Fig 37 Typical intraoral sources of autologous bone.

3.2.4 Crestal Augmentation

In both the maxilla and the mandible, onlay as well as interposition techniques are viable augmentation options (Fig 39).

In the posterior mandible, the sandwich osteoplasty technique has become established for vertical defects. The bone above the inferior alveolar nerve is split horizontally, displaced cranially, and fixed with a miniplate (Fig 40b). Although this procedure is considered established, the high rate of (temporary) nerve injury and the now-available alternative option of short implants tend to discourage this technique (Kamperos and coworkers 2016). In contrast, bone splitting for horizontal ridge augmentation combined with buccal apposition of replacement material is a good therapeutic option, especially in the maxillary premolar region (Fig 40a). In severe horizontal defects of the maxilla with some residual alveolar bone and a typical class III jaw relation, a Le Fort I osteotomy and maxillary advancement can be the method of choice. This allows rehabilitation of the hard and soft tissues and can be interpreted as a "split technique" (Fig 40c).

Crestal augmentation has been described in the past with cortical iliac crest and calvarial grafts (Figs 36a-b). Solid long-term data are also available for these procedures. However, the harvesting morbidity of these extraoral grafts is significantly higher than that of intraoral grafts (Fig 37), so the use of intraoral mandibular blocks has become more common as a primary option.

Currently, block techniques are increasingly being replaced by shell techniques (Figs 38 and 39). In particular, the prevalence of combined defects outside the bony envelope requires stable immobilization of particulate augmentation materials (autologous, xenogeneic, alloplastic), and rigid shells, meshes, and membranes are used for this purpose to ensure adequate shape and space maintenance (Table 1).

A special indication for maxillary crestal augmentation was reported by Caramês and coworkers (2022), who supported the augmentation procedure for facial soft-tissue support.

A 50-year-old female patient was referred for consultation and treatment following 20 years of complete edentulism in the maxilla and partial edentulism in the mandible (Figs 41a-c). The patient reported a history of periodontal disease and dental caries as the primary causes of her tooth loss. A bilateral sinus lift with concomitant placement of dental implants and horizontal augmentation was planned for the maxilla. An immediate loading approach was planned for the mandible.

Table 1 Selection of common "shells" for the stabilization of particulate materials.

Autologous	Allogeneic	Alloplastic materials	Xenogeneic materials
Autologous bone shells	Allogeneic cortical shells	Titanium mesh Polylactide shells PTFE membranes	Collagen membranes Xenogeneic bone laminae

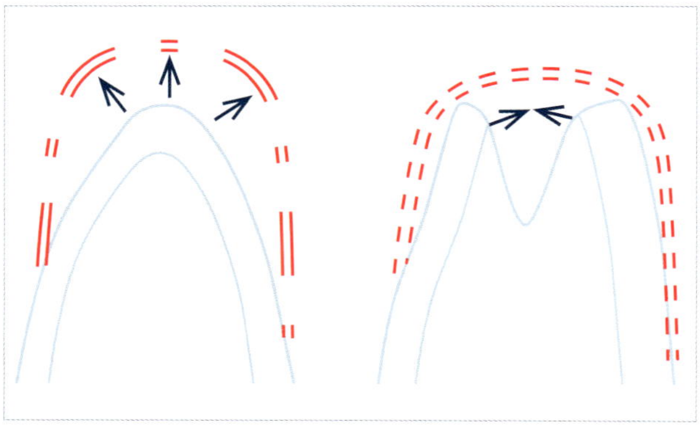

Fig 38 Onlay (left) vs. inlay (right) graft.

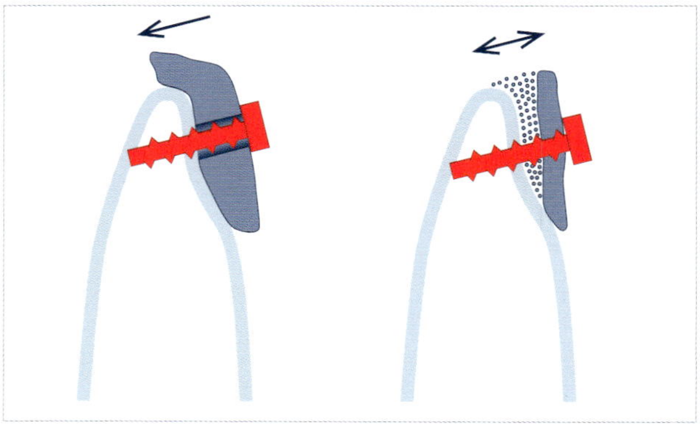

Fig 39 Onlay graft. Block vs. shell techniques.

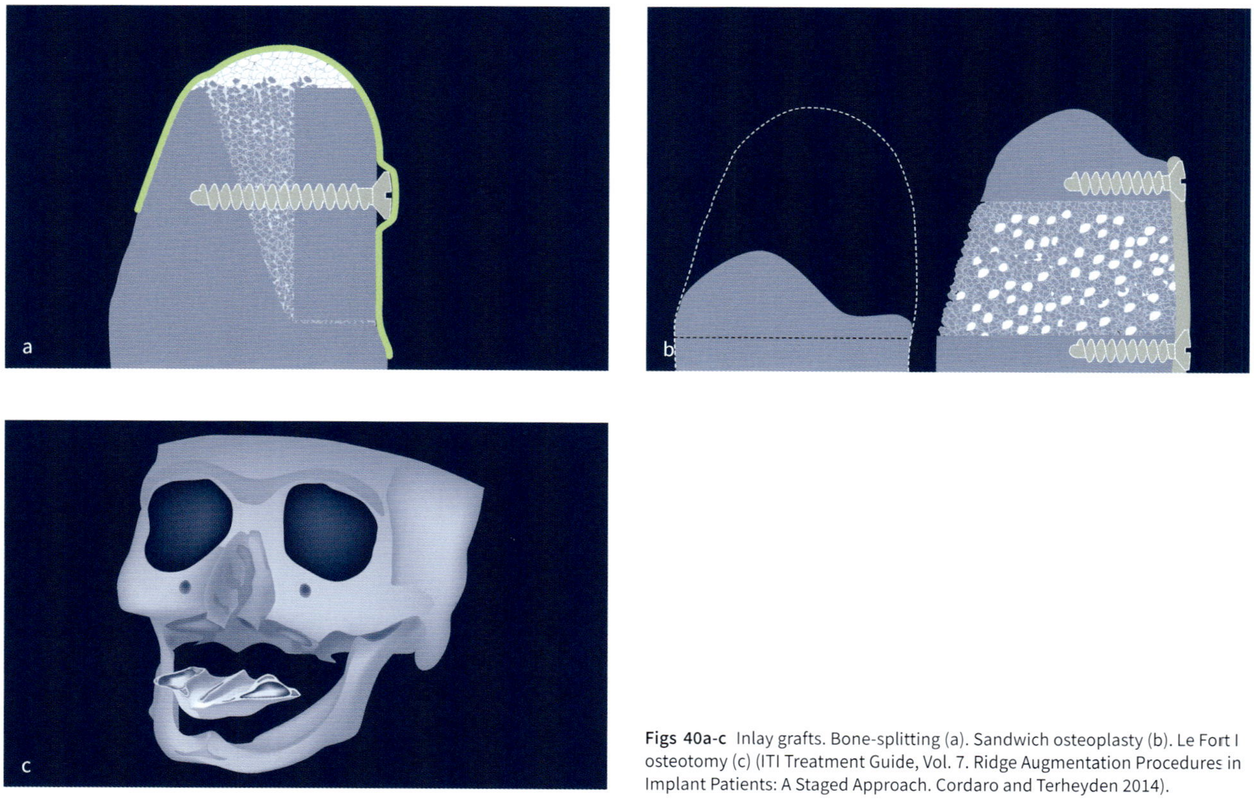

Figs 40a-c Inlay grafts. Bone-splitting (a). Sandwich osteoplasty (b). Le Fort I osteotomy (c) (ITI Treatment Guide, Vol. 7. Ridge Augmentation Procedures in Implant Patients: A Staged Approach. Cordaro and Terheyden 2014).

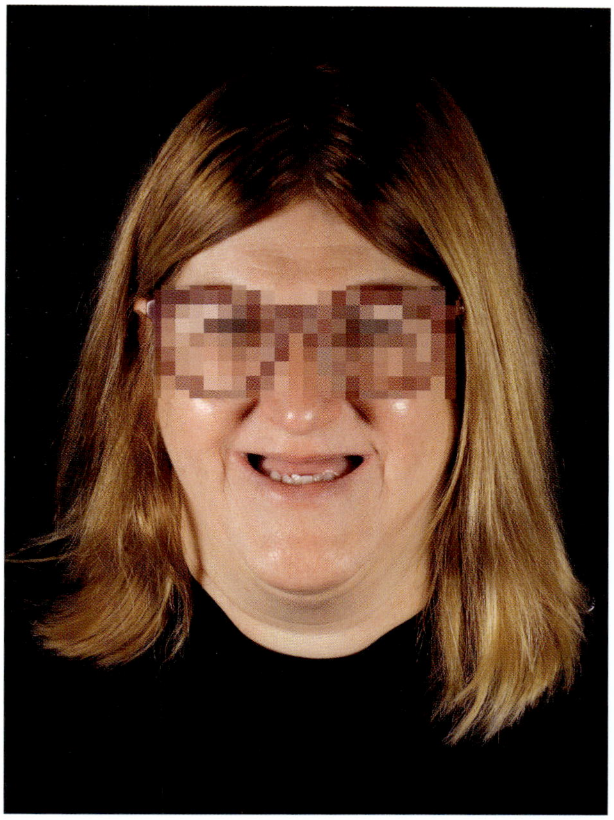

Fig 41a Preoperative smile without prothesis.

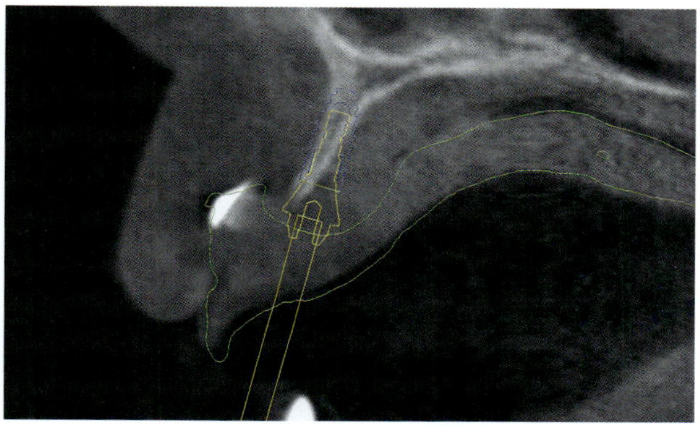

Fig 41b Virtual planning: 3.3-mm implant and its relation to the anterior crest of the maxilla.

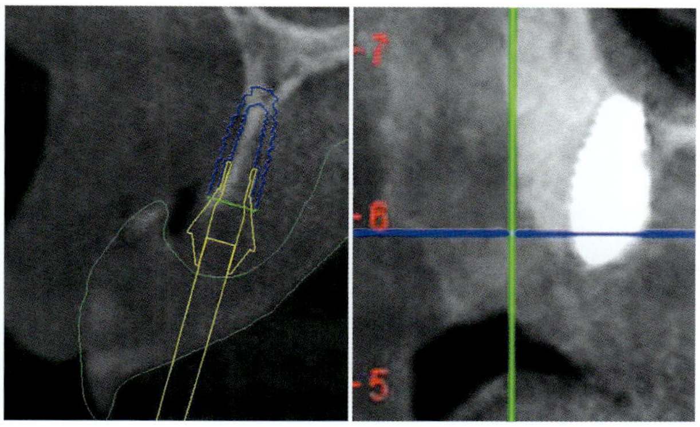

Fig 41c Six months follow-up after ridge augmentation.

A mixture of particulate xenograft and approximately 2 PRF membranes per 0.5 mg of biomaterial (50 : 50 ratio), and liquid fibrinogen was used to obtain a composite bone block. In the anterior zone, guided bone regeneration was performed to improve lip support and the emergence profile of the future fixed prosthesis by applying the previously prepared and shaped PRF/xenograft composite on the buccal plate of the premaxilla to restore bone volume. At the same time, eight implants were placed in the maxilla (Figs 42 and 43). After a provisional phase, the situation was restored with a monolithic zirconia restoration. At the 1-year follow-up visit, the peri-implant soft tissue showed no signs of inflammation, and there was no significant bone resorption around the implants (Figs 44 and 45).

The long-term stability of complex augmentations, particularly in the vertical dimension, has repeatedly been questioned. Case series have demonstrated the long-term stability of individual procedures. However, considerable experience is often required to achieve predictable results. It is also striking that the role of soft tissue in complex crestal augmentations is rarely discussed scientifically, despite clear evidence that the presence of an adequate peri-implant band of keratinized attached mucosa is a key to long-term success.

ACKNOWLEDGMENTS

Surgical and prosthodontic procedures

Prof Dr João Caramês – Lisbon, Portugal

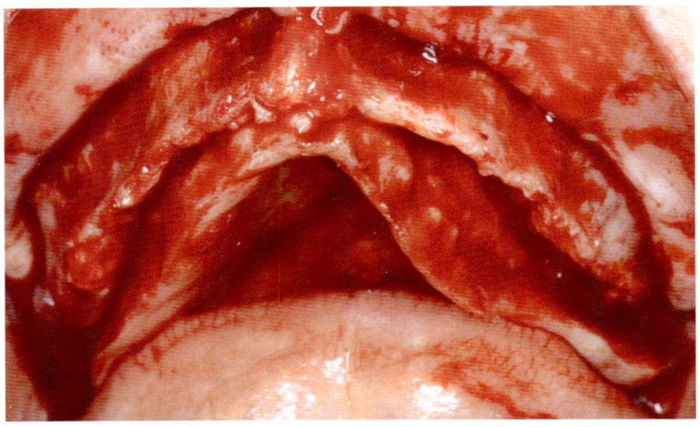

Fig 42a Maxillary surgery.

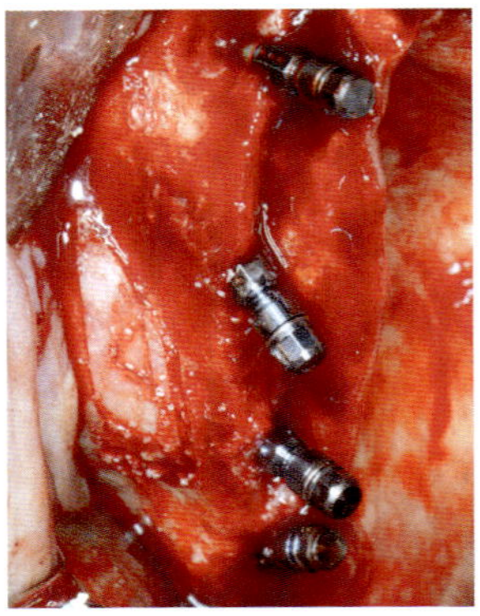

Fig 42b Implant position.

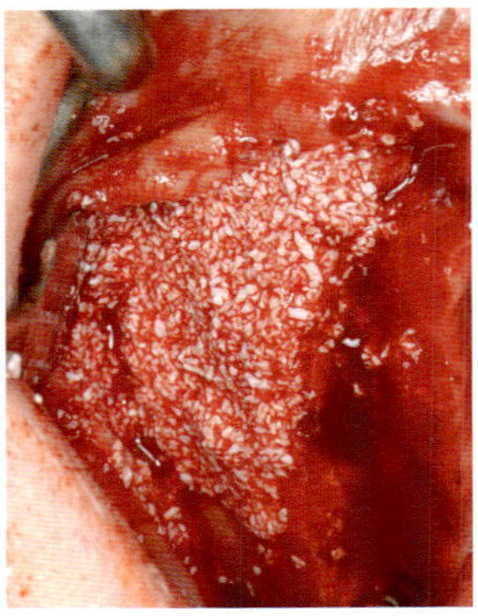

Fig 42c Xenogenic and autologous bone graft with PRF.

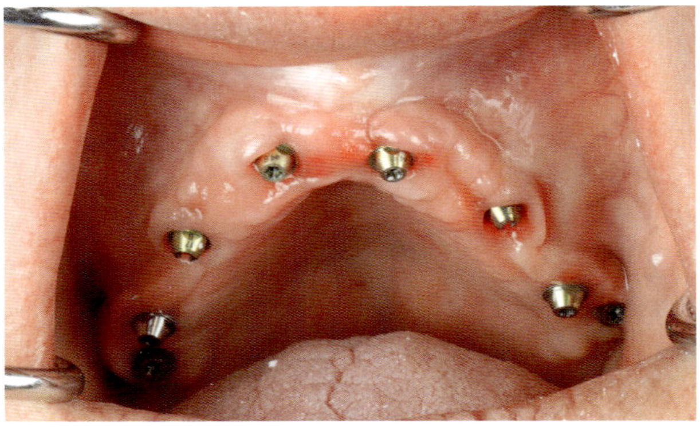

Fig 43 Intraoral situation 6 weeks after surgery.

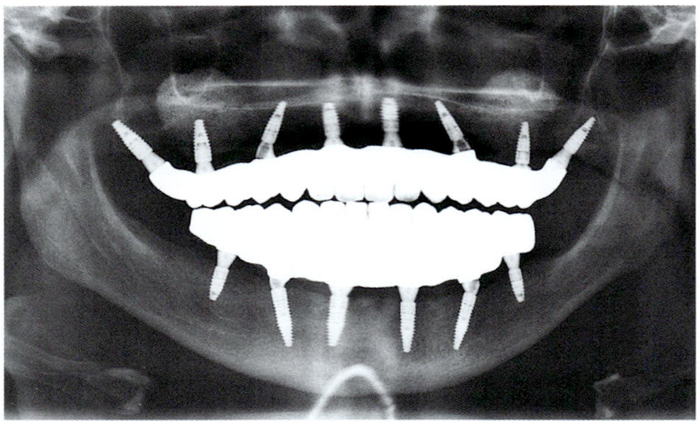

Fig 44 Final panoramic view.

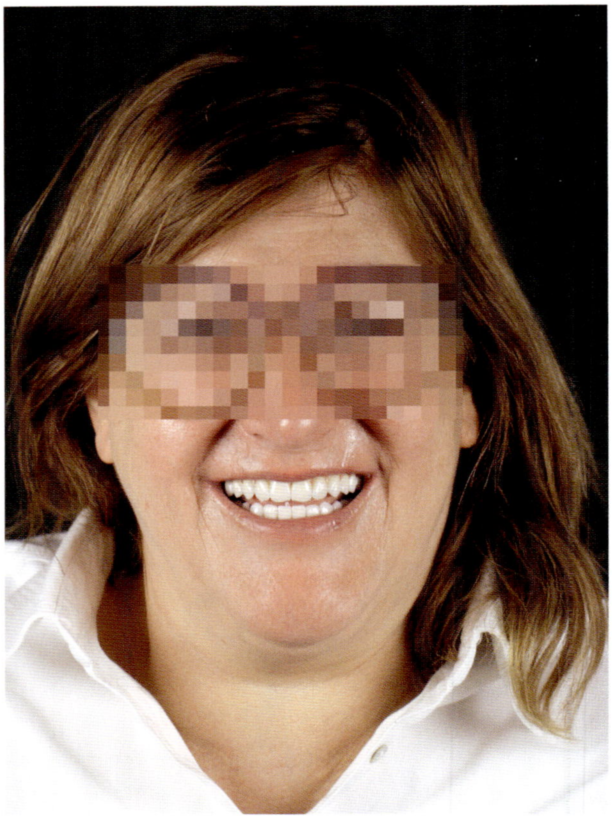

Fig 45 Final smile.

3.3 Loading Protocols in the Edentulous Jaw

S. Wolfart

Loading protocols are divided into immediate loading (delivery of the prosthesis within 1 week from implant placement), early loading (1 week to 2 months), and conventional loading (2 months or more) (Gallucci and coworkers 2014).

Whether immediate loading is possible in the edentulous jaw depends on the quality and quantity of the bone (e.g., the need for concomitant bone augmentation), the number of implants placed, and the type of restoration planned. A key factor for successful immediate loading is adequate primary stability of the implants of at least 35 Ncm (De Bruyn and coworkers 2014). Primary stability can be increased by using longer implants, adjusting drilling protocols, and using implants with "aggressive" thread patterns.

3.3.1 Immediate Loading with Removable Prostheses

EDENTULOUS MANDIBLE

Stoker and Wismeijer (2011) reported in a randomized clinical trial on the immediate loading of two implants connected by a bar to an overdenture in 124 edentulous patients. Two interconnected implants can be successfully loaded with a mandibular overdenture on the same day as implant placement with a high implant survival rate (99%). Only a few patients required additional relining of the overdenture (Stoker and Wismeijer 2011). These very good results were confirmed in a review published in 2014 by De Bruyn and coworkers (2014): The edentulous mandible can be immediately restored with two to four implants placed in the interforaminal region. The implants are restored with either splinted bars, or with non-splinted telescopic crowns or ball attachments. Implant survival rates are greater than 95% and marginal bone loss is less than 1 mm.

If only a single median implant is placed in the edentulous mandible and restored with a ball attachment, immediate loading is not recommended (Kern and coworkers 2018).

EDENTULOUS MAXILLA

The scientific evidence for immediate loading with an overdenture in the maxilla is limited. Only two studies were identified that successfully loaded four implants immediately with either a primary splinted bar (Pieri and coworkers 2009) or secondary splinted telescopic crowns (Eccellente and coworkers 2011). Therefore, claims regarding immediate loading with an overdenture in the edentulous maxilla should be interpreted with caution, due to insufficient data being available.

3.3.2 Immediate Loading with Fixed Long-Term Provisionals

EDENTULOUS MANDIBLE

With four to six implants, immediate loading in the edentulous mandible shows results comparable to conventional loading protocols (De Bruyn and coworkers 2014). For immediate loading of axially positioned implants in the anterior region combined with distally angled implants in the premolar region, implant survival and success rates are 93% and 91.7%, respectively, over an observation period of 10 to 18 years (Maló and coworkers 2019b).

EDENTULOUS MAXILLA

Immediate loading is also a viable treatment option for the maxilla, provided a sufficient number of implants are used. With six to eight implants, the failure rate is between 0% and 3.3%. The failure rate increases when the number of implants is reduced from six to four (De Bruyn and coworkers 2014). When only four implants are used, the concept of axially positioned implants in the anterior region combined with distally angled implants in the premolar region seems to be successful. The cumulative implant survival and success rates are 94.7% and 93.9% respectively, over an observation period of 5 to 13 years (Maló and coworkers 2019a).

3.3.3 Immediate Loading and dPROs

In terms of patient satisfaction, there is evidence that patients are more satisfied with immediate loading than with early or conventional implant loading. This is particularly true for full-arch fixed long-term provisional restorations (Gotfredsen and coworkers 2021; Donos and coworkers 2021). In general, patients who have been edentulous for a long time and are accustomed to wearing dentures are less likely to insist on an immediate restoration than patients who have recently lost their teeth and may never have worn a removable prosthesis.

3.4 Restorative Concepts

S. Wolfart

3.4.1 Functional Improvements with Prostheses

In terms of successful tertiary prophylaxis, it can be expected that rehabilitation of edentulous jaws with implant-supported restorations will contribute to the preservation of orofacial tissues such as the alveolar bone and jaw muscles when compared with conventional complete dentures or no treatment at all.

A systematic review and meta-analysis was conducted to examine the relevant data but was found to be inconclusive (De Souza and coworkers 2023). The main objectives of the analysis were alveolar ridge resorption and the thickness of the masseter muscle. The following clinical recommendations were derived from the 7th ITI Consensus Conference (2023):

Clinical recommendation 1
In edentulous patients, rehabilitation with a complete implant-supported fixed dental prosthesis or a removable implant-retained overdenture is beneficial to reduce alveolar bone resorption. The evidence does not favor one treatment modality over another. Regular maintenance appointments to ensure peri-implant health and occlusal stability of the prosthesis are also recommended to minimize alveolar bone loss (Schimmel and coworkers 2023).

Clinical recommendation 2
In fully edentulous patients, rehabilitations with complete implant-supported fixed dental prostheses or removable implant-retained overdentures are recommended to increase masseter muscle thickness compared to complete dentures. It is plausible to infer that this may have a positive effect on chewing (Schimmel and coworkers 2023).

Use this code to download the Proceedings of the 7th ITI Consensus Conference (2023)

3.4.2 Fixed Dental Restorations

NUMBER OF IMPLANTS AND RESTORATIVE APPROACHES
Implant-supported full-arch restorations in the edentulous jaw anchored on four to eight implants in the maxilla and mandible have been described in the literature. In rare cases, the use of ten implants per jaw has been reported. Many factors influence the decision on the number of implants. A systematic review has evaluated the surgical and prosthetic performance associated with the use of five or more implants compared with fewer than five implants (Polido and coworkers 2018). The following prosthetically relevant recommendations were derived from the 6th ITI Consensus Conference (2018):

Clinical recommendation 1
The final prosthetic plan should be considered when developing a surgical plan for implant treatment of edentulous arches. Factors to be considered include (Morton and coworkers 2018):

- Prosthesis material (see Chapter 3.4.2)
- One-piece or segmented prostheses (see Chapter 3.4.2)
- Esthetic factors (e.g., lip support, smile line)
- Condition of the opposing dentition
- Available space for the prosthesis
- Anatomy of the edentulous ridge (maxilla, mandible, bone volume and quality, anatomical limitations)
- Planned implant distribution and cantilever length (for fixed restorations)
- Space available for hygiene and maintenance (see Chapter 3.4.2)
- Patient preference and compliance

Clinical recommendation 2
A minimum number of four appropriately distributed implants are recommended to support a one-piece full-arch fixed prosthesis. However, the impact of future implant loss/complications on prosthesis support should

be considered when choosing implant number. Additional implants can provide options for fixed full-arch segmented prostheses (Morton and coworkers 2018).

Clinical recommendation 3
As part of a comprehensive plan, and when clinician skill and oral environment are favorable, the invasiveness of surgery can be reduced through utilization of improved implant materials, surfaces, and designs (short, narrow, tapered), prosthetic connections, and placement options (e.g., tilted implants) (Morton and coworkers 2018).

Clinical recommendation 4
The antero-posterior implant distribution should be maximized for full-arch fixed dental prostheses. When conditions allow, implants should be positioned axially. If anatomic limitations or prosthetic indications exist, the posterior implants can be intentionally tilted (Morton and coworkers 2018).

See Chapter 3.1 for a link to download the Proceedings of the 6th ITI Consensus Conference (2018)

RESTORATIVE MATERIALS

In addition to traditional metal-ceramic restorations, veneered or monolithic zirconia restorations are also currently under discussion.

The chipping rate of the veneering ceramic in veneered full-arch zirconia bridges is 35% within 5 years (Pieralli and coworkers 2018). Because of these high complication rates, monolithic zirconia restorations are currently preferred because they offer good esthetics and have a lower tendency to chip due to their monolithic design (Pjetursson and coworkers 2021). In addition, they are easy to integrate into a digital workflow and do not require any analog steps other than staining and bonding to a titanium base. However, their largely untested long-term performance is a clear disadvantage. Therefore, monolithic full-arch zirconia FDPs are not recommended due to insufficient data (Pieralli and coworkers 2018). If they are chosen as a treatment option, appropriate patient education regarding the unknown risks is necessary. Short-span FDPs used with a sufficient number of implants were covered, *mutatis mutandis*, by the 7th ITI Consensus Conference (2023), which provided the following clinical recommendations for short-span FDPs in the posterior region:

Clinical recommendation 1
In the posterior area, monolithic zirconia is recommended as the material of choice for implant-supported posterior multi-unit restorations in order to reduce technical complications such as ceramic fracture and chipping. The evidence supporting this recommendation is based on studies reporting on 3Y-TZP zirconia with a flexural strength > 1,000 MPa or multi-layered (3Y-TZP/5Y-TZP) alternatives (Derksen and coworkers 2023).

Clinical recommendation 2
The clinician and the dental technician need to be well-informed and should select the restorative material for every indication as a team. Even though zirconia is the best-documented ceramic material for posterior multi-unit restorations, it must not be forgiven that various types and generations exist. The significant differences in optical and mechanical properties have not all been validated in clinical studies (Derksen and coworkers 2023).

See Chapter 3.4.1 for a link to download the Proceedings of the 7th ITI Consensus Conference (2023)

FULL-ARCH OR SEGMENTED RESTORATIONS

Fixed restorations in the edentulous jaw can be either a one-piece full-arch fixed dental prothesis (FDP) spanning the entire jaw or, with a sufficient number of at least six implants, multiple short-span FDPs.

The latter solution of segmented FDPs consisting of multiple sections supported by six or more implants, offers higher prosthetic survival rates than one-piece full-arch restorations. This may be because the implants are placed in the molar region, avoiding cantilevers. The advantages of multiple short-span FDPs also include easier adaptation to divergent implants, easier achievement of a tension-free fit, a better combination of prosthetic materials, and relatively easy access for repairs (Derksen and coworkers 2023).

This is in contrast to the advantages of one-piece full-arch restorations, which are used primarily in patients with high vertical defects that require large areas to be covered with pink ceramics. In these cases, segmented restorations would result in long proximal contact areas that would include both the tooth and the pink ceramics. Such a proximal design extending through the pink aspects of the restoration is not only unesthetic and difficult to achieve from a technical standpoint, but it is also difficult for the patient to clean and should therefore be avoided whenever possible (Wolfart 2023).

TYPES OF RETENTION (CEMENTED VS. SCREW-RETAINED)

Full-arch restorations can be either cemented, screw-retained, or a combination of both. A review and meta-analysis by Sailer and coworkers (2012) shows generally high technical complication rates for fixed full-arch maxillary restorations. The complication rate is 63% for cemented restorations and 54% for screw-retained restorations. Combined with an average prevalence of peri-implantitis of 22% of patients overall (Derks and coworkers 2015), it becomes clear that predictable retrievability of full-arch restorations should be ensured in order to adequately manage any technical or biological complications. It can therefore be concluded that screw-retained restorations should be preferred to cemented restorations in full-arch situations.

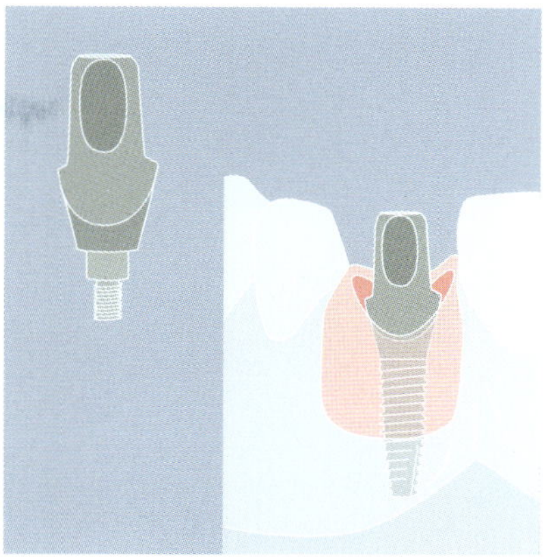

Fig 46 Custom CAD/CAM abutments are used to cement multiple short-span FDPs or one full-arch FDP in the edentulous jaw. Only these abutments allow for circular placement of the cement margin in the biologically acceptable slightly subgingival zone.

Cemented restorations: If multiple cemented short-span FDPs or a full-arch restoration are planned in the edentulous jaw, cementation should be performed on individualized CAD/CAM-fabricated abutments. Only these abutments allow proper placement of the cementation margin in the biologically acceptable supragingival or slightly subgingival zone. When the margin is placed more than 1 mm subgingivally, residual cement is missed 61% of the time; the risk of residual cement increases 3.6-fold compared with an epigingival cementation margin (Kim and coworkers 2023) (Fig 46). The insertion path and gingival emergence profile can also be optimally adapted to the respective clinical situation when using individual abutments.

Semi-definitive cementation should be aimed for (Wolfart 2023), with cement types that allow the restoration to be loosened by tapping in an emergency. Co-factors, such as abutment height (Mehl and coworkers 2012), preparation angle at the abutment and splinting, have a strong influence on retrievability and must be considered (Wolfart 2023). As these co-factors interact, particularly in the case of splinted restorations, the retrievability of full-arch restorations is no longer predictable. Therefore, there is always a risk that the restoration will have to be destroyed in an emergency.

Occlusally screw-retained restorations: The advantages of occlusally screw-retained restorations are predictable removability and low vertical space requirements (Fig 47). Removability facilitates repairs and oral hygiene. Disadvantages of occlusal screw-retained restorations include disruptive screw access channels, potential esthetic compromise, and effects on masticatory function. Other disadvantages include the difficulty of achieving a passive fit with splinted restorations and the fact that divergent implant axes and unfavorable implant positions often make occlusal screw fixation impossible.

Screw-retained abutments: Screw-retained abutments are used to achieve occlusal screw fixation in the presence of implants placed at different submucosal depths and with different angulations. These abutments are available with angulations of 17° or 30° (see Chapters 5.9 and 5.10 for detailed patient examples), and different gingival heights of 1, 2.5, 4, and 5.5 mm (Figs 48a-b).

The abutments are screwed directly onto the implants after implant placement or reentry and then remain in place. Angle correction and mucosal bridging allow a simplified impression technique at the abutment level. The impression posts are more parallel, and the connection between the abutment and the impression posts can be visually checked (as opposed to a bone-level impression). This also applies to the try-in and delivery of the final restoration. In addition, additional radiographs are not required due to the simplified verification of the accuracy of fit. Disadvantages of the screw-retained abutment concept include the additional gap between the abutment and the restoration, as well as the additional screw required, which is usually very short and delicate due to the design.

Angled screws: In edentulous cases, especially in the edentulous anterior maxilla, nearly parallel implant positions aligned with the occlusal surfaces are usually not feasible due to the anatomical position of the residual bone, which makes a purely occlusal screw connection almost impossible, especially for full-arch restorations In addition to the screw-retained abutment concept, systems with angled screws are helpful here (see Chapter 5.7 for a detailed patient example). In general, these systems require screwdrivers with rounded heads and specially designed retaining screws (Fig 49). The Straumann CARES screw-retained FDP offers segmented and full-arch FDPs in a grade 4 titanium and cobalt-chromium alloy for the prosthetic restoration of Straumann implants. Each screw channel can be individually angled up to 25° (Fig 50). The screws can be tightened at this angle with a torque of up to 35 Ncm.

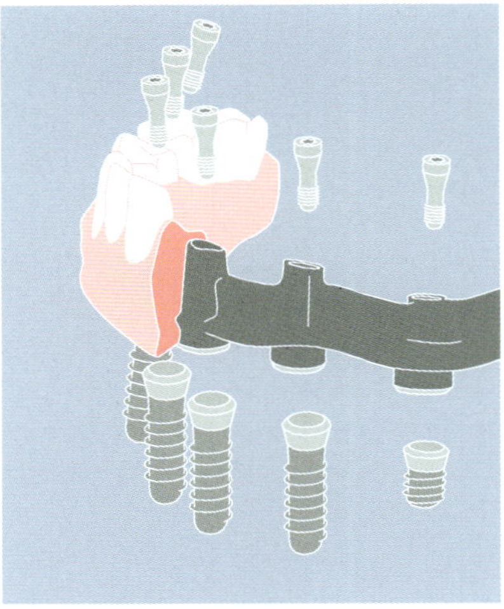

Fig 47 Occlusal screw retention is only possible without restriction if the implants are positioned according to the tooth axis and tooth position and the screw access channel exits centrally in the occlusal surface in the posterior region and orally in the anterior region.

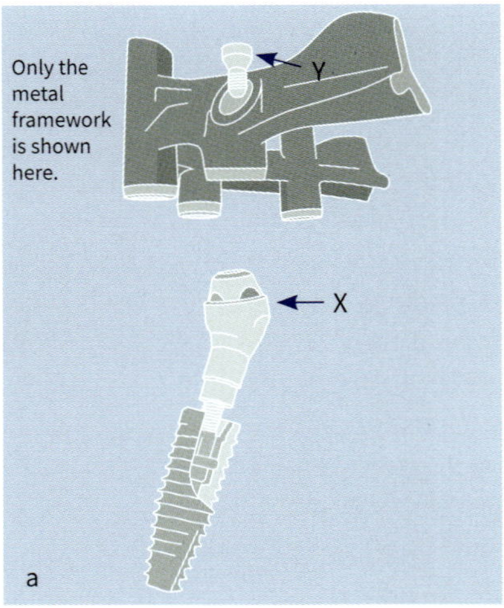

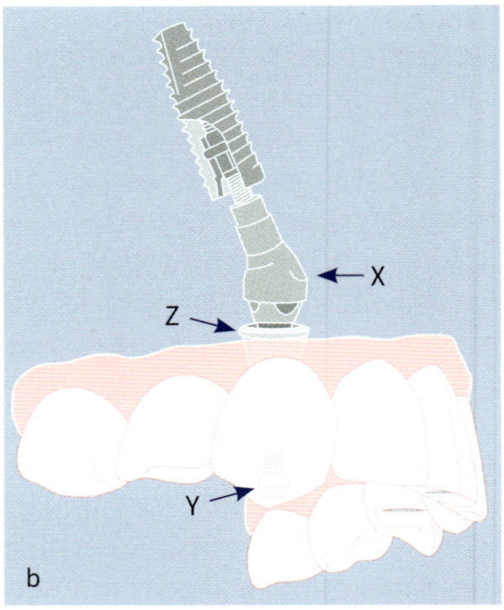

Figs 48a-b In the Straumann Pro Arch concept, screw-retained abutments (X) allow occlusal screw fixation even with implants positioned at different submucosal depths and angles. The angled abutment (X) is screwed directly onto the implant. The metal-ceramic (a) or all-ceramic (b) FDP is secured to the abutments with a second prosthetic screw (Y). In addition, a titanium base (Z) bonded to the all-ceramic FDP is required.

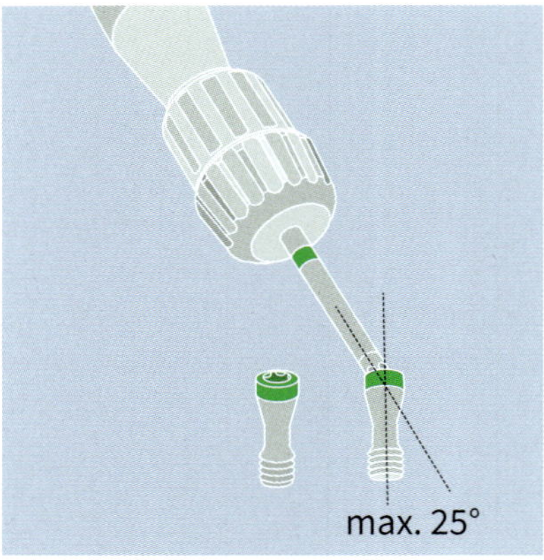

Fig 49 Retaining systems with angled screws (Straumann CARES screw-retained FDP system) require screwdrivers with rounded heads and specially designed retaining screws (possible angulation up to 25°).

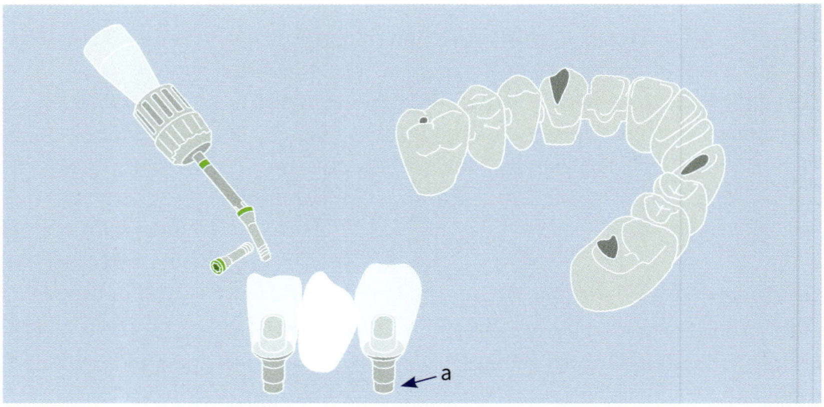

Fig 50 The Straumann CARES screw-retained FDP system offers segmented and full-arch FDPs in a grade 4 titanium and cobalt-chromium alloy. These frameworks are then veneered with veneering ceramics. Monolithic full-arch zirconia FDPs and multiple monolithic short-span FDPs are also possible in combination with special titanium bonding bases (a).

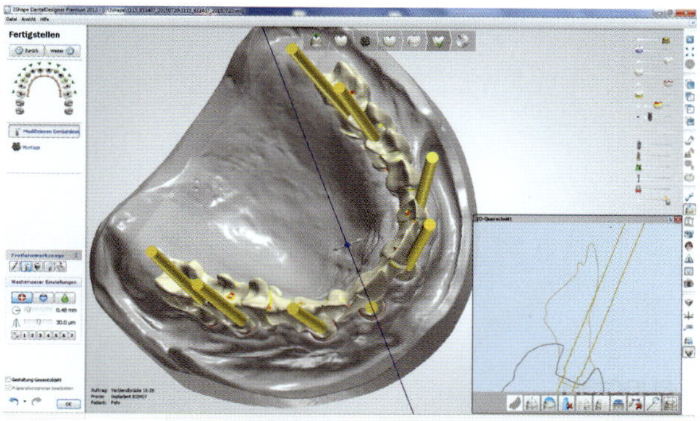

Fig 51 Full-arch framework planning with clear axial divergence of the implants (yellow cylinders) from the tooth axes. These must be corrected using a system with angled screws so that the screw access channels exit occlusally.

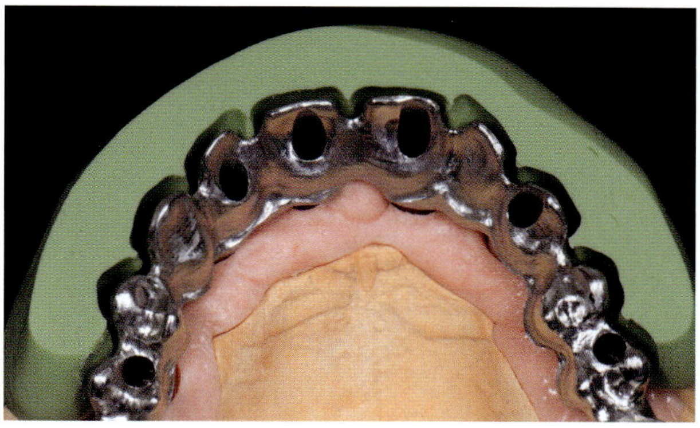

Fig 52 The milled framework (cobalt-chromium alloy) shows the occlusally and palatally corrected screw access channels. The key (green) of the wax-up reflects the estimated space required for the veneer.

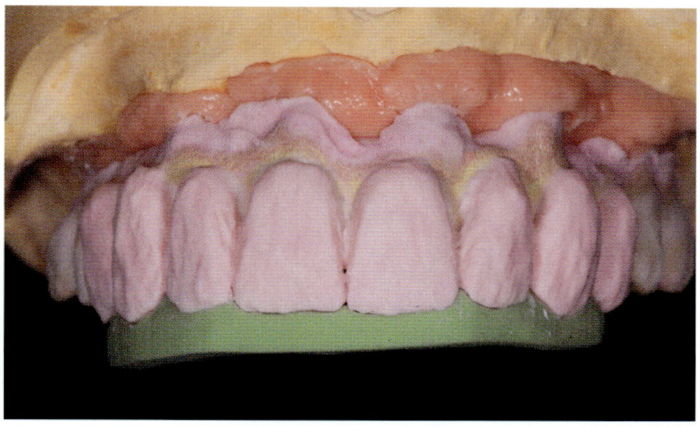

Fig 53 The white teeth and the pink gingiva are veneered simultaneously.

An angled screw is indicated when a straight screw access channel does not terminate occlusally in the posterior region or sufficiently far orally in the anterior region. An angled screw should also be considered when the screw access channel is too close to the lateral crown margins and a sufficiently thick ceramic layer cannot be achieved.

It is advisable to document the use of angled screws in the patient's implant identification card in case an external provider needs to perform emergency treatment.

The frameworks are fabricated from non-precious metals (CoCr or titanium) milled from a block in a CAM process or fabricated by selective laser melting (Figs 51 to 54a-b). The FDPs are then connected with screws directly at the implant level. There are some disadvantages to this concept. To ensure a safe insertion path for the restoration, the internal connections are always very short (Fig 54a) and have no anti-rotation device. With bone-level implants, the fit of the restoration on the implants must be checked deep within the mucosa. This can only be done with additional radiographs; the accuracy of this procedure is not always guaranteed because the connection can only be reliably checked if the radiographs are parallel to the implant-restoration connection. Once the metal-ceramic full-arch restoration has been completed, it is inserted, the prosthetic screws are tightened to 35 Ncm, and the screw access channels are sealed (Figs 55 and 56).

IMPLANT SURVIVAL IN FIXED RESTORATIONS

Implant survival as a function of implant number: A review of fixed implant-supported restorations in the *edentulous mandible* included 2,800 implants in 500 patients. The 10-year implant survival rate was 98% for rough implant surfaces and 97% for one-piece FDPs. Neither the number of implants (four or more) nor the anterior-posterior distribution of the implants had a significant effect on implant survival (Papaspyridakos and coworkers 2014a).

Retrospective data on 471 patients are available for *two anterior axial and two posterior tilted implants in the edentulous mandible.* Patients were followed for 10 to 18 years. The cumulative survival rate at 10 years for the definitive restorations is 98.8%. For the implants, the survival rate is 96.9% and the success rate is 95.9%. The average marginal bone loss at the implants was 1.7 mm at 10 years. The incidence of biological complications at the implant level is 11.8%. Technical complications occur both in provisional restorations with immediate loading (29.5%) and in permanent restorations (36.7%) (Maló and coworkers 2019b).

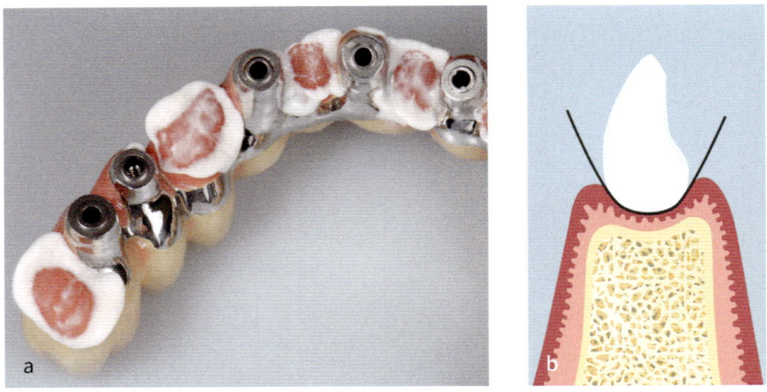

Figs 54a-b Pontic support: The thinly molded pontics areas (low-viscosity silicone material) show good congruence (a) with the corresponding alveolar ridge portions. The pontics rest on the alveolar ridge in an ovoid shape and are therefore easy to clean with dental floss (b).

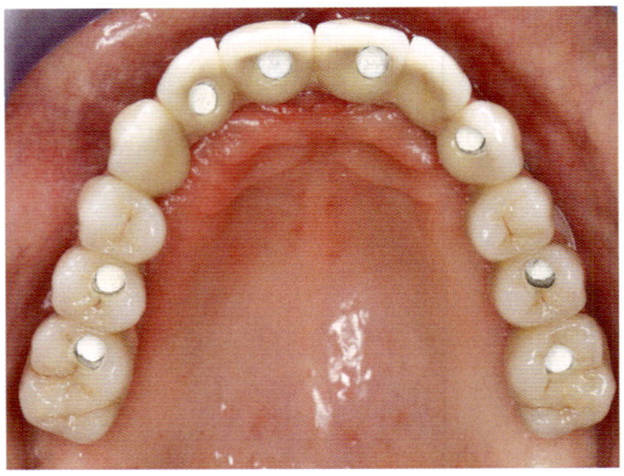

Fig 55 Occlusal view of the corrected screw access channel exits.

A review article on fixed implant-supported restorations in the *edentulous maxilla* summarized implant survival for FDPs supported by four to six implants. Implant survival was 97.5% after 5 years of observation and 95.0% after 10 years. The exact distribution of implants was not described in the studies reviewed. It was also not possible to determine how many of the restorations were supported by 4, 5, or 6 implants (Heydecke and coworkers 2012).

In the case of *two anterior axial and two posterior tilted implants in the edentulous maxilla,* data were available from a retrospective study of 1,072 patients. Long-term results were reported over a follow-up period of 5 to 13 years. The 10-year cumulative survival rate for the final restorations was 99.2%. For the implants, the survival rate was 96.0% and the success rate was 95.2%. The average marginal bone loss at the implants at 10 years was 1.7 mm. The incidence of biological complications at the implant level was 7.8%. Technical complications occurred in both provisional restorations with immediate loading (58.3%) and in final restorations (7.3%) (Maló and coworkers 2019a).

Implant survival in relation to implant inclination: Due to the different loading conditions, biomechanics and cleanability of tilted and straight implants, an accurate analysis of the survival and success rates of these implants is important before recommendations for appropriate treatment approaches can be made.

In this context, 17 non-randomized studies with more than 7,000 implants were included in a systematic review. The implant loss rate was 2.5% for straight implants and 2.4% for tilted implants after an average follow-up of 3 to 5 years. Thus, there was no difference in failure between tilted and straight implants. Similarly, peri-implant marginal bone loss was 1.27 mm on average for both straight and tilted implants. Therefore, no effect of implant inclination on implant survival or peri-implant bone loss was found (Apaza Alccayhuaman and coworkers 2018).

CLEANABILITY

Mucositis on implant-supported prosthetic restorations is often the starting point for extensive peri-implant inflammation, which can compromise implant success. The better the accessibility of the restoration in the area of the implants for oral hygiene, the less likely peri-implantitis will occur (Serino and coworkers 2009). Therefore, the cleanability of the fixed restorations plays a critical role in their long-term success. The most effective means of cleaning are special dental floss (e.g., Meridol Special Floss, Oral-B Superfloss) under the pontics (Figs 57a-b) and interdental brushes in the proximal region (Tuna and coworkers 2019). There must be sufficient openings for the interdental brushes proximal to the implants. The pontics should rest on the alveolar mucosa with an ovoid cross-section and be cleanable with special dental floss (Figs 54b and 57b).

3.4.3 Removable Restorations

Three retention systems have become established for anchoring removable implant-supported prosthetic restorations in the edentulous jaw, which must be weighed against each other in the individual patient case—ball attachments, bar attachments, and telescopic crown attachments. From the patient's point of view, both primary and secondary splinted (bar, telescope) and unsplinted (ball) attachments are equally effective and can be recommended (Schimmel and coworkers 2023).

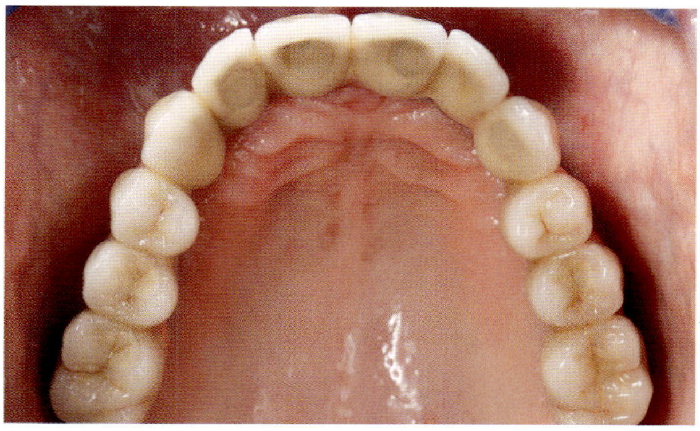

Fig 56 Screw access channels obturated with resin inlays.

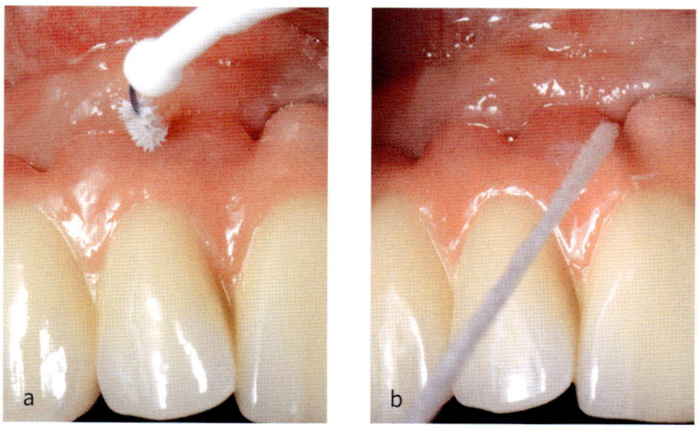

Figs 57a-b The most effective means of cleaning are interdental brushes in the proximal region (a) and special dental floss (e.g., Meridol Special Floss, Oral-B Superfloss) under the pontics (b).

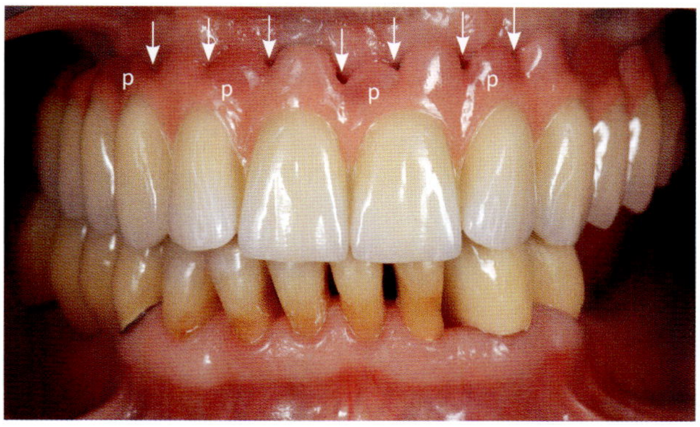

Fig 58 Frontal view 3 months after delivery. The openings for the interdental brushes (arrows) and the pontics (p) between are clearly visible.

BALL ATTACHMENTS

Ball attachments provide both implant and mucosal support for the prosthesis, which the patient perceives as slightly mobile. Ball attachments are simple and inexpensive to fabricate, require few treatment sessions, and result in low implant stress. It is important that implants are placed as parallel as possible and that vertical defects are not too large, as long levers and extra-axial forces can lead to overloading of the elements. Thanks to the latest developments in these systems, it is now possible to handle axial divergences of up to 60° according to the manufacturer (Wolfart 2023). Among the many representatives of ball attachments, two systems can be highlighted as examples due to their different functionality: a ball attachment (Dalbo Plus; Cendres + Métaux, Biel/Bienne, Switzerland) and the Novaloc attachment (Medentika, Institut Straumann AG, Basel, Switzerland) (Figs 59 and 60). They are different in shape and function of the abutment, the type of retention element, and the way in which differences in angulation between two implants can be compensated. For ball attachments, this is achieved by different positioning of the matrix on the ball, and for the Novaloc system, by certain design features of the matrix. The Novaloc system offers additional physical angle correction (Fig 60). The characteristics of each system are summarized in Table 2.

Restorations with ball attachments can require more follow-up visits to activate the attachments (Stoker and Wismeijer 2011). A recent systematic review showed that locators had fewer prosthetic complications than ball attachments (Prasad and coworkers 2024).

Novaloc attachments: The Novaloc attachment has a special surface coating (ADLC coating: amorphous diamond-like carbon). According to the manufacturer, this leads to improved hardness and sliding properties, which in turn should result in less abrasion on the abutment and less damage to the retention insert. Primary interimplant angle corrections of up to 40° can be achieved with the PEEK retention inserts (Fig 60). For implant axes diverging by more than 40°, a 15° angled abutment can be used to physically improve the axial divergence. According to the manufacturer, an axial divergence of up to 70° can be compensated.

Framework fabrication: Regardless of the type of ball attachment used, the removable prosthesis should always be reinforced with a non-precious metal framework in the area of the attachments to prevent fracture of the prosthesis in this structurally weaker area (Fig 61). Overall, the framework extends over the entire base of the prosthesis.

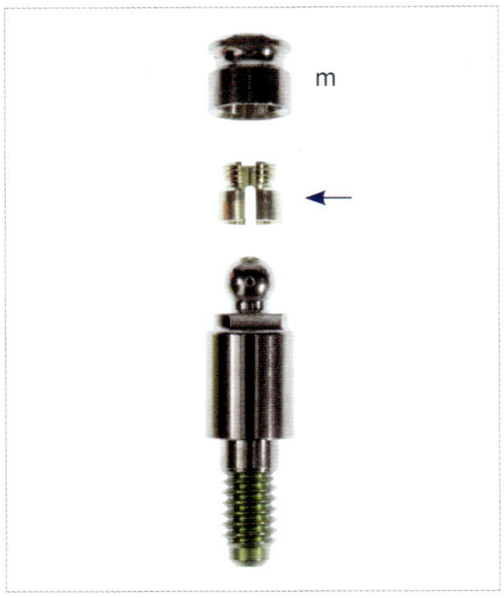

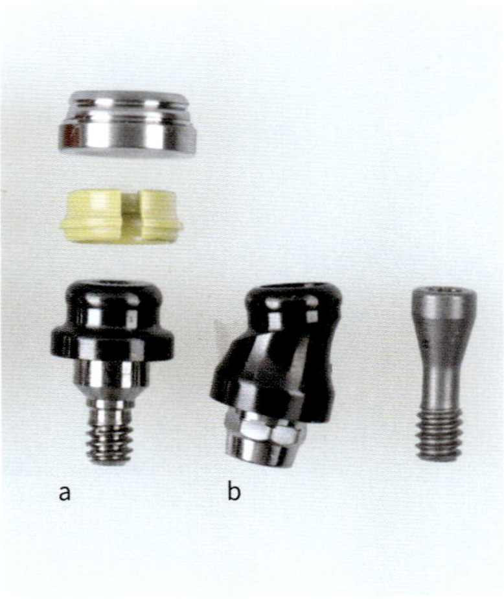

Fig 59 Ball attachment without physical angle correction. With the Dalbo Plus attachment, the retention ball is screwed onto the implant and the metal matrix is incorporated into the prosthesis. A lamellar retention insert (arrow), which can be activated by screwing in and out, is placed in the matrix (m).

Fig 60 Novaloc with physical angle correction: cylindrical attachment with undercut, a PEEK retention insert, and a metal matrix. It can be used as a straight attachment (a) or as a 15° angled attachment (b).

Table 2 Comparison of different ball attachments (modified from Wolfart 2023).

	Dalbo-Plus	Novaloc
Design	▪ Ball attachment (diameter 2.25 mm) screwed onto implant ▪ Titanium matrix with precious-metal lamellar insert (Elitor)	▪ Special titanium attachment screwed onto implant with special surface treatment (ADLC coating) ▪ Titanium matrix
Activation	▪ Activated by screwing in the lamellar insert: 2–12 N	▪ PEEK retention inserts in six different friction levels (extra-light to ultra-strong)
Compensation of axial divergence between implants	Angle correction: Without physical matrix angle correction between two implants: 20°	Physical angle correction: 15° angled attachment Additional angle correction between two implants: 40° Total possible angle correction between two implants: 70°
Patient example	See Chapter 5.1	See Chapters 5.2 and 5.3

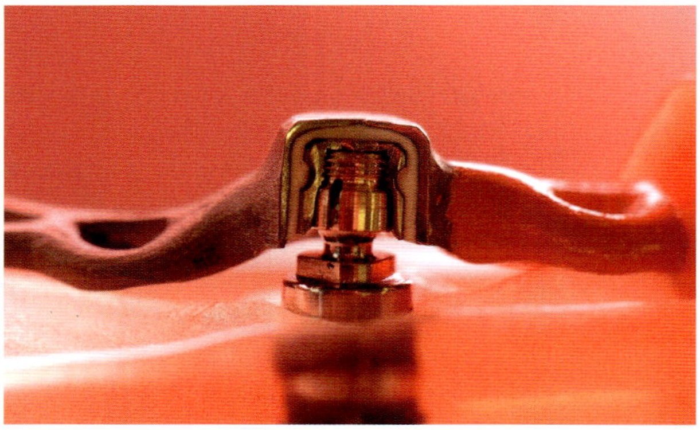

Fig 61 A non-precious metal framework is incorporated into the prosthesis to prevent fractures. The attachments (in this case Dalbo Plus) are adhesively connected to their housings. The metal framework is then covered with a pink opaque. (Image courtesy of R. Busch, Kiel, Germany.)

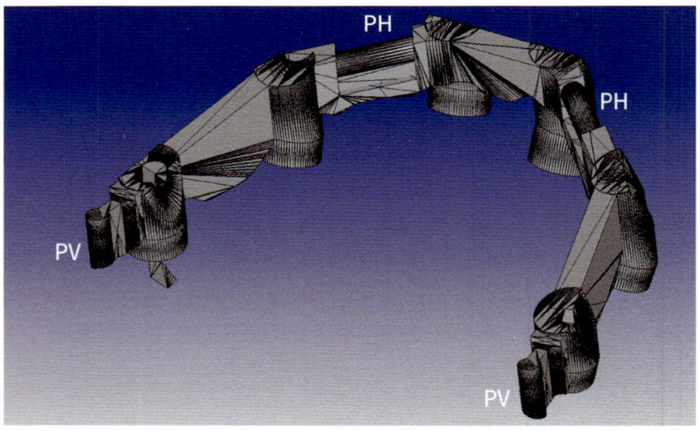

Fig 62 Construction of the parallel-milled titanium bar. Two terminal Preci-Vertix attachments (PV) and two horizontally aligned Preci-Horix attachments (PH) were incorporated as friction inserts.

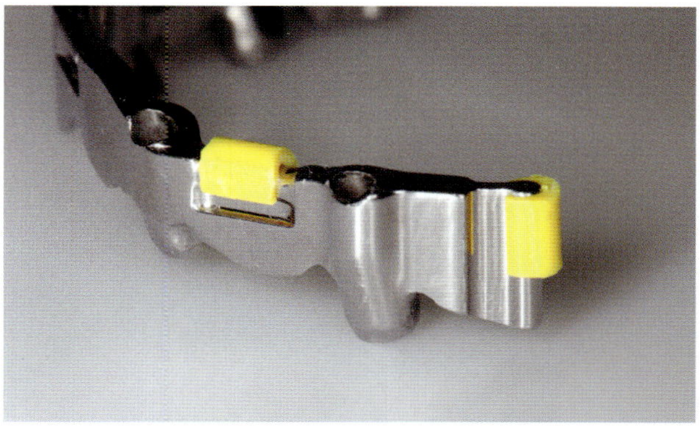

Fig 63 The design proposal is converted into the finished titanium bar by the milling center. Friction inserts (yellow) slid onto the Preci-Vertix and Preci-Horix attachments.

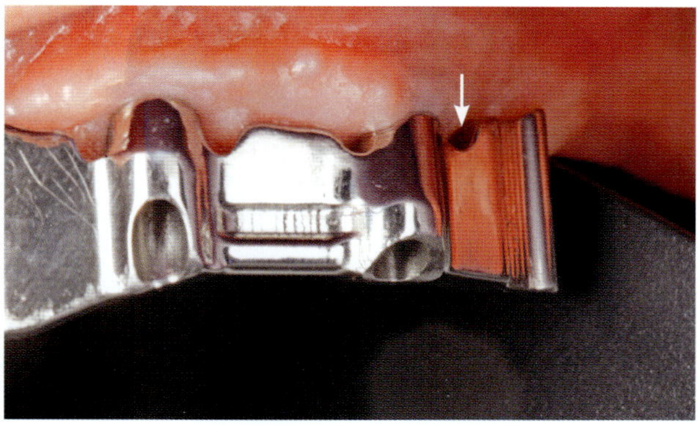

Fig 64 The bar rests on the mucosa in the area of the milled spacers, similar to an FDP pontic (cleanable with special dental floss, e.g., Oral-B Superfloss). Interdental brush guide surfaces are placed mesially and distally to the implants. Distally to the last implant, the brush guide is part of the attachment male (arrows).

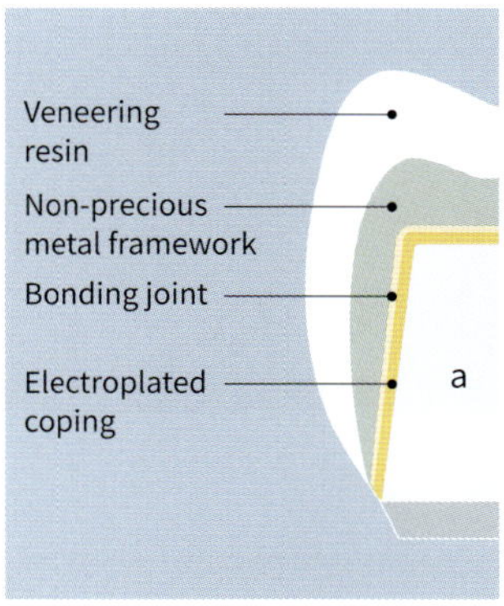

Fig 65 Schematic representation of the tapered (1° to 2°) abutments (a) and the telescopic crown, consisting of a fully veneered secondary framework into which the electroplated copings were adhesively bonded intraorally.

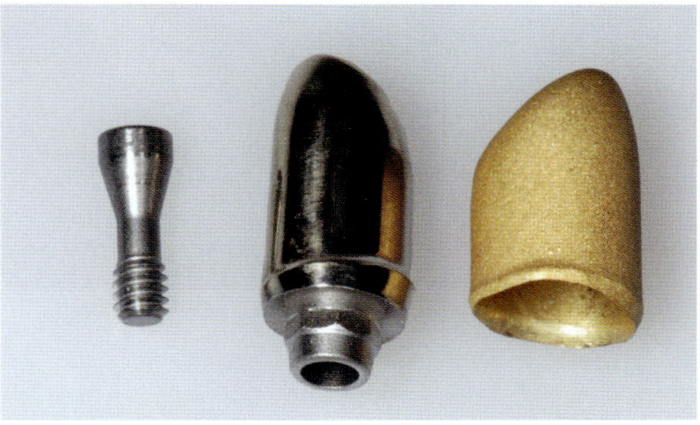

Fig 66 Tapered implant abutments (1 to 2°) and removed electroplated coping with a wall thickness of approximately 0.2 mm.

MILLED CAD/CAM BARS

Retention with a milled bar results in a rigid connection. A palate-free design of the denture base is possible. The bars are CAD/CAM-milled from titanium or a non-precious alloy in a milling center. Compensation for different implant axes is possible. Primary splinting reduces the load on each implant (see Chapters 5.4 and 5.5 for detailed patient examples).

The prosthesis is retained with friction inserts, such as the Preci-Vertix or Preci-Horix attachments (Fig 62). The retention force can be adjusted by providing different friction inserts, which can be replaced when worn. The male rod-shaped Preci-Vertix attachment is designed to be placed distal to the terminal implant. The friction insert consists of an elastic resin component and is held in a retention housing in the prosthesis by clamping action. The Preci-Horix attachment is the horizontal counterpart to the Preci-Vertix and is designed into the bar in the inter-implant regions (Figs 63 and 64).

For good cleanability, the bar rests on the mucosa in the area of the milled spacers, similar to a bridge pontic and should be cleaned in this area with special dental floss. Interdental brush guide surfaces are placed mesially and distally to the implants. Distally to the last implant, the brush guide is part of the attachment male (Fig 64).

TELESCOPIC CROWNS

Retention with telescopic crowns provides a functional sensation similar to that of natural teeth due to the rigid connection. Reduction of the denture base all the way to a straight bridge design is possible. In general, the load on the implants is high with this type of restoration (see Chapters 5.3 and 5.6 for detailed patient examples).

Electroplated telescopic crowns: In this type of restoration, after CAD/CAM fabrication of the titanium or zirconium implant abutment (convergence angle: 1° to 2°), a fine gold coping is electroplated directly onto the abutment (Diedrichs and coworkers 1991; Wirz and Hoffmann 1999; Wirz and Jäger

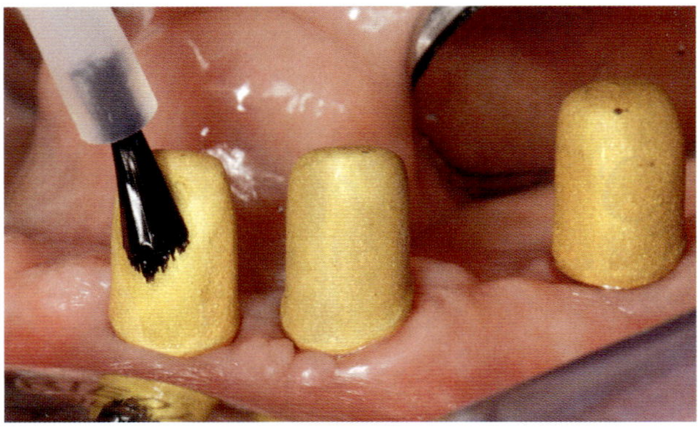
Fig 67 The abutments are finally screwed onto the implants. The electroplated copings are cleaned with alcohol in an ultrasonic bath, then placed and conditioned with a metal primer (e.g., Alloy Primer or Monobond Plus).

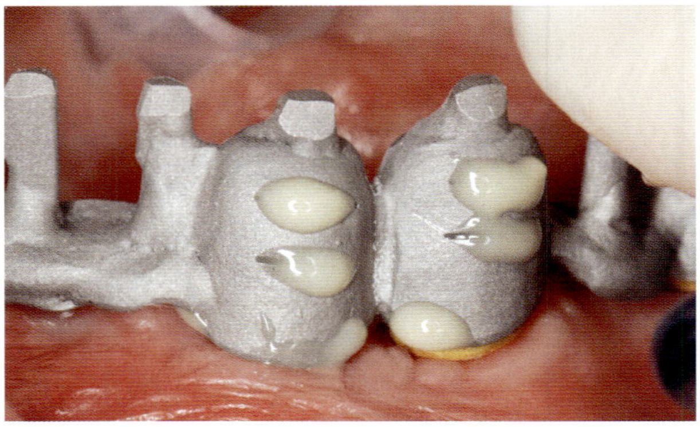
Fig 68 Intraoral bonding of the electroplated copings with a composite adhesive (e.g., Panavia 21). The non-precious metal framework surrounds the copings up to the margins, with slits for excess adhesive.

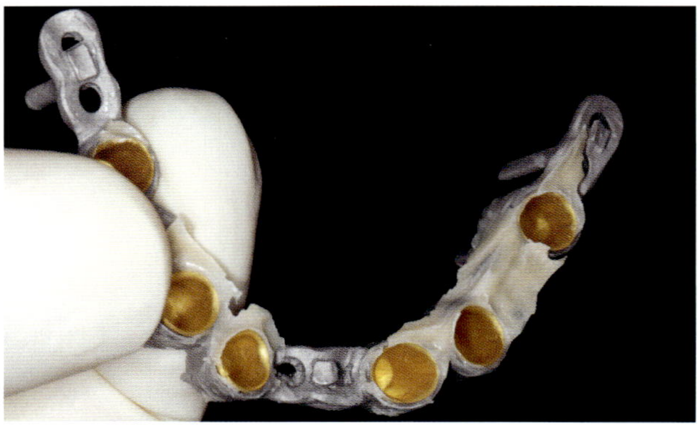
Fig 69 Adhesively bonded copings in the framework immediately after removal from the mouth.

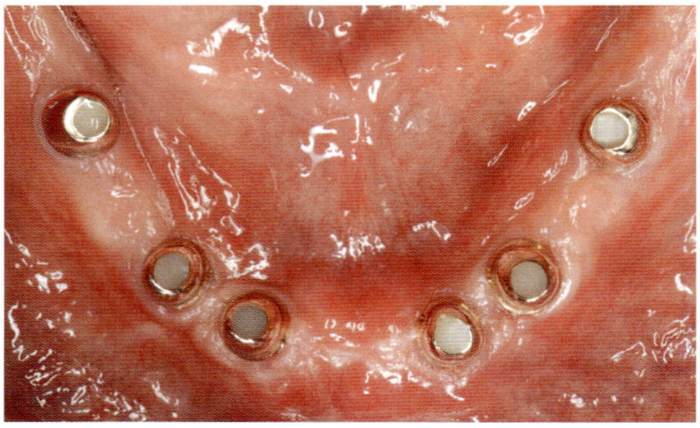
Fig 70 Top view of the implant abutments.

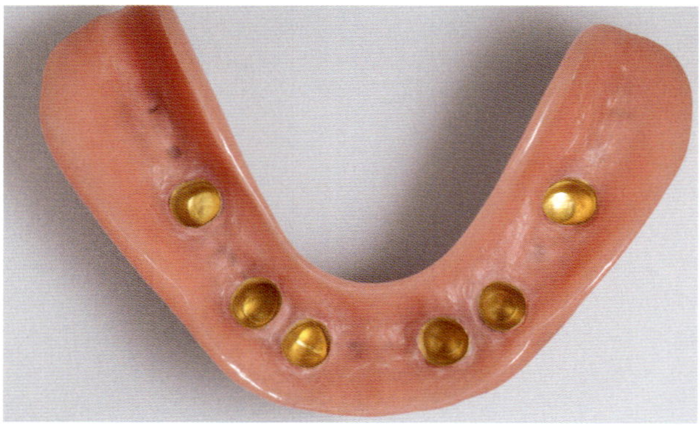
Fig 71 Basal view of the completed mandibular restoration.

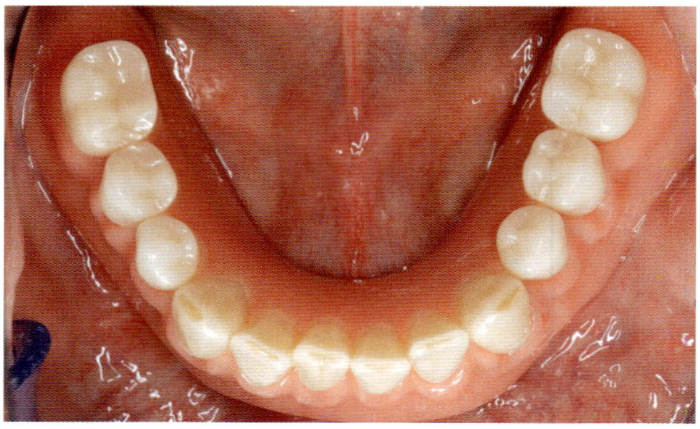
Fig 72 Treatment outcome 3 months after placement.

1998) (Figs 65 and 66). The thin electroformed coping is stabilized by being adhesively bonded into a non-precious secondary framework and acts as an intermediate crown.

It is important that the coping is completely surrounded by the secondary framework up to the marginal region. The accuracy of fit of electroplated copings is significantly better than that of cast telescopic crowns. The adhesive surfaces of the electroplated copings, which are covered with soft fine gold, result in a smooth glide when loosening and joining the prostheses (Kern and coworkers 2022). Intraoral bonding of the copings to the secondary framework eliminates the need for framework soldering and ensures a stress-free fit of the entire restoration—a so-called passive fit (Figs 67 to 72).

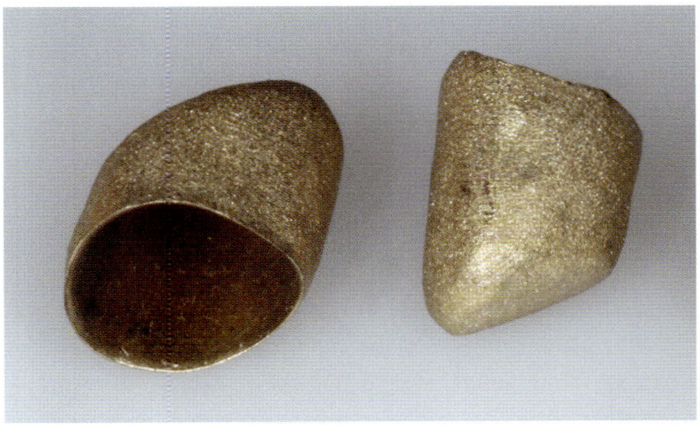

Fig 73 Intraoral bonding of classic telescopic crowns. Cast telescopic crowns (wall thickness approximately 0.5–0.7 mm, air-abraded rough surface).

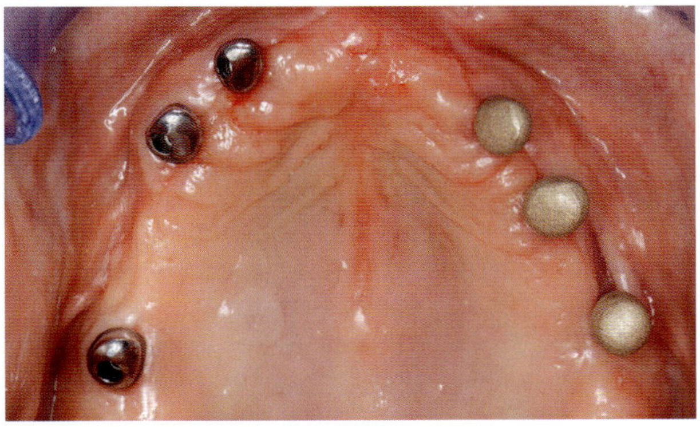

Fig 74 Screw-retained telescopic abutments. Telescopic crowns are already in place in the left maxillary quadrant.

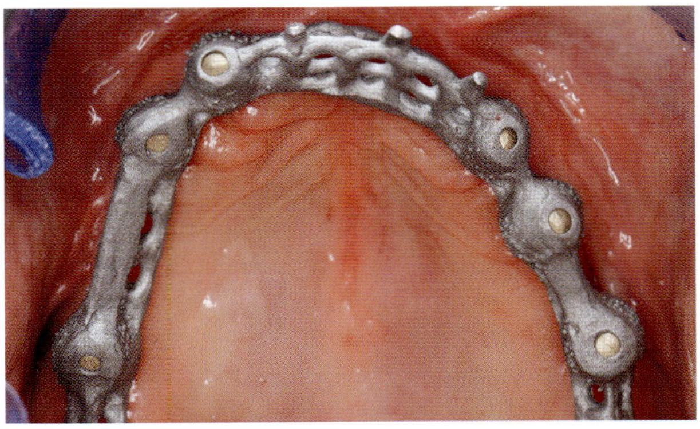

Fig 75 Try-in of the secondary framework on the telescopic crowns. The fit must be passive.

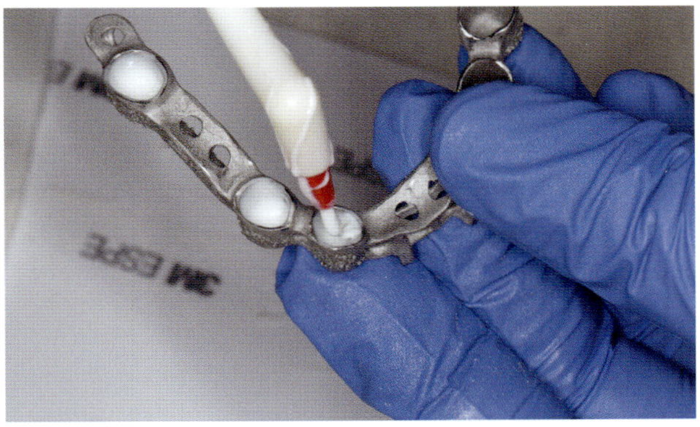

Fig 76 Filling the pretreated framework with resin adhesive.

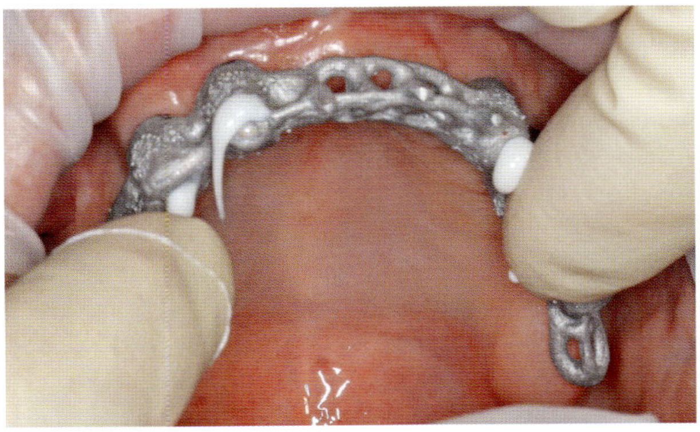

Fig 77 The framework is placed in its final position.

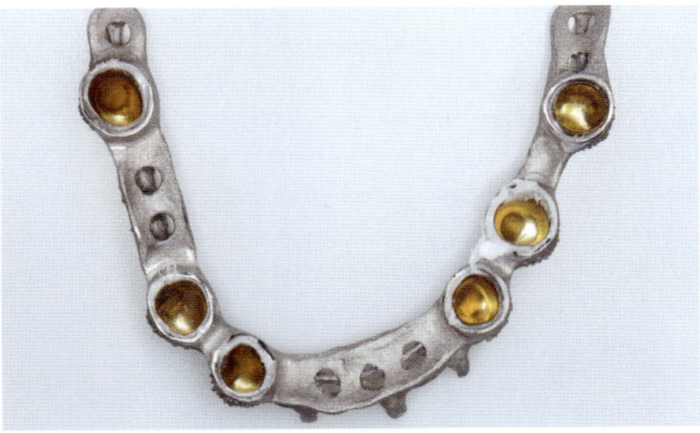

Fig 78 Basal view of the intraorally bonded framework.

Intraoral bonding of implant-supported classic telescopic crowns: Classic telescopic crowns are subject to inaccuracies due to the conventional fabrication process, which can lead to stresses between the implants when the prosthesis is inserted. To compensate for this, the implant-supported telescopic crowns can be bonded intraorally instead of being connected to the framework on the model in the laboratory (Wolfart 2023) (Figs 73 to 79).

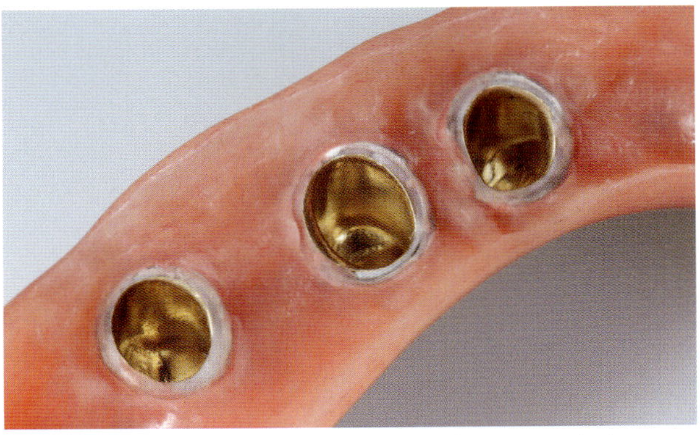

Fig 79 Detail of the basal surface of the finished telescopic prosthesis.

This procedure combines the proven long-term performance of classic telescopic crowns with the passive fit of electroplated telescopes. It should be noted, however, that due to the parallel-walled telescopic abutments, true angle correction is only possible within narrow limits. Abutments with a convergence angle of 1° are required for a reliable passive fit.

LONG-TERM PERFORMANCE OF THE PROSTHESIS IN RELATION TO THE NUMBER OF IMPLANTS

Long-term performance of ball and bar attachments: The effect of different numbers of implants in removable restorations on dental patient-reported outcomes (dPROs) is discussed in detail in Chapter 2.1.2. However, when considering the number of implants in relation to the expected long-term performance of the prosthetic restoration, the edentulous maxilla must be considered separately from the edentulous mandible because of the different anatomical situation.

The *edentulous maxilla* is more sensitive than the edentulous mandible in terms of the minimum number of implants required. For example, a maxillary overdenture supported by three or fewer implants has a 5-year implant survival rate of only 69.7%. This is significantly lower than for restorations on four implants (89.1%) (Kern and coworkers 2016). A minimum of four implants, whether splinted or unsplinted, is therefore strongly recommended (Di Francesco and coworkers 2019).

Four to six implants can be restored in the edentulous maxilla with ball attachments or Locators, bars, or telescopic crowns. Zou and coworkers (2013) compared these three systems with the following results: With four implants, all three systems show implant survival rates of 100% at 3 years and few technical complications. In a systematic review, splinted bars on at least four implants show higher implant and prosthesis survival (both more than 95% per year) than unsplinted attachments (balls, Locators, telescopic crowns) (Raghoebar and coworkers 2014).

The use of four or six implants for a bar-retained restoration was evaluated in a randomized controlled trial. At 5 years, there was no difference in prosthetic function or implant survival, which was close to 100% in both groups (Slot and coworkers 2019).

A systematic review of the retention of overdentures on mini-implants showed a mini-implant survival rate of 77% at 1.8 years. When the palate was covered by the overdentures, there was significantly less bone resorption than with dentures without palatal coverage. Overall, however, the survival rate of these implants was far below that of standard implants (Vi and coworkers 2021).

In the *edentulous mandible,* the retention of a prosthesis on two interforaminal implants is scientifically well documented and represents the standard of care for this indication (Schimmel and coworkers 2023; Feine and coworkers 2002). In a prospective clinical study with two interforaminal implants, bar, ball, and magnetic attachments were compared. The ball attachments showed the highest retention values and the best soft-tissue adaptation at 10 years. Denture stability and chewing comfort were rated better for the ball and bar attachments than for the magnetic attachments (Naert and coworkers 2004a). Regarding the implants themselves, all three groups showed an excellent prognosis with implant survival rates of 100% (Naert and coworkers 2004b). Other very promising ten-year results have been described for both ball attachments and round bars (Dolder bars) (Cune and coworkers 2010; Meijer and coworkers 2009).

If a patient's financial circumstances do not allow the use of two implants, the placement of a single central implant can also be considered. This concept has now been followed for more than 10 years in a pilot study and has shown good results without implant loss (Passia and coworkers 2019). A study with more than 150 patients confirms the success of this treatment concept, with an implant survival rate of 98.5% at 3 years, provided that the implant is allowed to heal without loading (Kern and coworkers 2018).

Long-term performance of telescopic crowns: Prostheses retained by telescopic crowns on at least four implants show slightly worse long-term implant performance than bar prostheses for the edentulous maxilla over a 5-year observation period (Raghoebar and coworkers 2014).

For the maxilla and mandible combined, implant survival rates for electroplated and classic telescopic crown-retained restorations are at least 85% and prosthesis survival rates without major complications are at least 80% at 5 years (Rammelsberg and coworkers 2014; Fobbe and coworkers 2019; Mori and coworkers 2019; Schwarz and coworkers 2014; Brandt and coworkers 2019).

The following major complications occurred with electroplated telescopic crowns after a mean follow-up of 3.4 years: loss of overdenture due to implant loss (3%), loss of electroplated telescope retention (3%), fracture or major revision of the prosthetic framework (7%). Less severe complications included mainly repairs to the veneer (23%), chipping or fracture of the denture base (17%), and detachment of the electroplated coping (10%). No complications occurred in 16 patients, 1 complication in 10 patients, 2 complications in 3 patients, and 3 complications in 1 patient (Schwarz and coworkers 2014).

IMPLANT SURVIVAL IN REMOVABLE PROSTHESES IN RELATION TO THE NUMBER OF IMPLANTS AND THE ATTACHMENT SYSTEM

High-quality comparative studies are available for the *edentulous mandible* that allow detailed comparisons between implant survival and different treatment approaches (Kern and coworkers 2016). All established attachment systems have 5-year survival rates above 90%. For example, the 5-year survival rate for a single central implant (supported by a ball attachment) is 92.1%. With two interforaminal implants the survival rate increases significantly to 98.4% and with four interforaminal implants to 99.5%.

When the restoration is supported by ball abutments, implant survival is 98.3% and 99.0% for bars. There is insufficient data to make a meaningful analysis of telescopic crown retained dentures.

Less detailed data are available for the *edentulous maxilla*. Here it can only be stated that implant survival at 5 years is 89.1% for removable restorations with at least 4 implants. When fewer than four implants are used, implant survival drops significantly to 69.7%. This suggests that a removable restoration supported by only two or three implants should be avoided in the edentulous maxilla.

CLEANSABILITY

As already described for fixed prostheses (see Chapter 3.4.2), the cleansability of implants and attachments, as well as the prostheses themselves, plays an important role in preventing the occurrence of peri-implant mucositis or peri-implantitis.

In this context, a clinical recommendation from the 6th ITI Consensus Conference (2018) provides the following observation: Patients have reported that they find it easier to maintain oral hygiene with an implant overdenture than with an implant-supported fixed restoration; therefore, the former may be preferable for certain patients (Feine and coworkers 2018).

See Chapter 3.1 for a link to download the Proceedings of the 6th ITI Consensus Conference (2018)

3.5 Prosthetic Management of Tissue Loss in the Edentulous Jaw

S. Wolfart

The first step in the management of soft-tissue and hard-tissue loss is to assess the extent of any defect in its spatial dimensions. The defect can be assessed clinically or radiographically. An additional clinically relevant estimate can be obtained with an ideally aligned set-up. Once this is translated into a clear radiographic template, the hard-tissue and soft-tissue loss can be thoroughly evaluated (Fig 1).

One of the goals of patient rehabilitation is to reconstruct the atrophied tissue. This is the only way to fully restore the patient's esthetics, function, and speech. The latter is often particularly urgent as many patients suffer from articulation deficits, as illustrated by the real-time MRI slices (Figs 80a-f). They impressively show the interaction between the tongue, the palatal aspects of the anterior teeth, and the epiglottis in the formation of certain consonants. In this respect, it is not surprising that patients with inadequate rehabilitation in this area show articulatory problems. These are particularly common with "S"-type sounds (sibilants) and can persist for years after the delivery of a restoration (Fonteyne and coworkers 2019).

There are essentially two ways to compensate for this tissue loss—surgically or prosthetically. Purely prosthetic treatment is possible to varying degrees, depending on the type of restoration. In general, better compensation can be achieved with removable palate-free overdentures than with fixed restorations. For example, the majority of patients who first received an implant-supported fixed restoration and then a removable overdenture in the edentulous maxilla chose the removable overdenture because of the better speech (articulation) function and ease of cleaning of the restoration (Heydecke and coworkers 2003).

3.5.1 Removable Restorations

The atrophied tissue can be fully compensated with the denture saddle. This compensation with pink denture acrylic can also be modified at any time during the wearing period until the best possible result for the patient is achieved. Since an overdenture is removed for oral hygiene, it can be in contact with the alveolar ridge over a large area. This creates the perfect transition between the residual ridge and the restored areas of the jaw. Even if further changes in the alveolar ridge occur during the follow-up period, adjustments can be made at any time by relining. The only disadvantage is the slightly reduced esthetics of the acrylic denture saddles.

3.5.2 Fixed Restorations

For reasons of oral hygiene, fixed restorations should not be saddle-shaped on the alveolar ridge. The largest possible contact area should only correspond to the shape of an extended, convex pontic. In addition, small openings must be provided mesially and distally of the implants to allow easy access for interdental brushes to ensure optimal cleaning of the restoration by the patient. A disadvantage of this is that the alveolar ridge can be fully reconstructed in the vertical plane but not in the horizontal or sagittal planes. All-ceramic restorations do not allow any major changes to the pink ceramic to compensate for tissue loss. Here, occlusally screw-retained fixed restorations with an acrylic base are advantageous because they are correctable.

A suboptimally designed palatal anterior region or openings for the interdental brushes can be a problem for articulation. Figs 80a-f show how sensitive the phonation process is in this area. In addition, the openings for the interdental brushes pose the risk of "hissing" noises accompanying the pronunciation of sibilants. Some patients even complain of saliva leaking through these openings.

Because of these problems it is recommended that fixed restorations, especially in the maxilla, be tested with a fixed long-term provisional. This acrylic provisional must match the planned definitive restoration exactly in all dimensions. If the patient is not satisfied with it, corrections can be made to it until the patient is comfortable. At the same time, it can

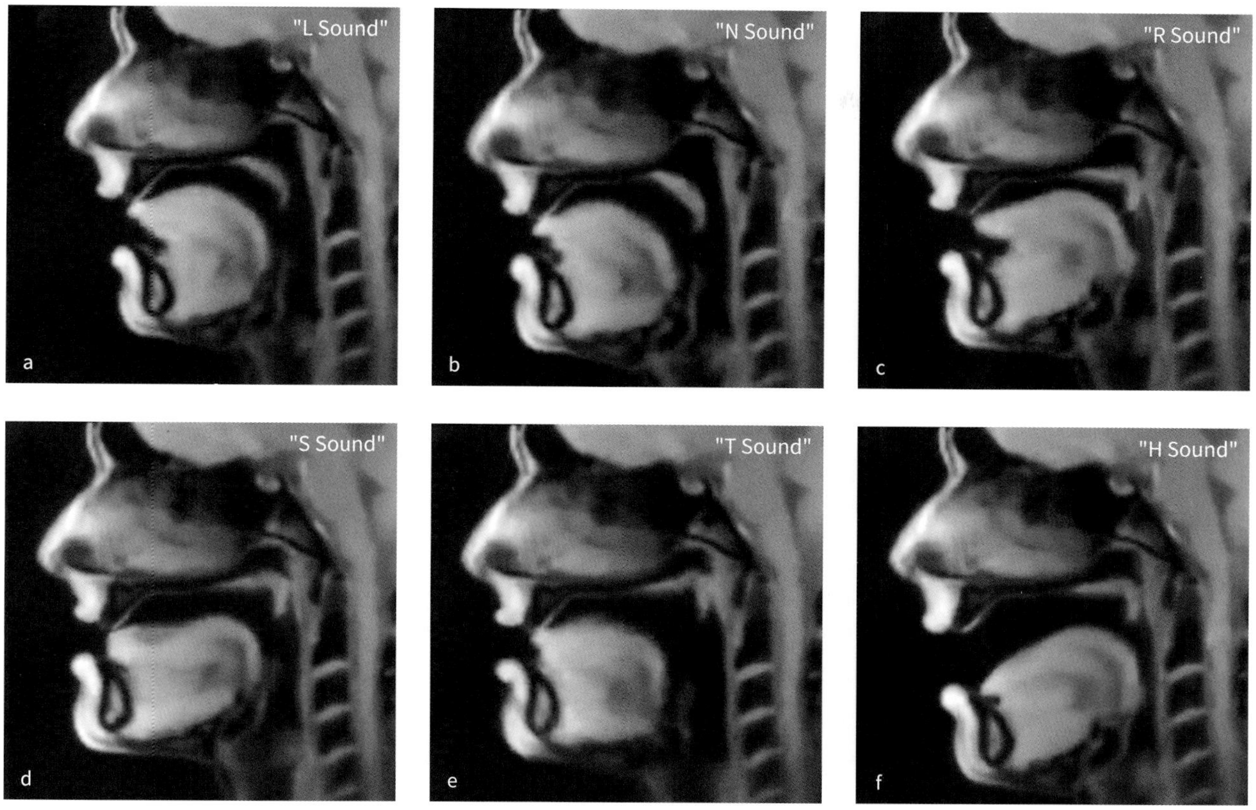

Figs 80a-f The role of the anterior palate and incisors in phonation. This area is particularly important for the articulation of the consonants "L," "N," "R," "S," and "T," as these still images from a real-time MRI clip clearly show. For other sounds, such as "H," this area is of little importance. (Image courtesy of Jens Frahm/ Max Planck Institute for Biophysical Chemistry, https://www.youtube.com/watch?v=6dAEE7FYQfc)

be determined whether the patient is able to clean the restoration adequately. If these trial adjustments do not result in a satisfactory solution, or if the patient is unable to clean and maintain the restoration adequately, a definitive fixed restoration should be avoided. In these cases, a removable palate-free overdenture is an alternative.

In this two-stage procedure with an initial long-term provisional, the additional cost of treatment must be weighed against the certainty of a successful outcome. Obviously, the patient must be made aware of this additional cost and the fact that it is significantly less than the cost of a failed complex full-arch restoration before treatment begins.

3.6 Treatment Options and Patient Profiles

S. Wolfart

The differential therapeutic consideration of the edentulous jaw is complex. Since there are several potential treatment modalities with good to very good long-term performance, the understanding of the patient's expectations, as well as important anatomical and general medical factors, is crucial. This information is compiled in the patient profile and then used in the decision-making process.

The first step is to determine whether the patient has expressed a clear preference for a fixed or a removable restoration.

In the case of a *removable restoration*, an informed decision must be made between a minimally mobile prosthesis and one with rigid retention. With the minimally mobile option, the patient never completely loses the feeling of wearing a denture, while the rigid option provides more of a "real teeth" feeling.

The minimally mobile retention option is realized with a simple ball attachment or Novaloc retentive element. It is contraindicated only in cases of extensive vertical bone loss requiring a prosthetic design with a pronounced vertical dimension. In these cases, the resulting high leverage on the ball attachments can lead to involuntary loosening and increased wear of the retention elements.

This problem does not occur with rigid retention, which can be achieved with parallel-walled milled bars or telescoping crown abutments. The passive-fit concept is preferred for telescopic prostheses and can be achieved with electroplated copings or by intraoral bonding of classic telescopic crowns. All types of restorations are usually fabricated as overdentures, which are palate-free when in the maxilla. With minimal vertical tissue loss and, critically, precisely positioned implants, telescopic prostheses can also be designed as removable "bridges," without a pink acrylic saddle (Wolfart 2023).

If a *fixed restoration* is desired, the amount of vertical and horizontal tissue loss is a critical factor in determining patient tolerance (see Chapter 3.5). The restoration should therefore be tested for function, phonetics, esthetics and cleanability using a fixed long-term provisional before the final restoration is fabricated. If the patient is not satisfied with this long-term provisional, the therapy concept can easily be changed to a rigidly supported removable restoration.

With removable restorations, any problems with lip padding, speech, sagittal and vertical position of the maxillary anterior teeth, and cleaning of the restoration, can be solved more easily than with fixed restorations. However, if the long-term provisional works well for 3 to 6 months, it can be converted to a definitive fixed restoration.

Due to the almost inevitable vertical and horizontal tissue defects mentioned above, it will almost always be necessary to work with both tooth-colored and pink ceramic. Once pink ceramic is used, segmented FDPs are usually impractical because the proximal contacts between the FDPs would have to pass not only through the white ceramics but also through the pink ceramics. This interruption of the pink portions always looks artificial and disconcerting. In addition, such overly long proximal contacts are difficult to adjust in the laboratory and almost impossible to clean. Therefore, a one-piece full-arch FDP is the primary recommendation in these cases. Due to bone resorption and the associated implant positions and angulations, strictly occlusally screw-retained FDPs (with straight screw access channels) are not realistic. In these cases, either the use of multi-unit intermediate abutments is required or angled screw retention should be aimed for (Wolfart 2023).

If cementation is planned, custom CAD/CAM titanium abutments are used, which ensure a maximum subgingival cementation margin of 0.5 mm. In general, retention with angled screws should be preferred to cementation to ensure safe removal of the restoration (Wolfart 2023).

For patients who cannot afford more than four implants and insist on a fixed restoration immediately after implant placement, and whose bone supply is sufficient for maxillary implant placement only anterior to the maxillary sinus, the treatment concept using anterior axial and posterior angled implants is a valuable option. It avoids extensive two-stage bone augmentation with long treatment times and removable provisional prostheses. Patients with a terminal residual dentition who are unfamiliar with removable prostheses are particularly attracted to this treatment option. The promise of avoiding the removable provisional speaks for itself.

These treatment options are presented in Table 3 based on the appropriate patient profile.

Table 3 Treatment options considering the appropriate patient profile.

Example of a suitable patient profile* (details of the seven main factors are discussed in Chapter 2.1.3).		low – high ▪ Resilience ▪ Function ▪ Retention ▪ Esthetics ▪ Tissue loss ▪ Financial options ▪ Risk 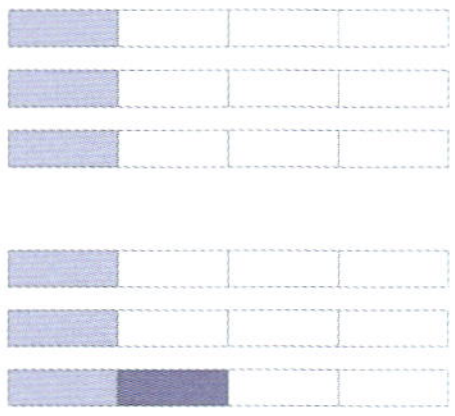	low – high ▪ Resilience ▪ Function ▪ Retention ▪ Esthetics ▪ Tissue loss ▪ Financial options ▪ Risk 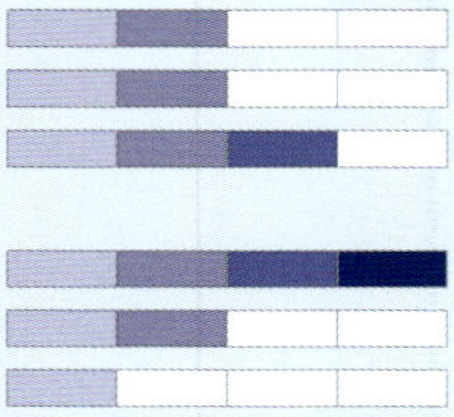
Additional information		See Chapters 5.1 to 5.3 for detailed patient examples	See Chapters 5.4 and 5.5 for detailed patient examples
Design		Stud attachments (e.g., ball attachment, Locator, Novaloc)	Parallel-milled bar (CAD/CAM)
Number of implants		4–6 maxillary 1–4 mandibular	4–6 maxillary 4 mandibular
Implant details	**Standard implant**	+	+
	Angled implant		+
	Reduced-diameter implant	+ (min. 2 implants mandibular)	+
	Mini implants	+ (min. 4 implants)	
	Short implants	+ (min. 4 implants)	+
	Zygomatic implant		+ (Ahlgren and coworkers 2006)
Technical details		Overdenture Stud attachments Metal framework with resin base/ Acrylic denture teeth	Overdenture Retention elements (e.g., Preci-Vertix/ Horix) Metal framework with resin base/ Acrylic denture teeth
Degree of difficulty according to the SAC Classification in Implant dentistry ** (Dawson and coworkers 2022)		Straightforward	Advanced/ Complex
Long-term performance		Very good	Very good

* The "esthetics" factor is not considered here, as it is not relevant for assignment to the treatment options.
** The classification includes tissue loss, accessibility, time of loading, esthetic risk, type of provisional restoration, presence of parafunctions, and the intended occlusal concept (Dawson and coworkers 2022).

	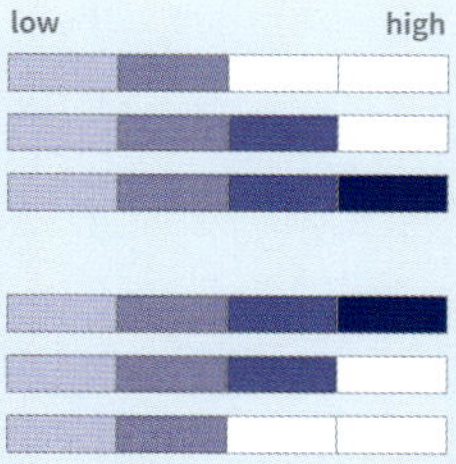 ▪ Resilience ▪ Function ▪ Retention ▪ Esthetics ▪ Tissue loss ▪ Financial options ▪ Risk	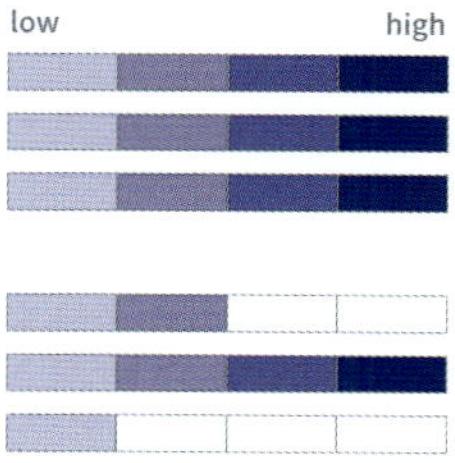 ▪ Resilience ▪ Function ▪ Retention ▪ Esthetics ▪ Tissue loss ▪ Financial options ▪ Risk		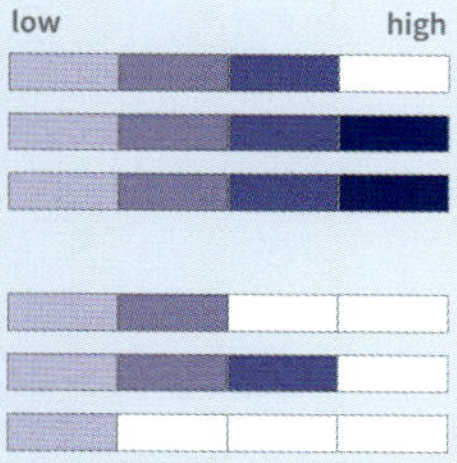 ▪ Resilience ▪ Function ▪ Retention ▪ Esthetics ▪ Tissue loss ▪ Financial options ▪ Risk
	See Chapters 5.3 and 5.6 for detailed patient examples	See Chapters 5.7 to 5.10 for detailed patient examples		Patient with terminal residual dentition, reduced bone availability, does not tolerate a removable temporary restoration, wants the shortest possible treatment time and has limited financially means
	Electroplated/classic telescopic crown (both adhesively bonded intraorally, passive fit)	Full-arch FDP/ segmented FDP, screw retained abutments or angled screws	Full-arch FDP/ segmented FDP, cemented	Pro Arch concept, immediate implant placement/ intermediate screw retained abutments/ Screw retained restoration
	4–6 maxillary 4 mandibular	4–8 maxillary 4–8 mandibular	4–8 maxillary 4–8 mandibular	4–6 maxillary 4 mandibular
	+	+	+	+
		+	+	+
		+	+	
		+	+	
	+ (Landes and coworkers 2009)	+	+	+
	Overdenture or "bridge" design Metal framework with resin base/ Acrylic denture teeth	Metal-ceramics CAD/CAM-milled non-precious framework + milled implant connection geometry (fully veneered) OR Monolithic zirconia with special Ti base abutments (adhesively bonded)	Metal-ceramics CAD/CAM-milled non-precious framework (fully veneered) OR Monolithic zirconia both with CAD/ CAM custom Ti abutments	Resin-veneered non-precious CAD/ CAM framework, PMMA veneer or denture teeth Angled prefabricated intermediate abutments Occlusally screw-retained
	Advanced/ Complex	Advanced/ Complex	Advanced/ Complex	Complex
	Very good	Very good	Very good	Very good

3.7 Needs for future research

S. Wolfart

3.7.1 Personalized Medicine in Implant Surgery

The future of implant surgery, particularly for patients with pre-existing conditions, presents significant opportunities but also raises several unresolved questions. As we move toward more personalized approaches in medicine, the development of implants that can adapt to the unique biological and immunological profiles of each patient is becoming a critical area of research. However, the long-term stability of implants in individuals with chronic diseases such as diabetes, osteoporosis, or autoimmune disorders remains an open question. Can we develop materials and designs that not only integrate well with compromised tissues but also adapt to the progressive nature of these diseases?

In addition, while minimally invasive surgical techniques continue to evolve and reduce immediate postoperative complications, their long-term effectiveness in maintaining implant stability in these patients is still under investigation. Another pressing question is how we can further modulate the immune response to prevent implant problems. Current immunomodulatory strategies are promising, but they are far from being fully understood or universally applicable.

The future holds the potential for breakthroughs in biomaterials, regenerative techniques, and patient-specific solutions, but the challenge is to integrate these innovations into a comprehensive treatment plan that ensures implant durability and functionality for decades. Ultimately, long-term studies and clinical trials are needed to answer these questions and bridge the gap between current technology and the ideal of fully stable, personalized implants for patients with underlying health problems.

3.7.2 Patient-Related Data (dPROs)

There is still a great need for research on patient-related data. While quality of life is assessed using validated instruments, patient satisfaction is assessed using only a common-sense concept of satisfaction (Messias and coworkers 2022). There is also a need for economic analysis with a cost-benefit assessment, including the cost of follow-up care. In particular, randomized clinical trials (RCTs) comparing removable and fixed restorations are needed. This is the only way to conclusively assess the effect of treatment on dPROs and oral function. Future RCTs should use dPROMs with sufficient psychometric properties to ensure high methodological quality and comparability. For example, the use of the OHIP questionnaire should be the minimum standard for the collection of dPROs.

3.7.3 Digital Workflow

The combination of various digital technologies, such as CBCT in conjunction with superimposed STL surface data from intraoral scanners, improves the accuracy of our planning and the predictability of surgical and prosthetic treatments. The continuous development of new hardware and software systems means that there is a constant continual need for their evaluation through research. This is also true for the resulting ever-changing digital workflows. Research is needed to integrate the individual digital modules into a complete digital workflow so that implantology and implant prosthetics of the edentulous jaw can be performed within a consistent, practical digital workflow.

It is striking that analog impressions are still the gold standard in the field of implant prosthetics of the edentulous jaw even though optical impressions can now ensure at least the same accuracy as the analog impression technique. To become practical, digital impressions, face scans, augmented reality, dental design software, and digital articulator systems must be linked, and their accuracy and practicality in the overall workflow must be evaluated. The concept of an all-digital workflow is currently being tested in the field of fixed prosthodontics; however, high-quality research is needed to transfer these findings to removable, implant-retained prostheses.

3.7.4 All-Ceramic Restorations

In the area of fixed restorations for the edentulous jaw, research is needed on monolithic or microveneered all-ceramic restorations. RCTs are needed to evaluate different types of monolithic zirconia (e.g., 3Y-TZP zirconia, multilayer 3Y-TZP/5Y-TZP), restoration designs (short-span FDPs, full-arch FDPs, cantilever FDPs) and differences in unit numbers.

Comparisons between restorations with prefabricated titanium bases and custom-made titanium abutments, restorations with angled screw-retained systems and angled intermediate abutments will also be evaluated. In addition to long-term outcomes and ongoing technical and biological complications, esthetics and other dPROs should be analyzed, and cost and time efficiencies should be reported.

4 Follow-Up and Complications

S. Wolfart, B. Al-Nawas

4.1 Maintenance and Prosthetic Complications

S. Wolfart

The good to very good long-term performance of implant-supported overdentures and fixed restorations in the edentulous jaw over a period of 5 to 10 years has been demonstrated in many review articles (Tsigarida and coworkers 2021; Del Fabbro and coworkers 2022) with a focus on implant survival and implant success. It is generally accepted that biological and technical (mechanical) complications are a routine occurrence (Papaspyridakos and coworkers 2012) and should therefore be anticipated.

Implant-related biological complications primarily refer to alterations in implant osseointegration and to inflammatory processes in the peri-implant soft and hard tissues. "Technical complications" is a collective term for mechanical damage to the implant, implant components, or superstructures. While these events do not necessarily result in failure of the implant or restoration itself, they are significant in terms of repair effort, time, and cost to the clinician and patient. Few studies have attempted to estimate the associated costs (Messias and coworkers 2022).

Timely patient education about the need for maintenance and regular follow-up appointments is critical for long-term treatment success and the prevention of complications (Papaspyridakos and coworkers 2012; Assaf and coworkers 2017).

4.1.1 Fixed Restorations

NATURE AND INCIDENCE OF COMPLICATIONS

Several types of complications can be observed in edentulous patients with implant-supported fixed restorations consisting of metal frameworks combined with acrylic or ceramic veneers. A systematic review (Papaspyridakos and coworkers 2012) found a total of 653 complication events in 281 restorations, with a mean observation period of 9.5 years. The proportion of complication-free restorations was 29% at 5 years and 9% at 10 years. The most common complications are summarized in Table 1. This table shows that biological and technical complications occur continuously and frequently over time due to fatigue and stress.

Table 1 Overview of complications associated with fixed implant-supported restorations in the edentulous jaw (data from Papaspyridakos and coworkers 2012).

	Type of complication	Estimated occurrence at 5 years	Estimated occurrence at 10 years
Biological	Peri-implant bone loss > 2 mm	20.1%	40.3%
	Hypertrophy or hyperplasia of soft tissues	13.0%	26.0%
	Inflammation below the restoration	5.6%	11.3%
Technical	Veneer fracture/chipping	33.3%	66.6%
	Loss of obturation of the screw access channel	22.9%	45.8%
	Replacement of all resin teeth	16.2%	32.4%
	Screw loosening	10.4%	20.8%
	Wear of the resin teeth	10.0%	20.0%
	Framework fractures	4.9%	9.8%
	Conversion to an overdenture	2.5%	5.0%
	Conversion to a complete denture	0.7%	1.4%
	Patient dissatisfaction	1.8%	3.6%

CLINICAL EXAMPLE: COMPLICATIONS AND MAINTENANCE EFFORT OF A FIXED RESTORATION (FOLLOW-UP: 5 YEARS)

As an example of a typical follow-up, a patient with 6 implants at sites 17, 16, 14, 23, 25, and 26 was presented. The one-piece CAD/CAM non-precious metal framework was veneered with pink and tooth-colored ceramics. The FDP was occlusally screw-retained with an angled screw system, and the screws

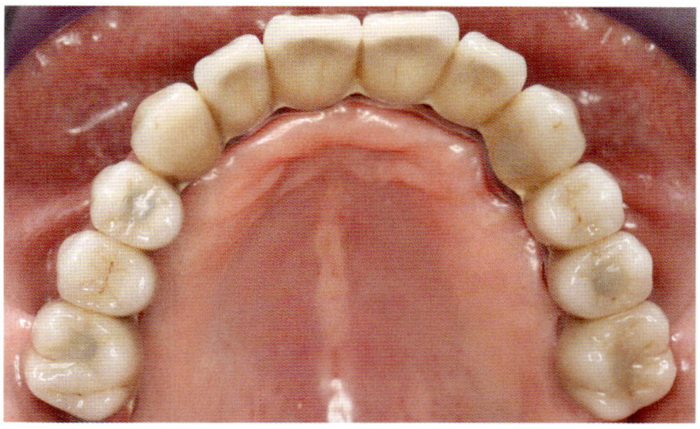

Fig 1 Delivery: Occlusally screw-retained full-arch metal-ceramic FDP for implants at sites 17, 16, 14, 23, 25, and 26. Screw access channel obturated with PTFE tape and a restorative composite resin.

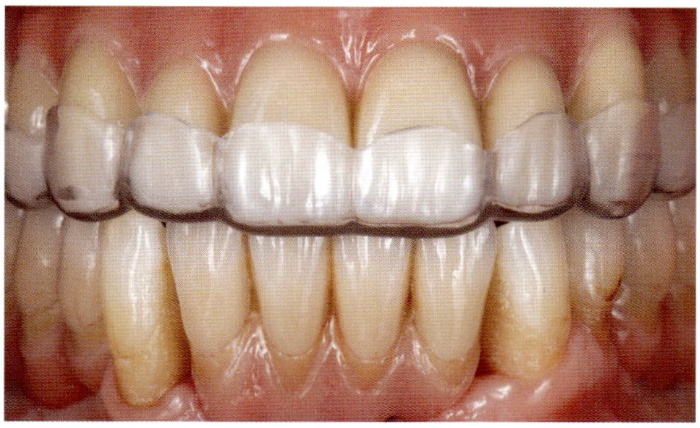

Fig 2 Follow-up at 7 days: Delivery of a night guard (1.5 mm thick).

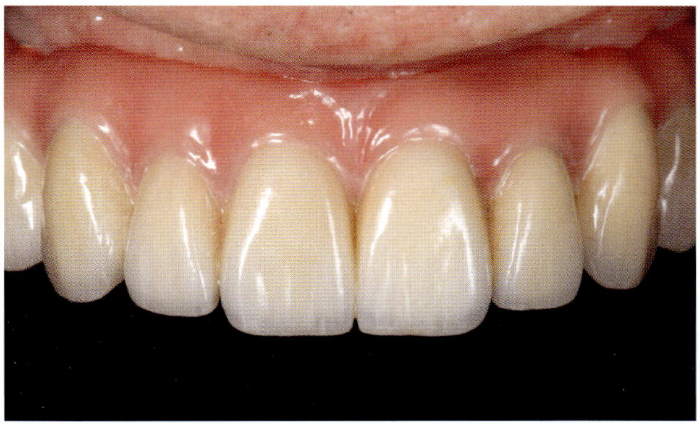

Fig 3 Follow-up at 6 months: Interdental plaque was removed as part of professional cleaning.

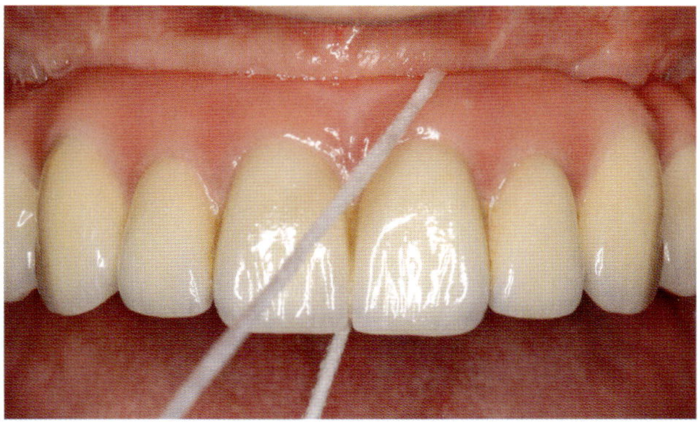

Fig 4 The patient was again given detailed instructions to improve oral hygiene at home.

were tightened to the manufacturer's recommended torque. The screw access channels were obturated with PTFE tape and a restorative composite (Fig 1). A 1.5-mm vacuum-formed acrylic splint was placed 7 days later as a night guard to protect the ceramics from chipping caused by bruxism (Fig 2).

Follow-up at 6 months: The patient presented with a clear need for improvement in home oral hygiene (Fig 3) and was instructed accordingly. He was also re-instructed on the use of interdental brushes and the use of special dental floss (e.g., Oral-B Superfloss; Procter & Gamble, Belmont, CA, USA) to clean the interdental surface and pontic areas (Fig 4). The occlusion was also evaluated. In static occlusion, the contact points were evenly distributed (Fig 5). There was bilateral anterior/canine guidance in lateral excursions. No adjustments were required.

Follow-up at 1 and 2 years: No abnormalities.

Follow-up at 3 years: The patient had not worn his night guard for 3 months. Chipping of tooth 11 had occurred a few weeks earlier (Fig 6). The restoration was repaired with a mesial corner build-up using a restorative composite. The correction was performed under the protection of a rubber dam. The fractured ceramic veneer was pretreated with hydrofluoric acid (Porcelain Repair Kit; South Jordan, UT, USA) for intraoral application. Silane was applied and the filling was placed and polished (Fig 7).

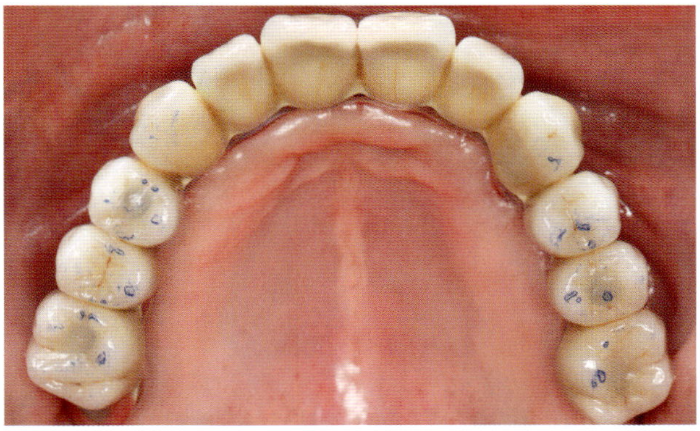

Fig 5 The occlusion showed an even distribution of static occlusal contacts and anterior/canine guidance. No adjustments were necessary.

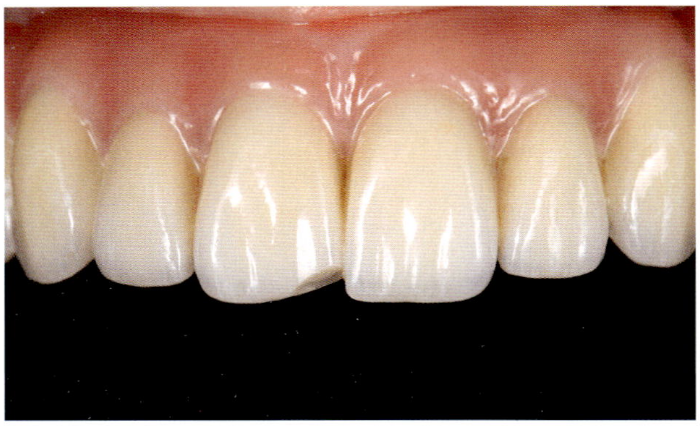

Fig 6 Follow-up at 3 years: Chipping had occurred a few weeks earlier. Repair under rubber dam protection with intraoral hydrofluoric acid and silane.

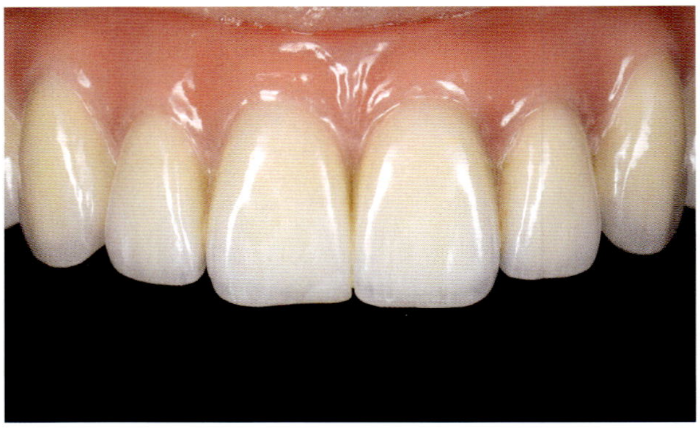

Fig 7 Mesial corner built up with a restorative composite and polished.

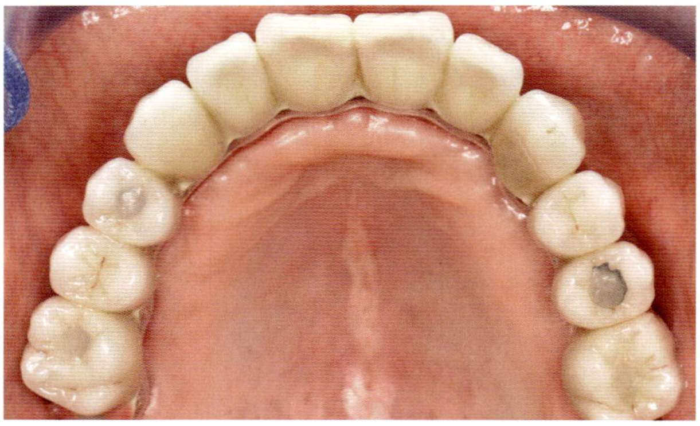

Fig 8 Follow-up at 5 years: Occlusal view showing discoloration at the screw access channels.

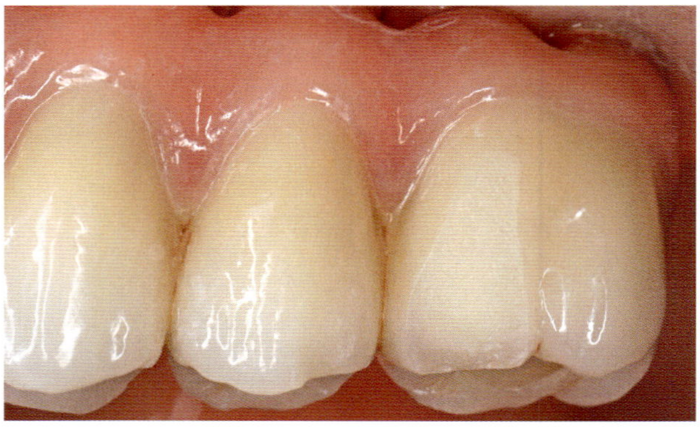

Fig 9 Buccal chipping of the veneers at sites 25 and 26. Both areas were smoothed and polished.

Follow-up at 4 years: No abnormalities.

Follow-up at 5 years: The top view shows the discolored plug of the screw access channel at site 25. In addition, buccal chipping had occurred on teeth 25 and 26. These teeth were simply smoothed and polished in the same session. The patient was reminded to wear his night guard regularly (Figs 8 and 9).

4.1.2 Removable Restorations

NATURE AND INCIDENCE OF COMPLICATIONS

Various complications or maintenance procedures may be associated with implant-supported mandibular or maxillary overdentures. Prosthetic maintenance requirements range from simple repairs to the replacement of the attachment or the fabrication of a new prosthesis. Selected complications and the associated treatment options for various therapeutic interventions are listed in Table 2.

The types of possible complications and their incidence depend on several factors such as the prosthetic design, retention system (ball attachments, Novaloc, bar, telescopic crowns, or magnets) and materials used, as well as the quality of the prosthesis in terms of occlusal design and congruency of the saddles with the alveolar ridge. Because of these multiple factors, it is not possible to provide average incidence rates for individual complications. There is also no evidence that any one implant design or retention system is superior to others (Assaf and coworkers 2017).

Kim and coworkers (2016) demonstrated that the most common procedure at follow-up was the activation or replacement of friction inserts. This was most commonly required for magnetic attachments. Inconsistent results were seen for ball attachments compared to bar attachments (Kim and coworkers 2012). The need to adjust the retention elements increased sharply between the first year after insertion and the 5-year follow-up. For example, matrices had to be activated in 18% of cases and replaced in 14% of cases. After 5 years, the frequency of these procedures increased to 47% and 57%, respectively (Çehreli and coworkers 2010).

To reduce the incidence of these complications, patients should be enrolled in a structured follow-up and a standard-

Table 2 Implant overdenture complications and treatment options.

Items to evaluate	Possible complications	Treatment options
Retention of the overdenture	Inadequate retention of the overdenture	Replace entire abutment and/or matrix
		Replace retention elements (e.g., friction inserts, clips)
		Activate existing retention inserts
	Abutment fractures (e.g., ball, bars, bar extensions)	Replace or refabricate
Denture base	Insufficient saddle congruence with alveolar ridge	Reline denture base
Denture saddles	Fractures of parts of the denture base	Replace denture base
Framework structures	Framework fractures with denture fracture	Replace/repair denture
Denture teeth	Severe wear of the denture teeth	Replace resin denture teeth and correct vertical dimension
	Loss of denture teeth from the denture	Correct individual denture teeth
	Chipping of resin veneer	Replace/renew veneer
Screws connecting implants and retention elements	Screw loss or fracture	Replace screws and tighten to the manufacturer's recommended torque
Implants	Implant fractures	Remove implants (see "Implant loss" for further action)
	Implant loss	Reimplant, rework, or refabricate the restoration

ized protocol should be followed (Assaf and coworkers 2017). This would include the following points:

- Inspection of the peri-implant soft tissue for signs of inflammation or peri-implant bone resorption, including probing.
- Professional supra- and subgingival (if necessary) cleaning of the implants, implant components, and overdenture.
- Patient education regarding home oral hygiene and other maintenance tasks. This regular information is necessary for long-term treatment success and to avoid complications.
- Verification of static and dynamic occlusion.
- Inspection of the prosthetic components (teeth, saddles) for defects.
- Inspection of the retention elements, activation of the retention elements, or replacement of the friction elements if necessary.
- Inspection of the dentures for relining needs and relining if necessary.
- Determination of the follow-up interval.

CLINICAL EXAMPLE: COMPLICATIONS AND MAINTENANCE OF A LOCATOR-SUPPORTED OVERDENTURE (FOLLOW-UP: 10 YEARS)

The patient was rehabilitated 10 years previously with an overdenture supported on four interforaminal implants. The patient wished to retain her remaining tooth 38 despite more than 50% attachment loss. This tooth was integrated into the restoration with a cast clasp that had a purely retentive function (Figs 10 to 16).

The maxilla was restored with a new complete denture, which allowed for optimal vertical dimension and occlusal plane alignment. At delivery, a bilaterally balanced occlusion was provided (Fig 14) to accommodate the weakest part of the rehabilitation, namely the maxillary complete denture. During placement, different friction levels of the Locator system were tested to determine the most appropriate retention strength of the overdenture (Figs 15 and 16).

Follow-up at 6 months: The patient felt that the retention of the prosthesis was very good. Static and dynamic occlusion showed a sliding movement in maximum intercuspation. The prostheses were re-registered with a supporting-pin

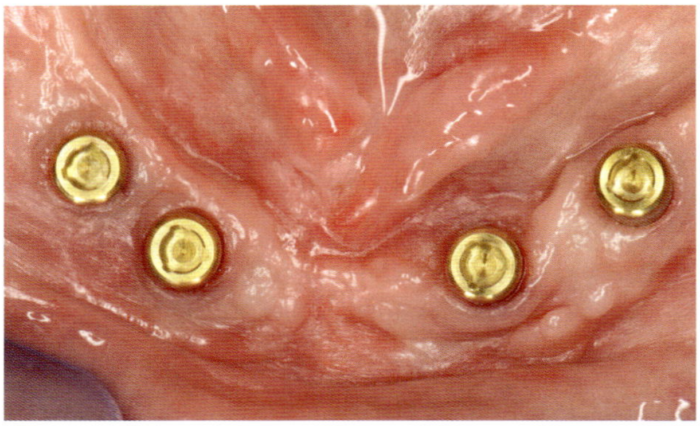

Fig 10 Delivery: Four interforaminal implants with Locators.

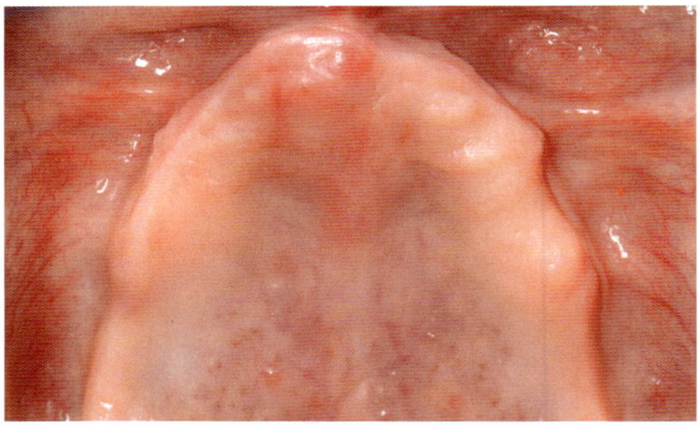

Fig 11 Maxilla restored with a complete denture because the patient had nc problems with one.

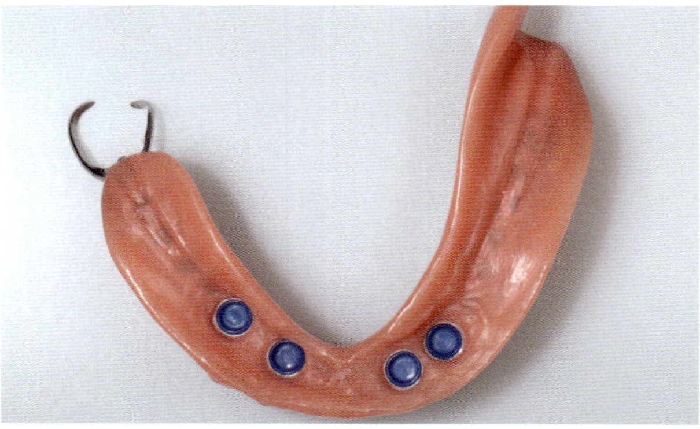

Fig 12 Implant-supported overdenture supported by a metal framework, with tooth 38 supported by a clasp.

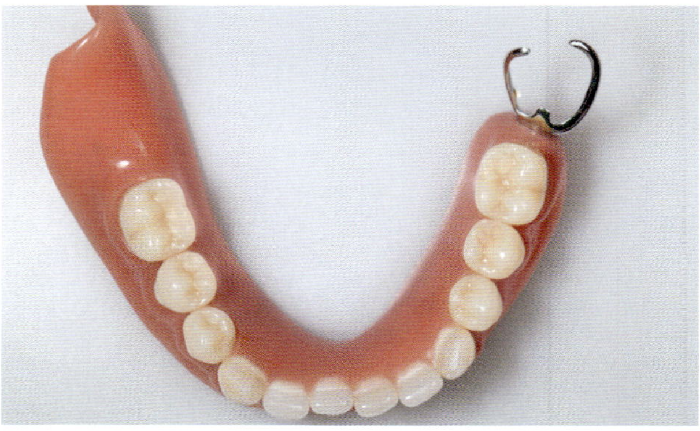

Fig 13 Occlusal view of the overdenture

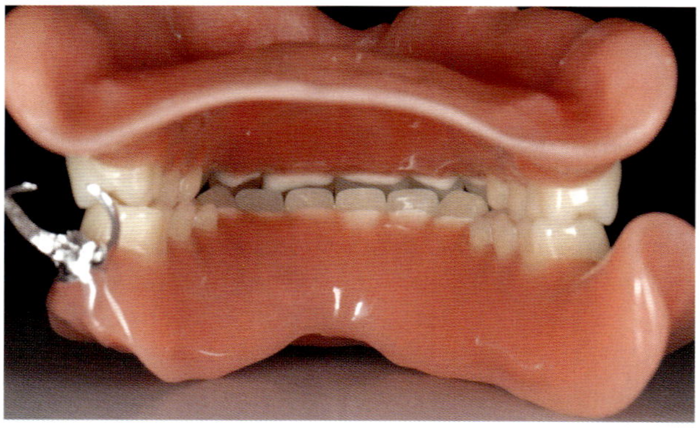

Fig 14 Bilateral dynamic occlusion.

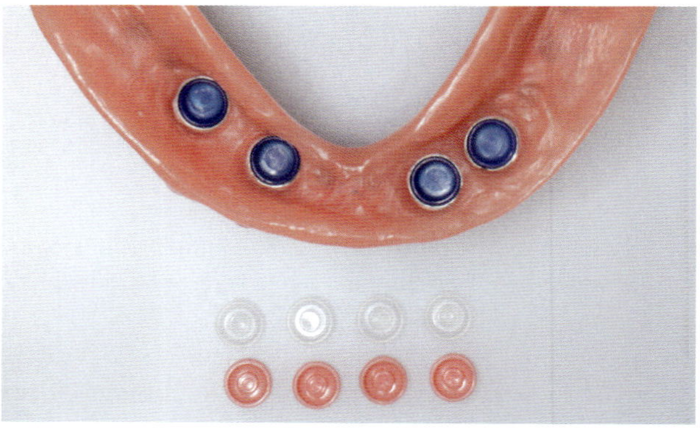

Fig 15 Different friction elements were tested together with the patient to determine the most appropriate retention strength (central punches were removed from the friction elements to facilitate insertion and removal).

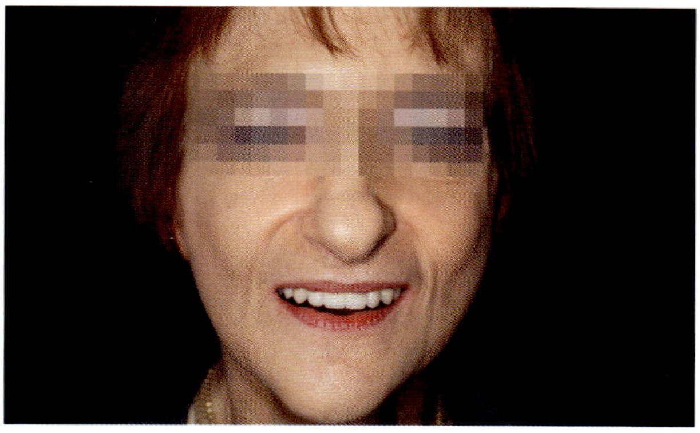

Fig 16 The patient's smile after delivery.

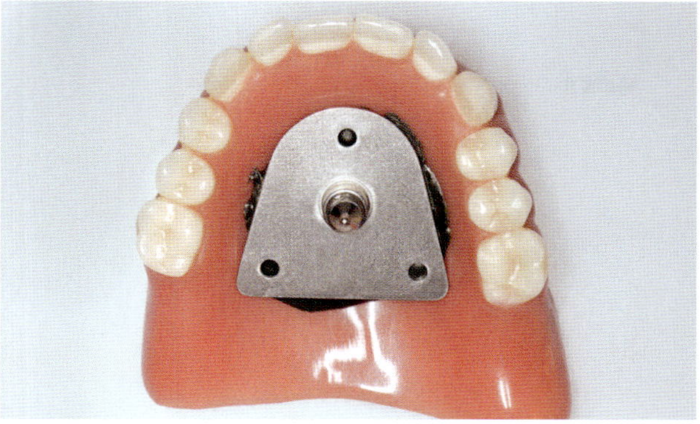

Fig 17 Follow-up at 6 months: Static occlusion with a slight sliding movement. Bilateral occlusion not properly supported. Bite re-registration with a supporting pin.

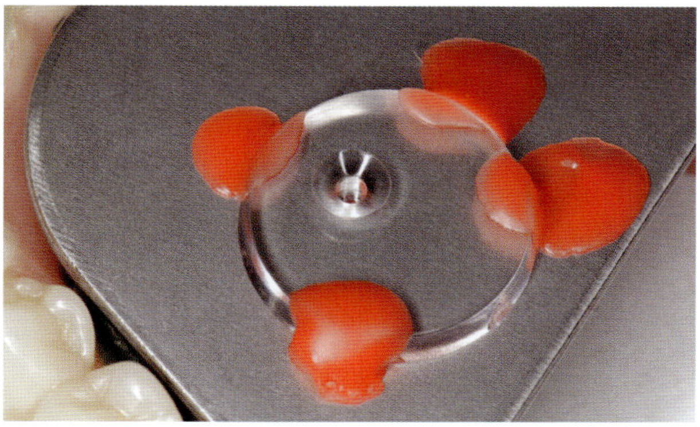

Fig 18 Plastic platelet with positioning aid for the support pin (hole), positioned and attached with adhesive wax.

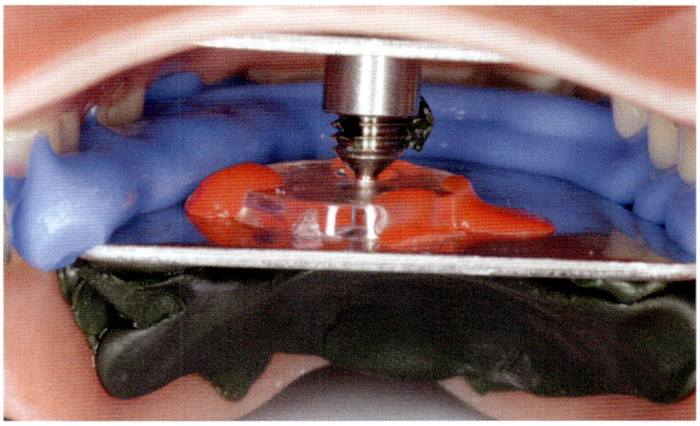

Fig 19 Keyed registration of the static and dynamic occlusion with blue resin (LuxaBite, DMG, Hamburg, Germany).

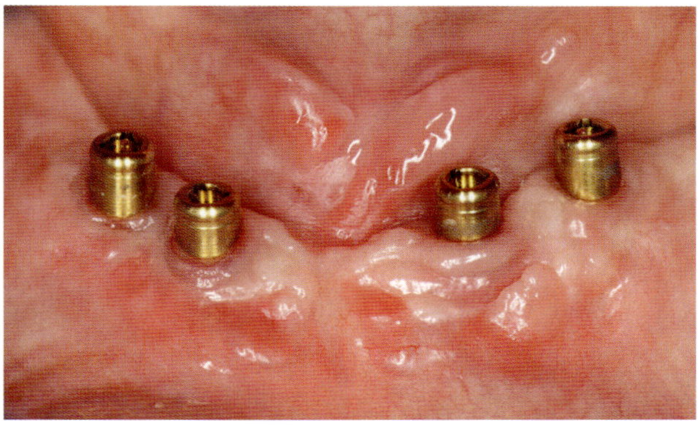

Fig 20 Follow-up at 12 months: First signs of wear on the Locators. Peri-implant soft tissue free of inflammation.

bite registration (Figs 17 to 19). The static and dynamic occlusion were then adjusted by the dental laboratory.

Follow-up at 12 months: First signs of wear were visible on the Locators (Fig 20). No other treatment was required.

Follow-up at 2 years: No significant findings, except that the friction of the overdenture had decreased slightly.

Follow-up at 3 years: The mandibular overdenture showed a need for relining as indicated by the routinely performed Fit Checker test. The friction elements showed inadequate retention. A relining impression was taken with zinc oxide-eugenol paste, the denture was relined in the dental laboratory and the friction elements were replaced at the same time (Fig 21 to 23a-b). The overdenture was reinserted on the same day.

Follow-up at 4, 5, and 6 years: No significant findings. The Locators were cleaned supragingivally, and the overdenture was cleaned in the ultrasonic unit.

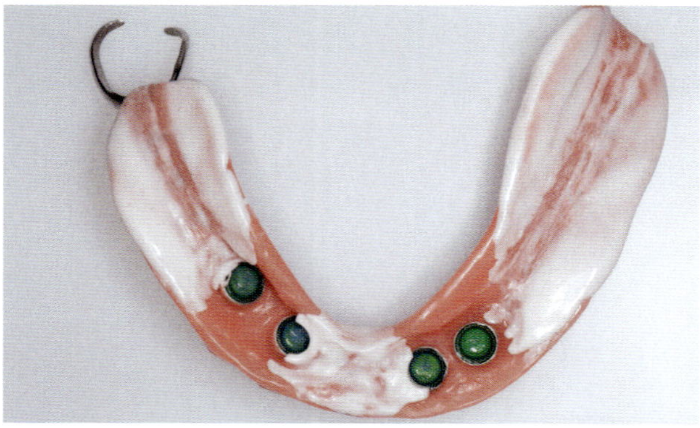

Fig 21 Follow-up at 3 years: Decreased friction of the Locators. The Fit Checker test showed a clear need for relining (thick Fit Checker areas).

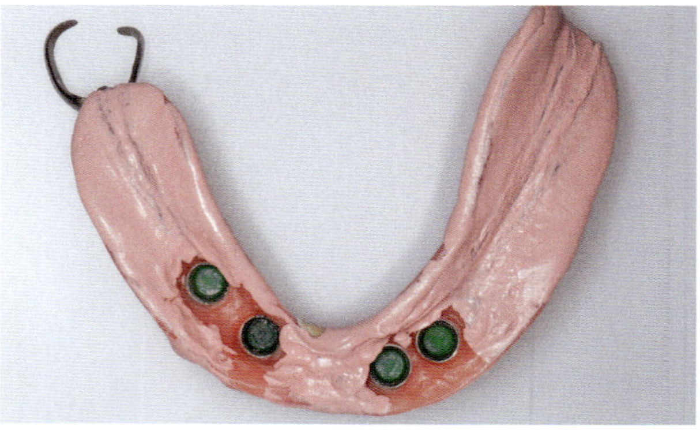

Fig 22 Implant-retained prosthesis relined with zinc oxide-eugenol paste.

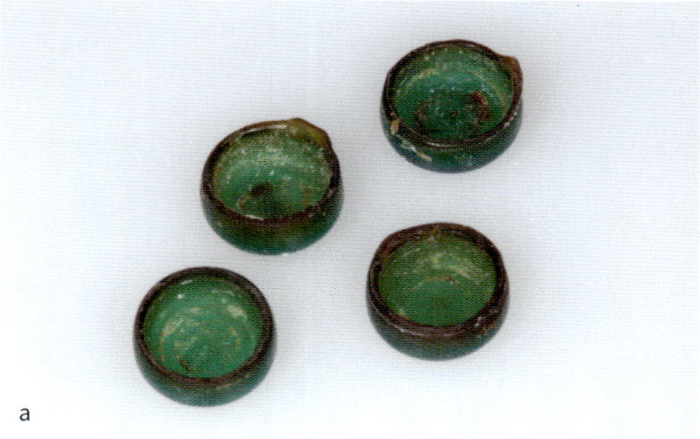

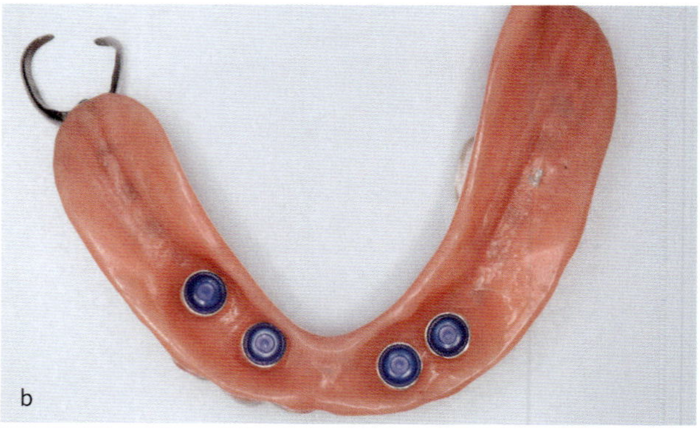

Figs 23a-b Worn retention elements removed from the prosthesis (a). New elements were replaced in the dental laboratory at the time the relining was performed (b).

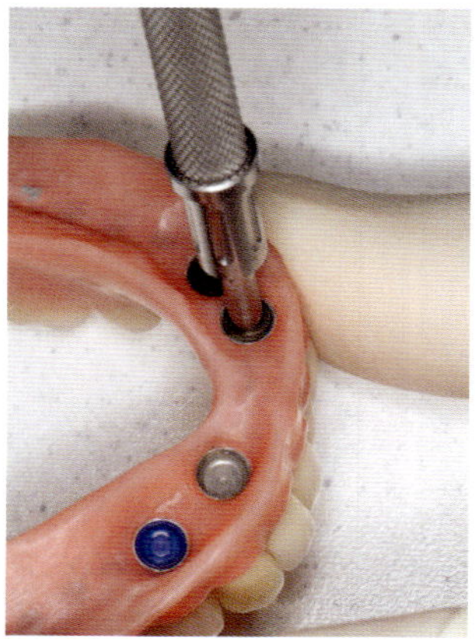

Fig 24 Follow-up at 7 years: Insufficient friction. This time, the retention elements were replaced chairside.

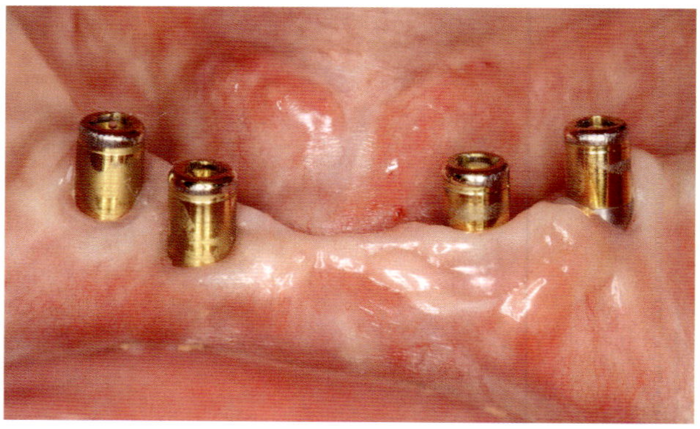

Fig 25 At the same time, the Locators again showed more pronounced signs of wear. Peri-implant soft tissue free of inflammation.

Follow-up at 7 years: The retention of the prosthesis was again too low, but there was no need for additional relining. In the meantime, the Locators had developed further signs of wear. In addition, the soft tissue around the implants had retracted or changed. However, the peri-implant probing depths were still unremarkable and there was little bleeding on probing. The retention elements were replaced directly at chairside (Figs 24 and 25).

Follow-up at 8 ***years:*** Due to increased wear on the Locators, friction on the elements was again greatly reduced. The elements were replaced again.

Follow-up at 9 years: Retention was again inadequate, and the Locators showed extreme signs of wear (Fig 26). Therefore, the Locators themselves were replaced with the successor model, the Locator R-Tx. According to the manu-

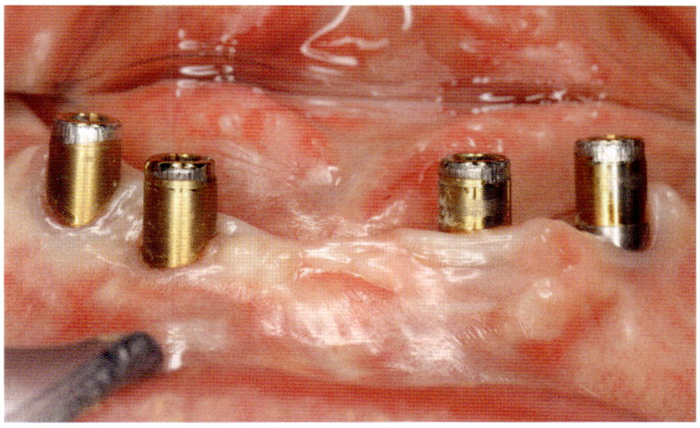

Fig 26 Follow-up at 9 years: Insufficient retention. Extremely worn Locators. Peri-implant soft tissue free of inflammation.

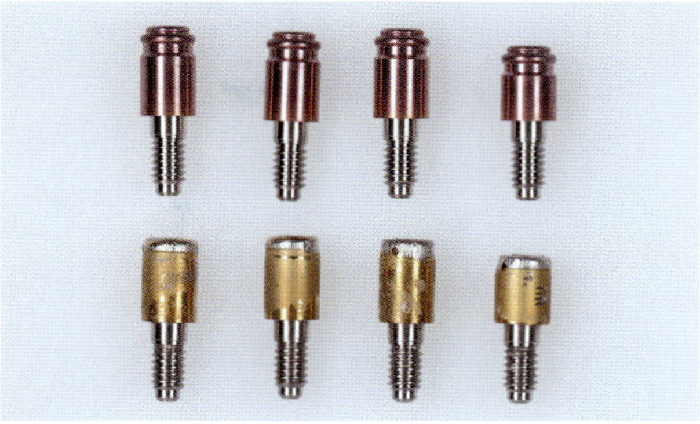

Fig 27 Removed Locator elements compared with the current Locator R-Tx. Identical dimensions allow for easy replacement.

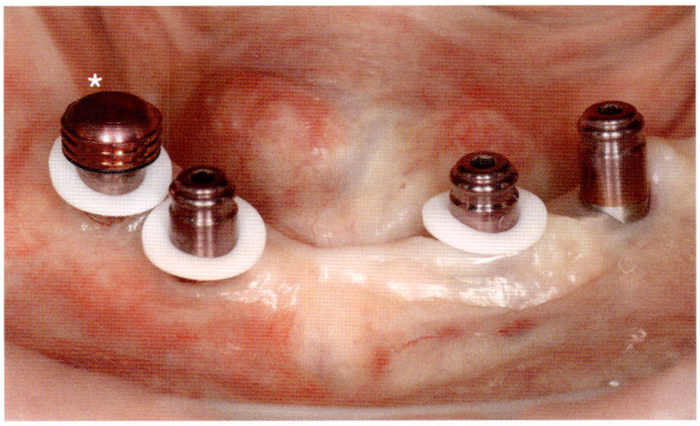

Fig 28 Locators screwed in with the implant-specific torque. Installation of the white block-out rings supplied. Locator matrix housing (*) already attached.

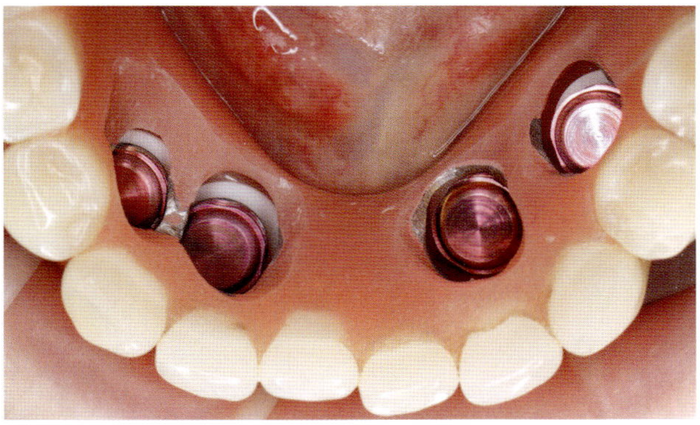

Fig 29 The overdenture must be able to be inserted in the final position with the matrix housings in place.

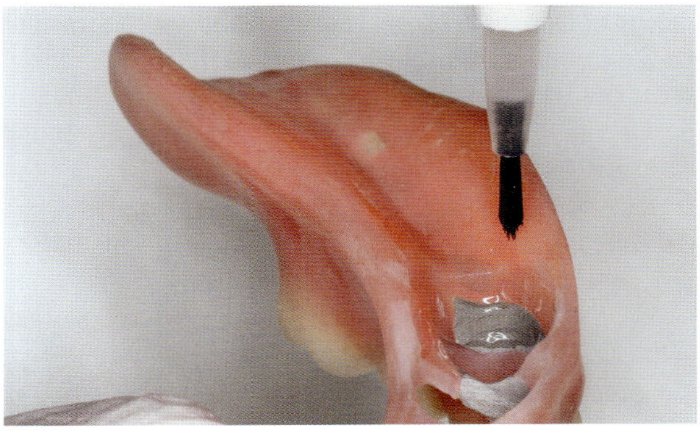

Fig 30 Conditioning of the denture base: air abrasion with alumina (2.5 bar, 50 μm), followed by activation of the resin with a primer (e.g., Glaze and Bond).

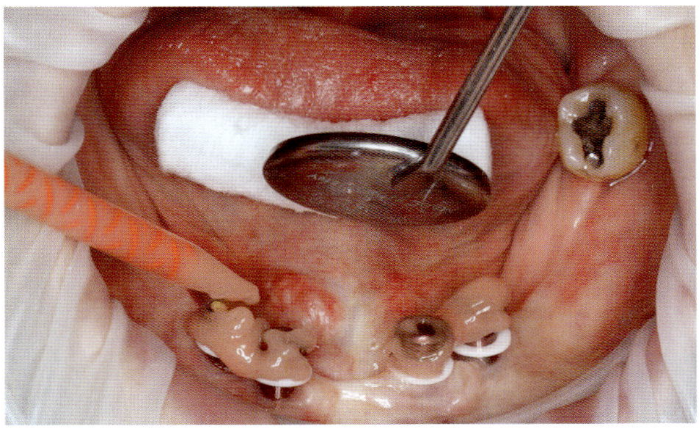

Fig 31 The composite material is applied directly to the undercuts of the matrices. The composite-filled overdenture is then placed on top.

facturer, the newly developed Locator has a harder surface coating. Due to the approximately conical basic shape and a swivel function of the retention insert in the matrix, this Locator can compensate for greater divergence between the implants and is also said to be more resistant to wear. The restoration was rebuilt according to the previously described protocol (Wolfart 2023). The worn classic Locators were removed (Fig 27), the new R-Tx Locators of identical dimensions were screwed in and the matrices were polymerized into the existing prosthesis (Figs 28 to 33). As the final position of the prosthesis may change during this conversion process, it was necessary to check the final fit of the denture base with flow silicone. A definitive relining was then performed (Figs 34 and 35).

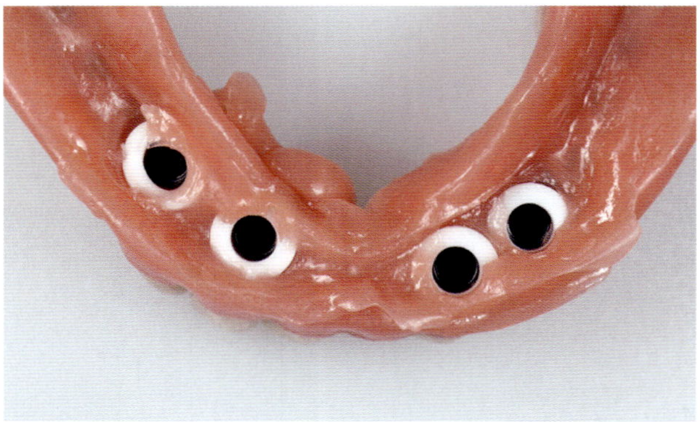

Fig 32 Removal of the block-out rings. The composite material has only flowed under the rings in a few areas. The restoration can be safely removed even after the composite has set.

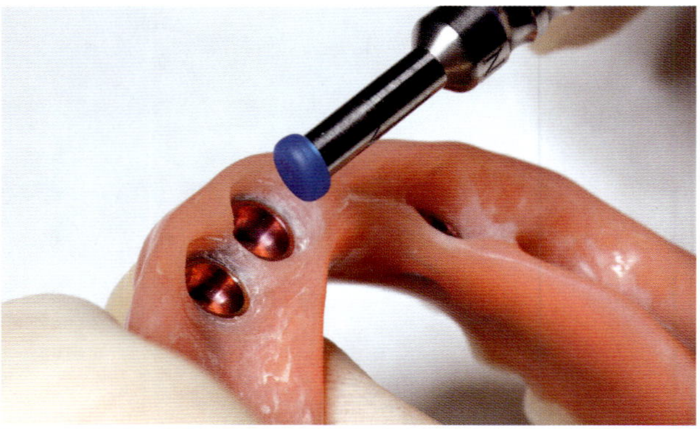

Fig 33 Retention inserts with special tooling.

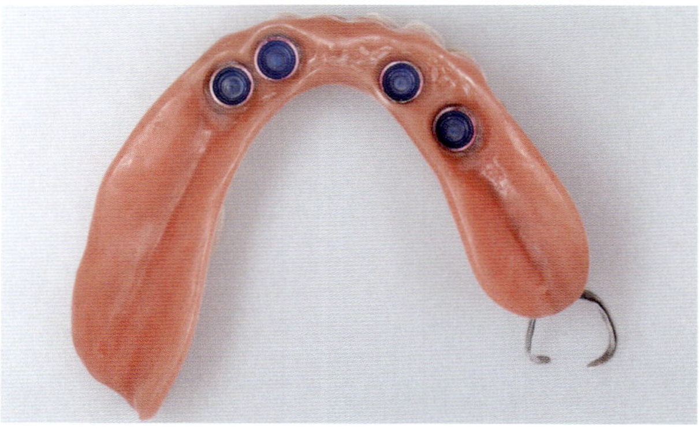

Fig 34 Completed relined and finished prosthesis (basal view).

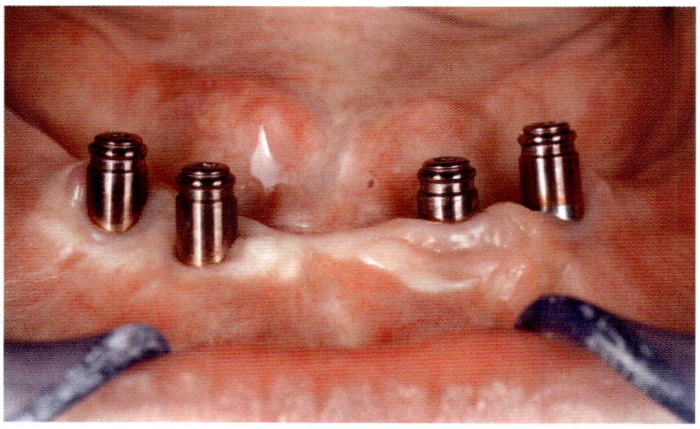

Fig 35 Frontal view of the definitively connected Locators.

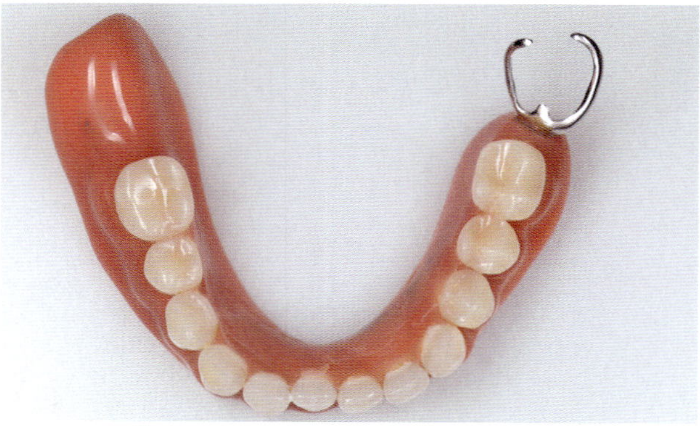

Fig 36 Follow-up at 10 years: Wear of the occlusal surfaces after 10 years (compare with Fig 13)

Follow-up at 10 years: The patient had no complaints. After 10 years, the occlusal surfaces of the acrylic teeth now showed considerable wear (Fig 36). As the patient was doing very well, no further procedures were planned for the time being.

CLINICAL EXAMPLE: COMPLICATIONS AND MAINTENANCE OF A CAD/CAM BAR-SUPPORTED OVERDENTURE (FOLLOW-UP: 10 YEARS)

Based on a diagnostic set-up, a parallel-milled titanium bar with two Preci-Vertix terminal attachments and two Preci-Horix horizontal attachments (both Alphadent, Waregem, Belgium) fabricated by CAD/CAM. The bar rested on the gingiva between the implants, similar to a pontic rest. There were small openings on the side of the implants to allow guided cleaning of the implants with interdental brushes. The overdenture itself has a palate-free design and consists of a continuous non-precious metal framework with a protective plate in the area where the “S” sounds are articulated to minimize thickness in this sensitive area and not compromise speech function. At delivery, the bar was screwed directly onto the implants and tightened to the manufacturer’s recommended torque. Only the two Preci-Vertix attachments and the central Preci-Horix attachment were provided with yellow friction elements to ensure adequate retention (Figs 37 to 41).

At the follow-up appointments every 6 months, the prosthesis was regularly cleaned in an ultrasonic unit. The probing depths at the implants and the bleeding index (BOP) were recorded. When necessary, the bar components were also cleaned subgingivally with a plastic curette (Figs 42 and 43).

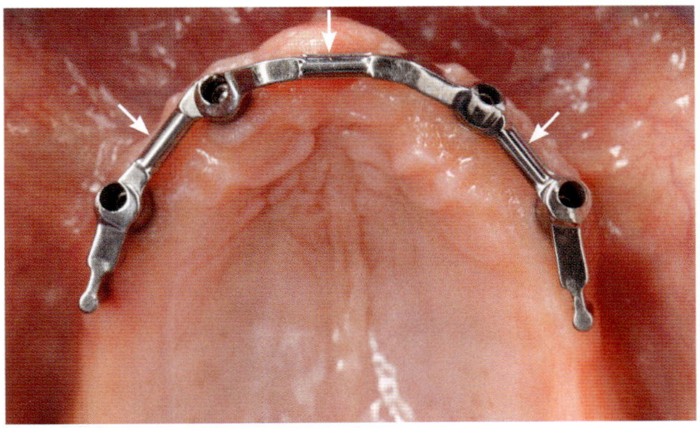

Fig 37 Delivery of the CAD/CAM-fabricated titanium bar with Preci-Vertix terminal and three Preci-Horix attachments (arrows) to an 83-year-old patient.

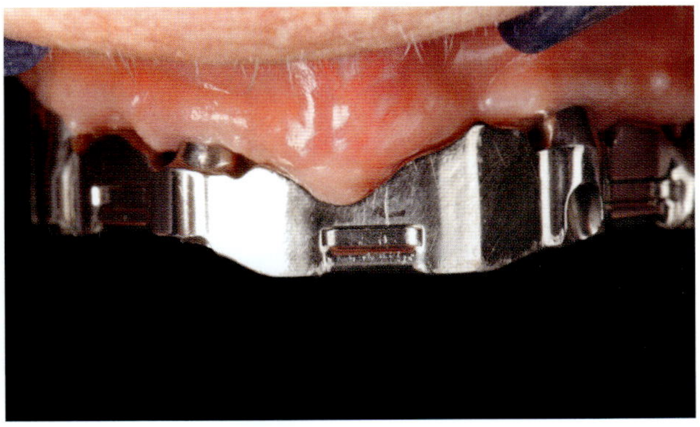

Fig 38 Frontal view of the bar with pontic-like support and openings for the interdental brushes.

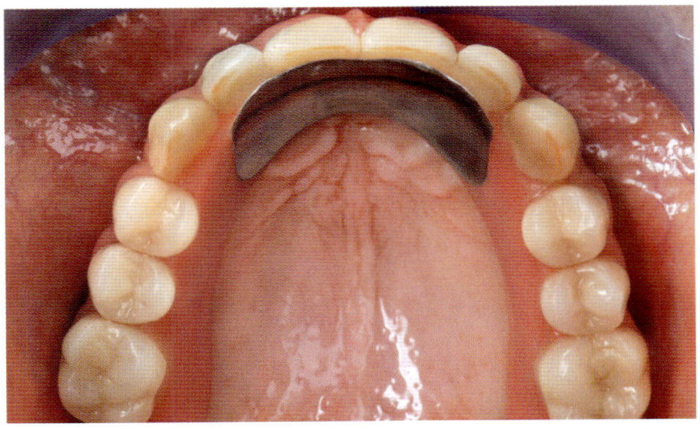

Fig 39 Occlusal view of the palate-free prosthesis with posterior protective plate to keep the area above the bar as thin as possible in this sensitive articulation area (speech function).

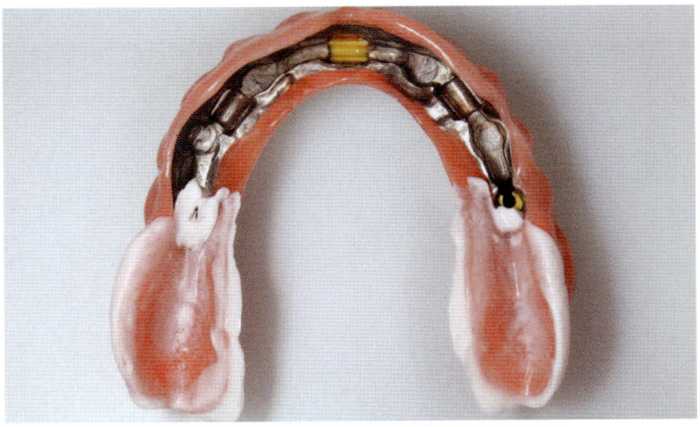

Fig 40 Verification of the very good congruence between the denture saddles and the alveolar ridge. Good retention was achieved with only three friction elements. The other clip positions were left for use in later years.

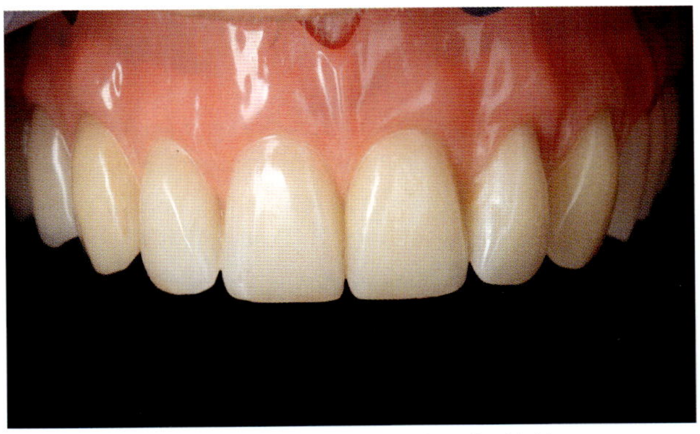

Fig 41 Frontal view of the prosthesis with labial acrylic shield to compensate for labial tissue loss and provide adequate lip support.

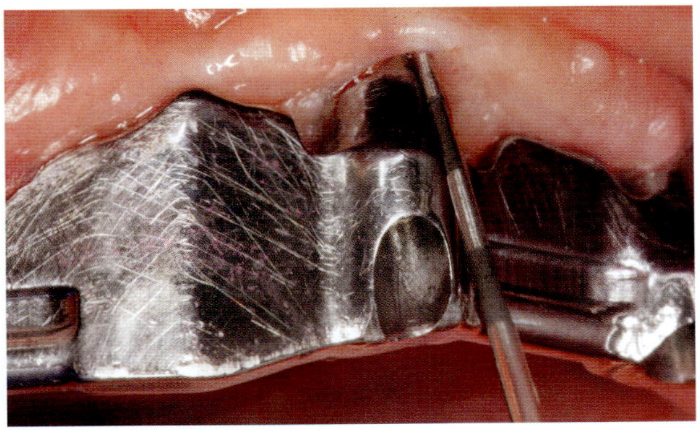

Fig 42 Regular 6-monthly follow-up visits with inspection of the peri-implant tissues.

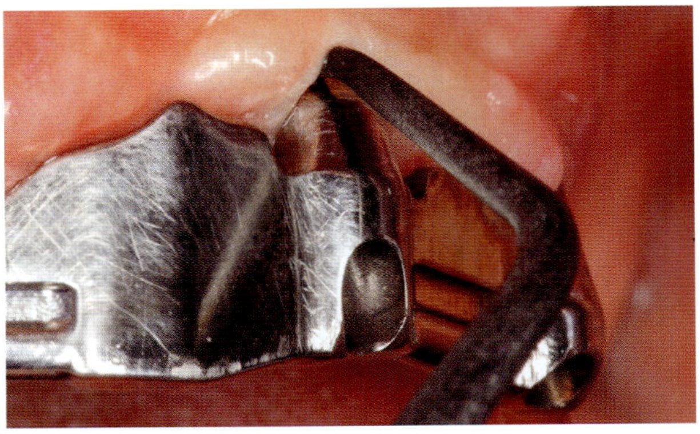

Fig 43 If necessary, subgingival cleaning of the bar with plastic curettes.

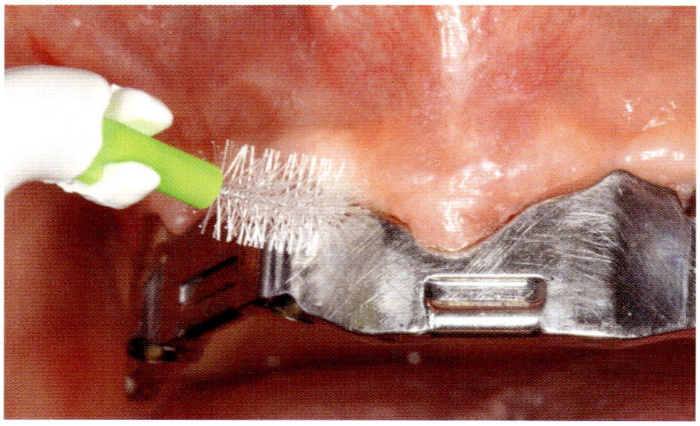

Fig 44 Re-instruction of the patient regarding the use of interdental brushes.

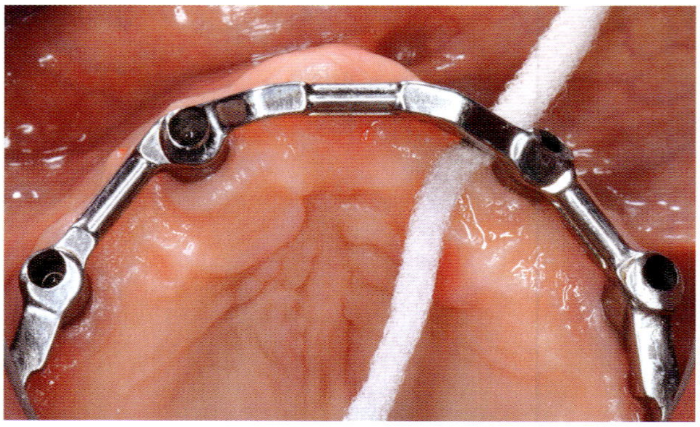

Fig 45 Re-instruction of the patient regarding the use of special dental floss.

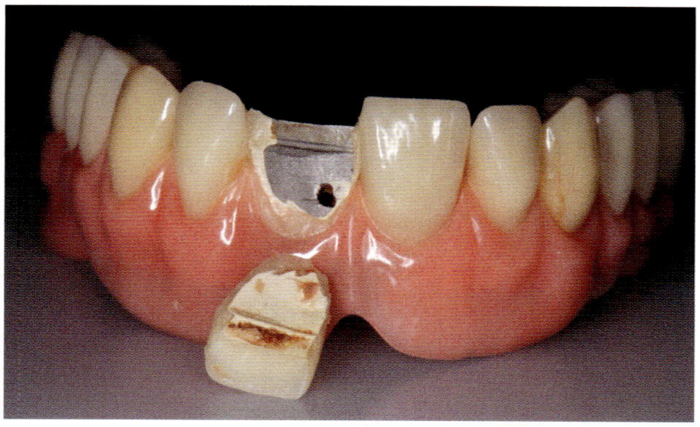

Fig 46 Follow-up at 3 years: The denture had been dropped into the sink during cleaning and a denture tooth had broken out of the denture. The damage was repaired by the dental laboratory on the same day.

The bar was cleaned with fine polishing paste and brushes, as well as interdental brushes and special dental floss. The patient was regularly instructed on home oral hygiene again (Figs 44 and 45).

Follow-up at 3 years: The denture had been dropped in the sink during cleaning and a denture tooth had broken out (Fig 46) but was replaced by the dental laboratory on the same day.

Follow-up at 4 and 8 years: Friction inserts were replaced or added.

Follow-up at 10 years: The patient was now 93 years old and continued to attend her biennial follow-up appointments. After 10 years of use, the bar and the prosthesis itself showed signs of wear. The prosthetic teeth were also heavily abraded (Figs 47 to 51), but this did not bother the patient in any way. Overall, she had no functional, speech, or esthetic limitations due to her dentures. The fact that only minimal follow-up care was required over the years also contributed greatly to her reported good quality of life (Fig 52).

Use this code to watch a highlight video with the patient reporting on her satisfaction with the treatment.

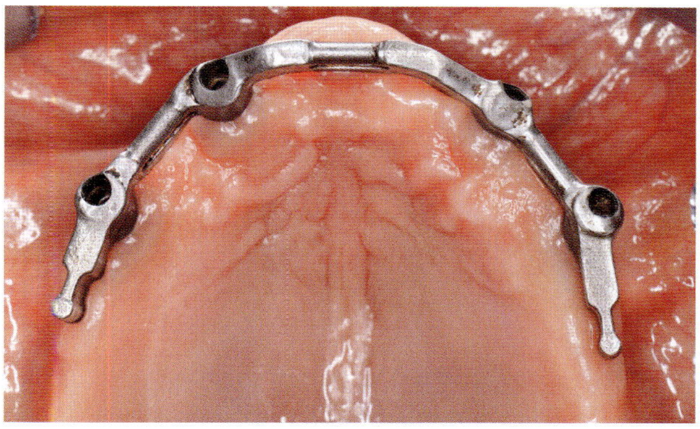

Fig 47 Follow-up at 10 years: Occlusal view of the bar showing signs of wear.

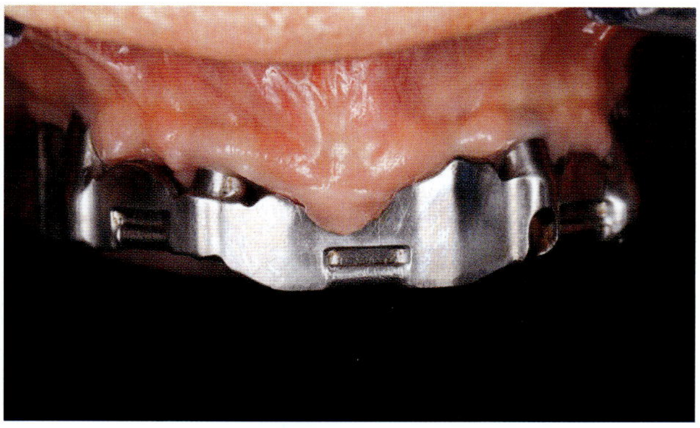

Fig 48 The labial view shows inflammation-free peri-implant tissue and no proliferation in the mucosal area. Signs of wear were also evident from this perspective.

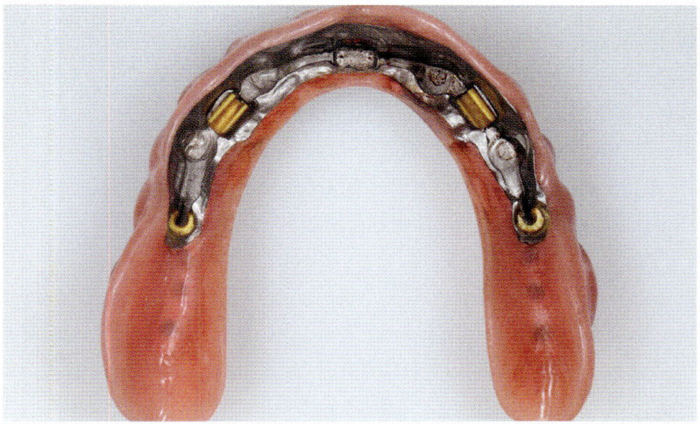

Fig 49 Basal surface of the overdenture with yellow friction elements. The central element had come loose and was lost a few weeks earlier, but without any limitation for the patient.

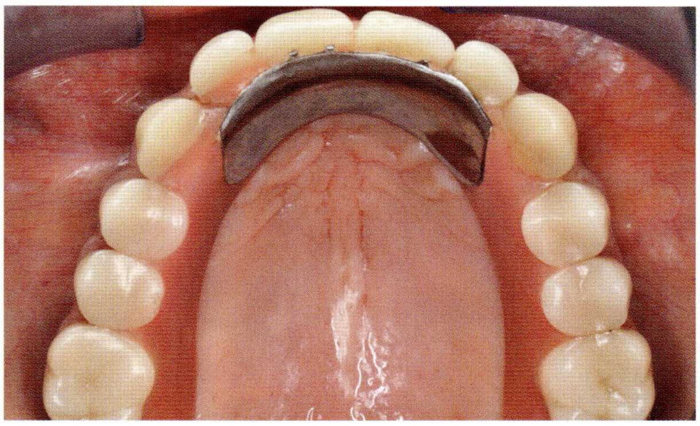

Fig 50 Prosthesis with clear signs of wear and denture teeth with severe wear.

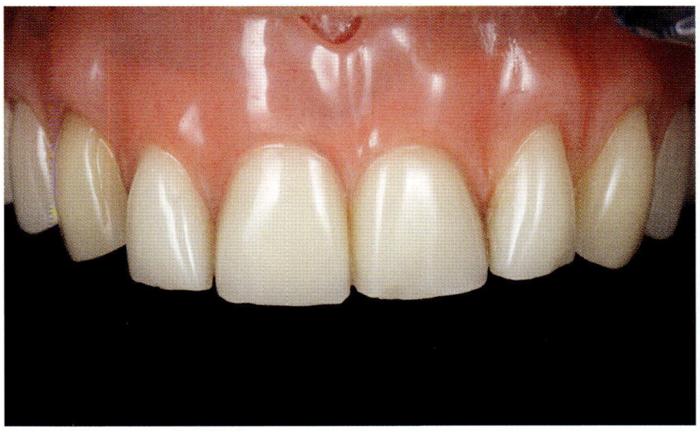

Fig 51 Abrasion was also evident in the labial view.

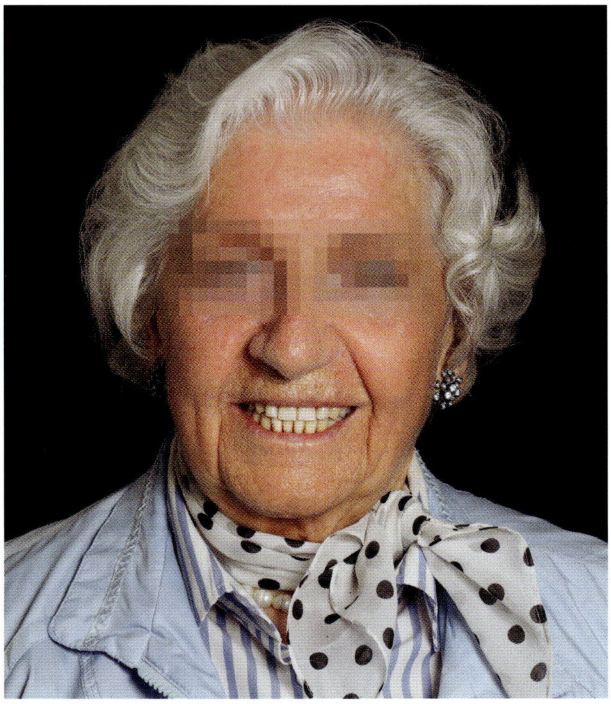

Fig 52 Follow-up at 10 years: The patient, now 93 years old, was very satisfied with the restoration and experienced a significant improvement in her quality of life compared to the complete denture she had worn previously for many years.

4.2 Biological Complications

B. Al-Nawas

Biological complications are rarely recorded systematically over a longer period of time. Often only retrospective analyses are available. Therefore, it is not possible to determine the exact prevalence or incidence. Given the heterogeneity of possible complications and the tendency to publish positive results, there is a risk of underreporting biological complications (Table 3).

4.2.1 Biological Implant Complications

Peri-implant mucositis and peri-implantitis as typical biological complications were defined by the AAP/EFP in 2017. Until then, heterogeneous definitions had been used (Berglundh and coworkers 2018) (Table 4).

A history of periodontitis, smoking, poor oral hygiene, and lack of peri-implant keratinized tissue are recognized risk factors for the development of peri-implant disease (Heitz-Mayfield and coworkers 2018). The open question remains as to how to treat patients who are losing their terminal dentition due to periodontitis. Some authors see an indication for an immediate fixed implant-supported restoration (Maló and coworkers 2014), while others emphasize the beneficial long-term effect of supportive periodontal therapy for retaining the teeth of this high-risk group (Heitz-Mayfield and coworkers 2016).

The presence of keratinized mucosa around implants is a well-recognized protective factor against biological problems (Sanz and coworkers 2016). This aspect draws attention to incision design during implant placement and second-stage surgery. Incision designs should always focus on increasing the stability of keratinized soft tissue around implants. If the lack of keratinized mucosa is associated with pathological changes, its dimensions can be surgically augmented using autologous grafts or soft-tissue substitutes.

Table 3 Overview of common biological complications.

Relation to implant/restoration	▪ Mucositis ▪ Soft-tissue hyperplasia ▪ Buccal soft-tissue dehiscence, lack of fixed mucosa
Relation to augmentation measures	▪ Resorption of the graft ▪ Sinus lift with chronic sinusitis/aspergillosis
Relation to general medical situation	▪ Limited ability to care for the restoration ▪ Affected bone physiology (radiation, antiresorptives) ▪ Bone necrosis

Table 4 Case definitions in daily clinical practice for peri-implant health, peri-implant mucositis, and peri-implantitis.

Peri-implant health	Peri-implant mucositis	Peri-implantitis
No BoP	BoP	BoP
No bone loss*	No bone loss*	Bone loss*

* Beyond crestal bone-level changes due to initial bone remodeling

Mucosal hyperplasia is also a typical peri-implant soft tissue finding in patients with removable dentures. These lesions are often difficult to treat and can lead to long-term infectious complications of the implant. Again, stable keratinized soft tissue around the implants is considered a protective factor. Control of smoking habits and good oral hygiene are patient factors that influence soft-tissue health.

4.2.2 Relationship with Augmentative Measures

The long-term stability of augmentation is always controversial. Resorption of the graft has been observed clinically, especially in complex vertical augmentations. This can result in exposed rough implant surfaces and peri-implant inflammation.

A rare but serious consequence of sinus lift surgery can be chronic sinusitis even years later, and aspergillosis in the presence of foreign material. In this case, surgical revision is unavoidable.

4.2.3 Relationship to the General Medical Situation

The general condition of edentulous patients in particular may change over the years. Deterioration in motor skills or in visual acuity may mean that independent maintenance of the denture is no longer fully successful. Some authors advocate prostheses that can be "converted" from fixed to removable. However, it is still unclear whether removable prostheses are actually advantageous in such situations.

It is not uncommon for antiresorptive drugs to be administered to elderly edentulous patients for osteoporosis or as part of oncological therapies, which may adversely affect bone physiology. Peri-implant infections can lead to bone necrosis. Special attention must be paid to these initially painless lesions.

5 Clinical Case Presentations

Patients looking for improved prosthesis retention with minimal effort

5.1 Single Midline Implant in the Edentulous Mandible Without Augmentation

M. Kern†

PATIENT CHARACTERISTICS AND PATIENT PROFILE
In July 2006, a 66-year-old edentulous woman received new complete dentures in both the maxilla and mandible at the Department of Prosthodontics, Propaedeutics and Dental Materials (University of Kiel, Germany). Both dentures had a perfect fit and met high dental standards (Figs 1a-b and 2a-b). To reduce the risk of fracture of the mandibular denture, it was reinforced with a mesh CoCr framework.

While the patient was satisfied with the esthetics of both dentures and with the function of her maxillary prosthesis, she was not satisfied with her mandibular prosthesis due to lack of retention during speech and chewing. She had quit smoking 1 year earlier, but she had lost her last teeth due to periodontitis and suffered from some allergies, particularly to penicillin, nickel, and nuts, but was otherwise healthy.

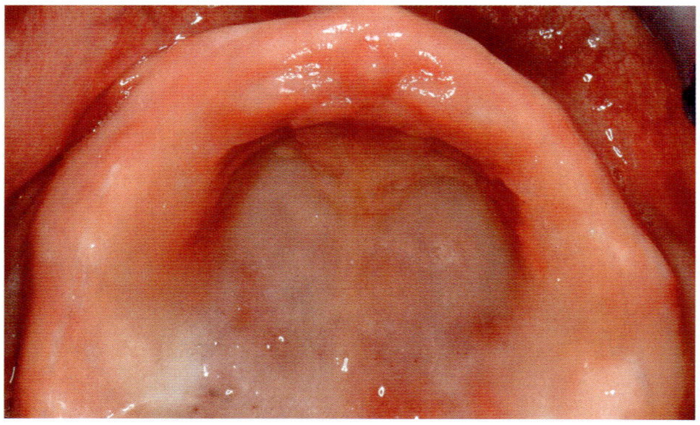

Fig 1a The edentulous maxilla.

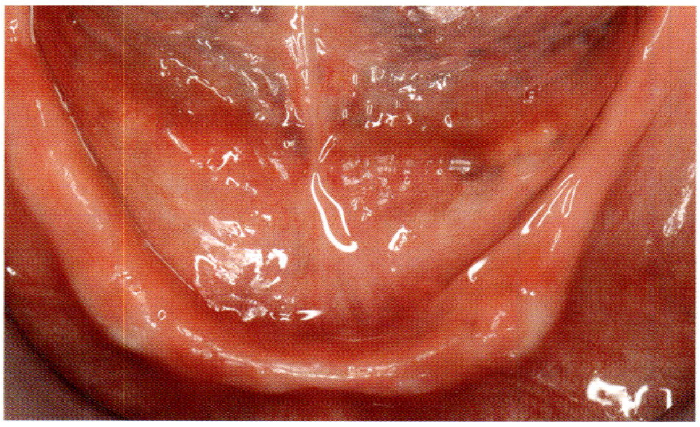

Fig 1b The edentulous mandible.

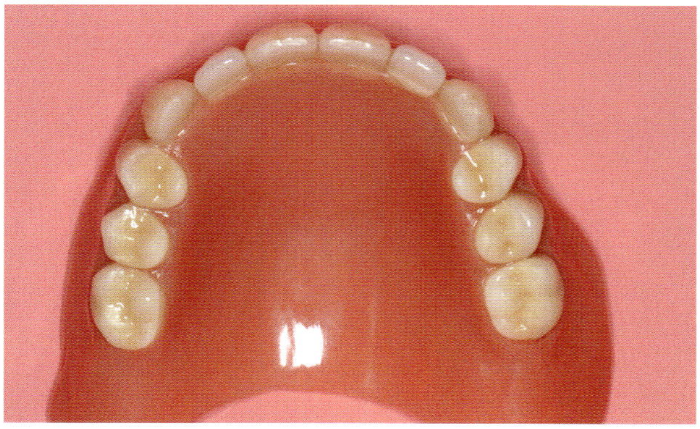

Fig 2a The maxillary denture.

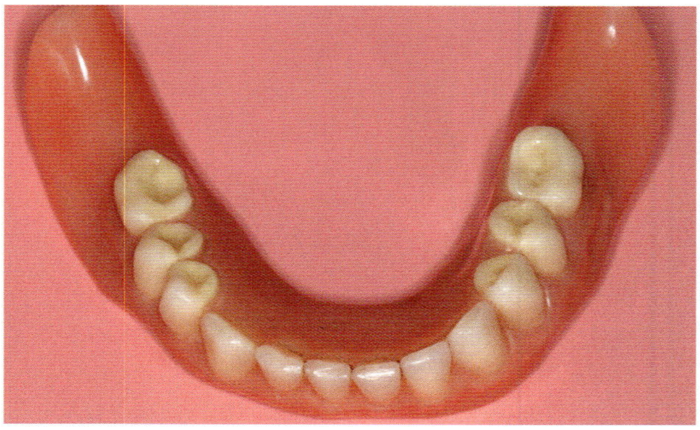

Fig 2b The mandibular denture.

Based on this information and the clinical evaluation described below, the following patient profile (Fig 3) can be derived for this patient (for more information about patient profiles, see Chapters 2.1.3 and 3.6).

CLINICAL EVALUATION AND TREATMENT PLAN

The patient's financial resources were limited and she could not afford the gold-standard therapy described at the 2002 McGill Consensus Conference with two implants in the edentulous mandible to retain her denture (Thomason and coworkers 2012). The patient was informed of the treatment option of placing a single midline implant in the mandible as minimal therapy to improve retention of the mandibular denture. A first clinical study with a single mandibular implant in a geriatric patient population over 5 years showed a remarkable improvement in oral comfort and function with an overdenture. Although a mean marginal bone loss of 1.42 ± 0.56 mm was observed, no implant was lost over an observation period of 5 years (Cordioli and coworkers 1997). In addition to the experimental nature of this treatment option, no specific risks were identified in this first clinical study of a single mandibular implant used for overdenture retention.

After discussing this treatment option with the patient, it was agreed that a titanium screw-type implant 3.8 mm in diameter would be placed in the mandibular midline to retain and stabilize the mandibular denture with a ball attachment. Although the patient was informed about the benefits of using two or more implants to better stabilize her removable prosthesis, or to place a fixed prosthesis with four or more implants (Kern and coworkers 2016), the patient insisted on the single-implant treatment option because she could not afford more implants but was not satisfied with the retention of her mandibular prosthesis. Therefore, she gave her informed consent to receive a single implant as a low-cost implant treatment (de Souza and coworkers 2022; Hartmann and coworkers 2020). No lateral augmentation was to be performed to improve the alveolar ridge width in order to contain associated risks. Therefore, it was agreed to reduce the height of the alveolar ridge to accommodate a 3.8 mm implant.

For pre-implantation diagnostics, a hole was drilled in the center of the prosthesis base to accommodate a ball bearing as a reference object for radiographic scaling, which was temporarily fixed with wax during radiography. The panoramic radiograph showed the reference object together with the metal framework of the mandibular denture and was suitable for determining the anterior mandibular height (Fig 4).

SURGICAL PROCEDURES

After local anesthesia, a midcrestal incision was made along the edentulous ridge from 33 to 43 with additional short vertical relieving incisions at both ends. A full-thickness flap was then elevated and the alveolar ridge from 32 to 42 was shortened by 2 mm to allow a 3.8 mm implant to be completely surrounded by bone.

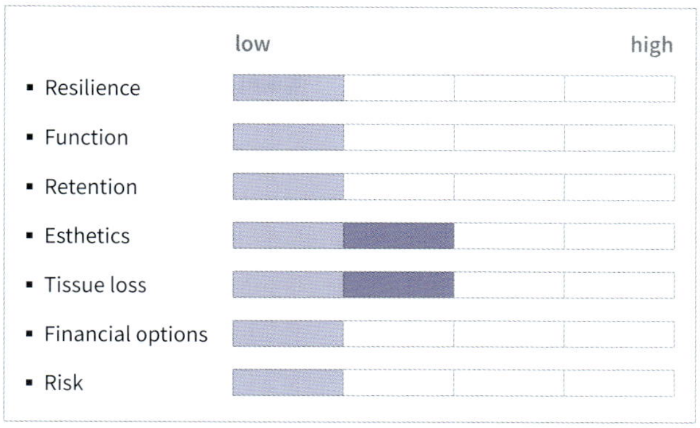

Fig 3 Patient profile.

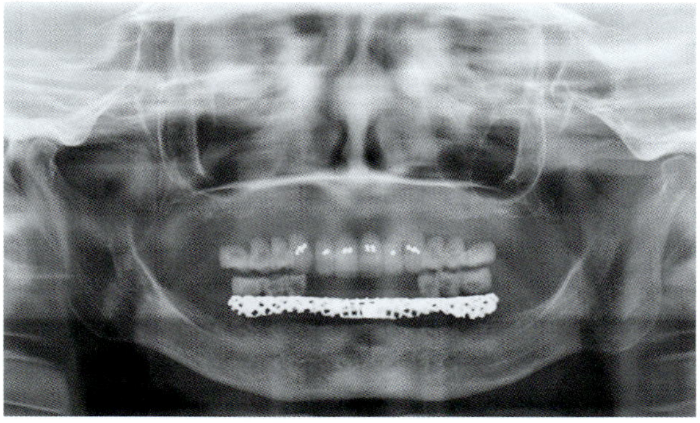

Fig 4 Panoramic radiograph with measuring ball fixed in the existing mandibular denture with metal framework.

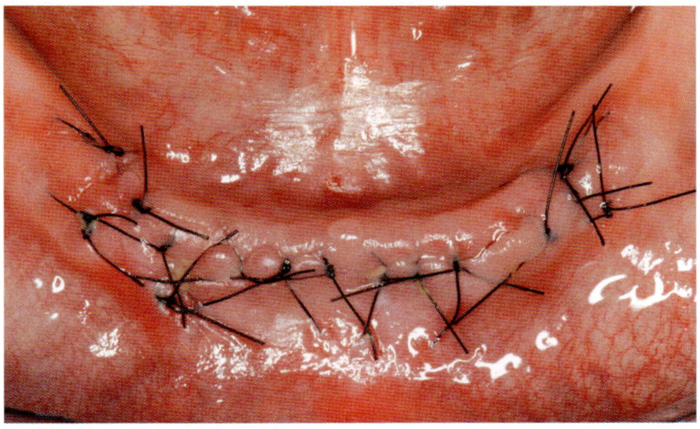

Fig 5 Wound closure with (Supramid 5.0, Resorba, Nürnberg, Germany).

A titanium screw implant (Screw-Line, diameter 3.8 mm, length 13 mm; Camlog Biotechnologies, Basel, Switzerland) was placed according to the manufacturer's standard protocol. Implant stability was measured using the Periotest device (Medizintechnik Gulden, Modautal, Germany) with a PTV (Periotest value) of −1. In addition, the implant stability quotient (ISQ) was measured using resonance frequency analysis (RFA) with an ISQ of 75 (Ostell, Gothenburg, Sweden). Tension-free primary wound closure was achieved for submerged healing (Fig 5) and a control panoramic radiograph

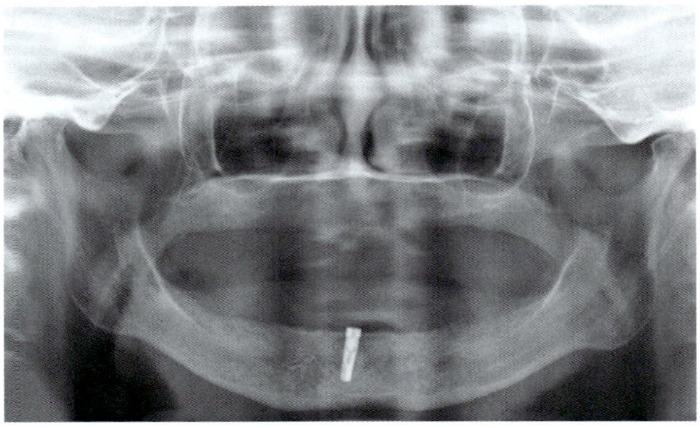

Fig 6 Control panoramic radiograph after insertion of the midline implant.

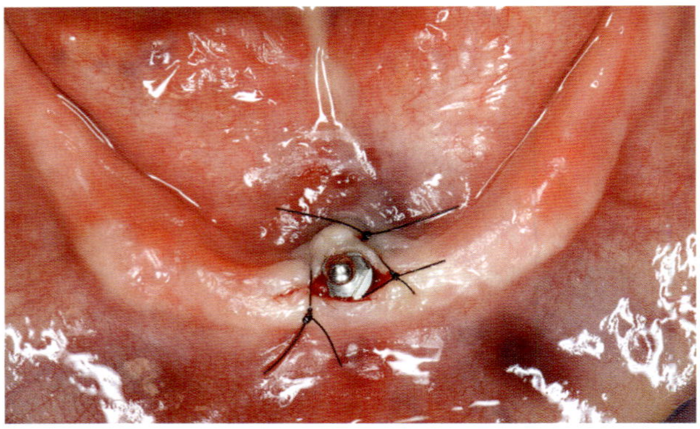

Fig 7 Inserted ball attachment after uncovering the implant.

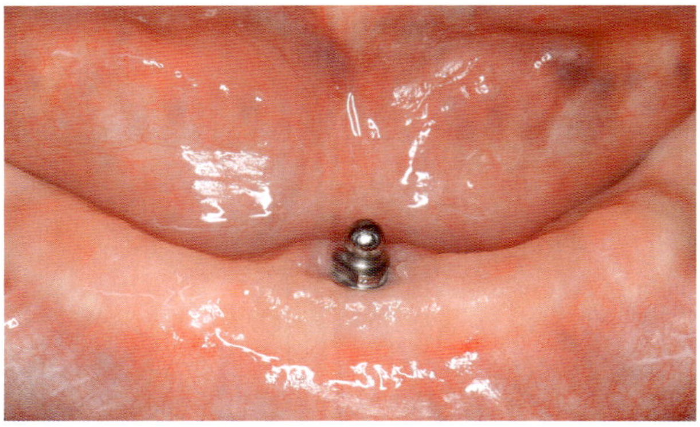

Fig 8 The midline implant 3 weeks after healing.

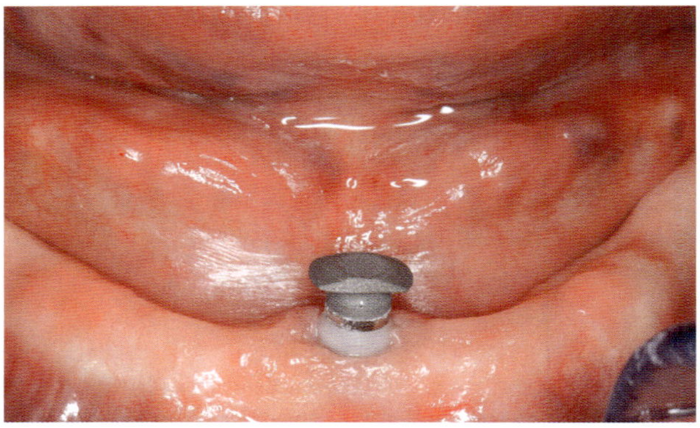

Fig 9 The connected ball attachment with its elliptical housing conditioned for bonding. The white nylon ring secured the upright position of the matrix.

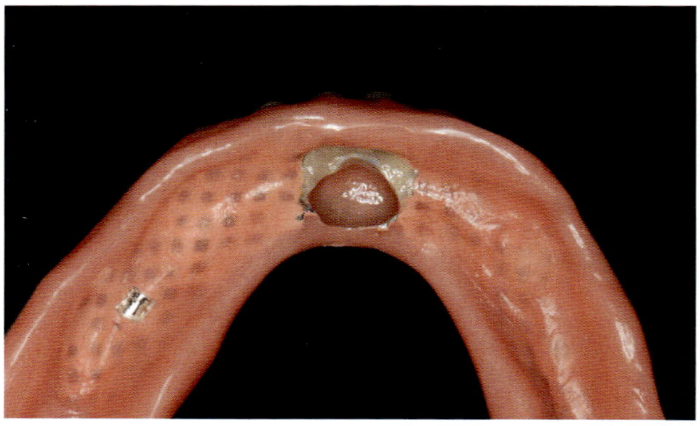

Fig 10 The cavity in the center of the denture was adapted to the size of the matrix housing and conditioned for adhesive bonding of the matrix.

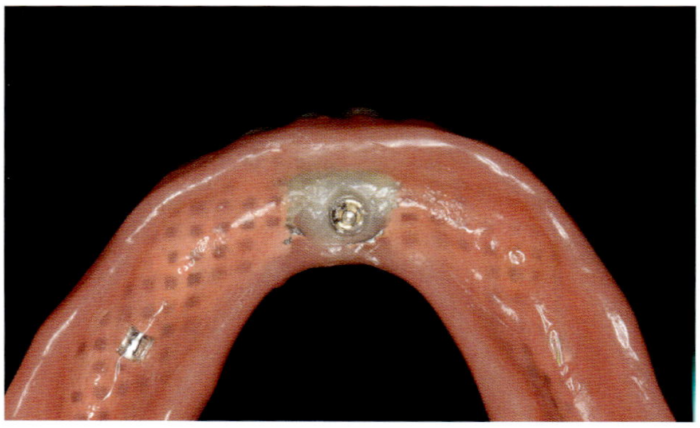

Fig 11 View of the denture with the ball attachment matrix inserted.

was taken (Fig 6). The mandibular denture was relieved in the wound area and relined with soft resin (Softliner; GC, Tokyo, Japan) to minimize pressure on the wound. Sutures were removed 10 days later.

Due to the patient's personal circumstances, the implant was uncovered 6 months after implant placement through a small incision without flap elevation and a ball abutment (gingival height 1.5 mm; Camlog) was screwed into the implant (Fig 7). The prosthesis was trimmed in the area of the ball and provisionally lined with soft resin (Softliner; GC).

PROSTHETIC PROCEDURES

Following a healing period of 3 weeks, the soft resin was removed and the cavity was slightly enlarged to allow the elliptical matrix housing of the ball attachment (Dalbo Plus elliptic; Cendres + Métaux, Biel/Bienne, Switzerland) to fit without interference (Figs 8 to 10). The prosthetic resin was conditioned with a resin primer (Glaze & Bond; DMG, Hamburg, Germany), while the matrix housing was tribochemically coated with silica and silanized (Rocatec; 3M ESPE, Seefeld,Germany). The matrix housing was then bonded into the mandibular denture (Fig 11) using a provisional crown and bridge resin (Luxatemp; DMG).

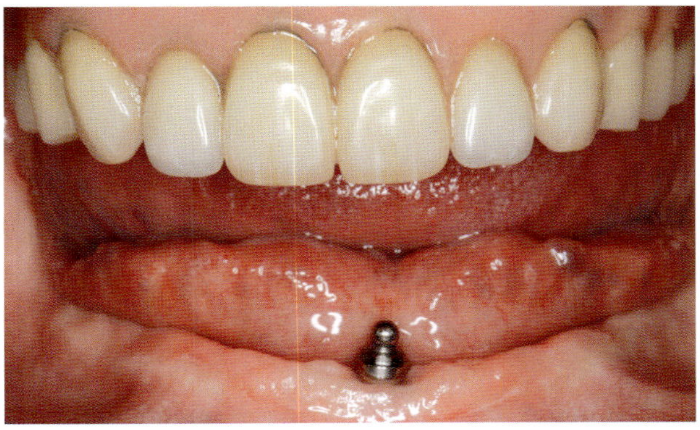

Fig 12 View of the ball attachment opposing the maxillary denture after 5 years (2011).

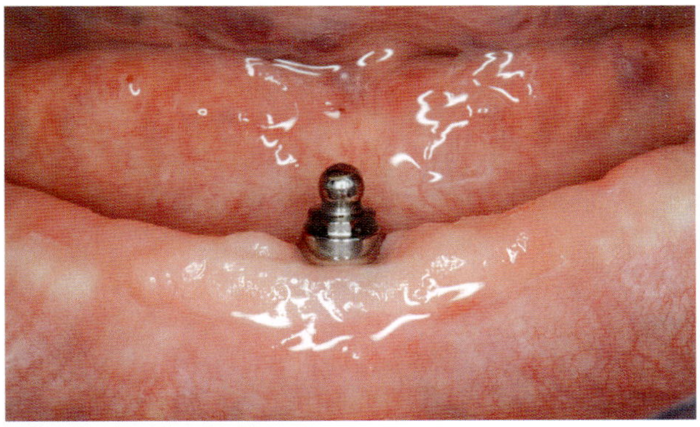

Fig 13 Close-up of the ball attachment at 5 years.

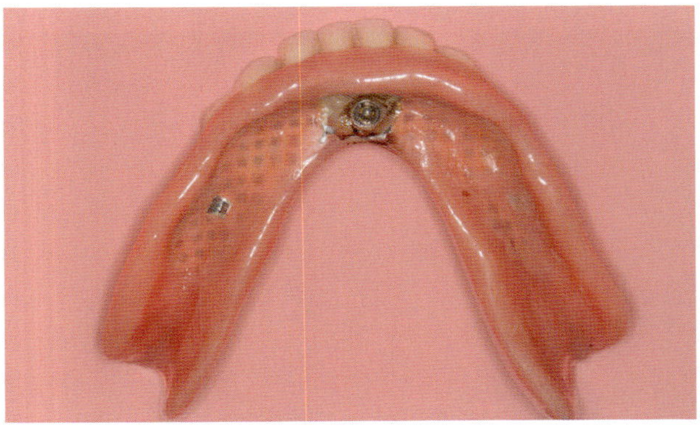

Fig 14 The denture base at 5 years. Some wear at the matrix of the ball attachment.

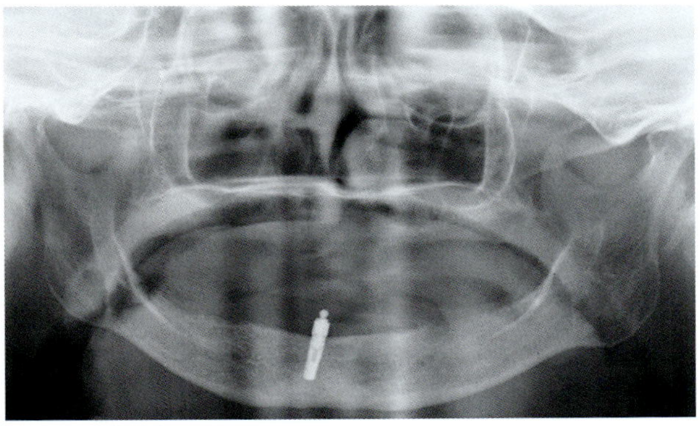

Fig 15 Panoramic radiograph at 5 years revealing moderate bone loss around the midline implant.

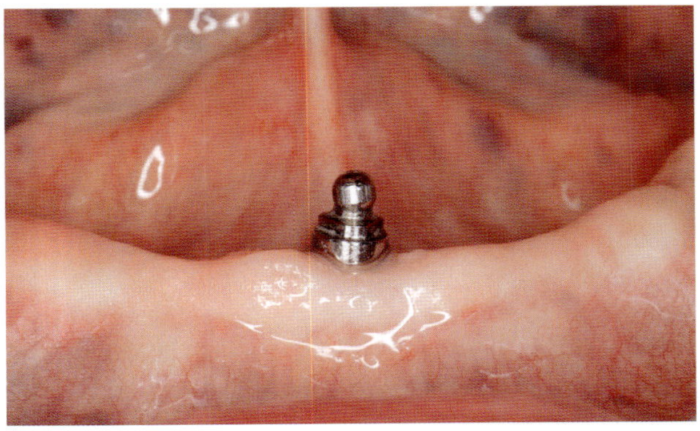

Fig 16 Close-up of the worn ball at 16 years (2022).

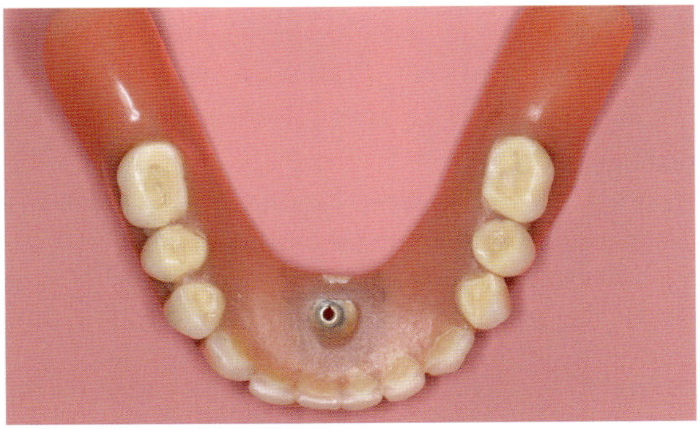

Fig 17 The mandibular denture after 16 years. Some wear at the teeth and loss of the matrix cover.

FOLLOW-UP AND PATIENT SATISFACTION

The patient was very satisfied with the improved retention and stability of her mandibular denture and was recalled at least once a year until November 2022 (Figs 12 to 21). In addition to the activation and replacement of the matrix, a fracture of the prosthesis resin occurred in the area of the ball attachment after 7 years, which was repaired on the day of the appointment. After 16 years, the ball attachment and matrix were replaced due to severe wear and damage resulting in complete loss of function (Figs 16 to 21).

Use this QR code to watch a highlight video with the patient reporting on her satisfaction with the treatment.

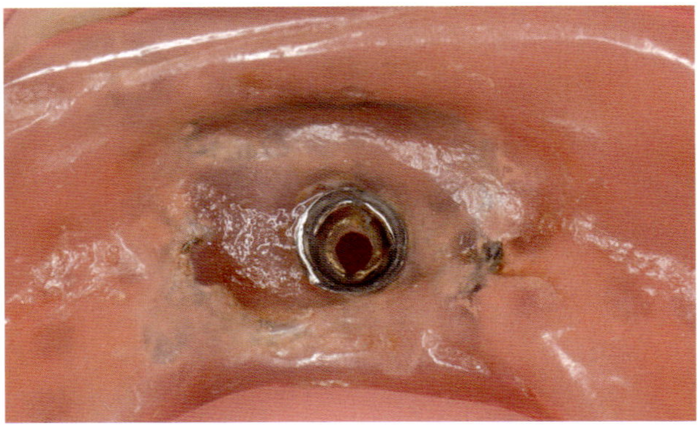

Fig 18 View of the denture with the worn and damaged ball attachment matrix. Two of the four retention lamellae have been lost and two are severely deformed, resulting in a complete loss of retention.

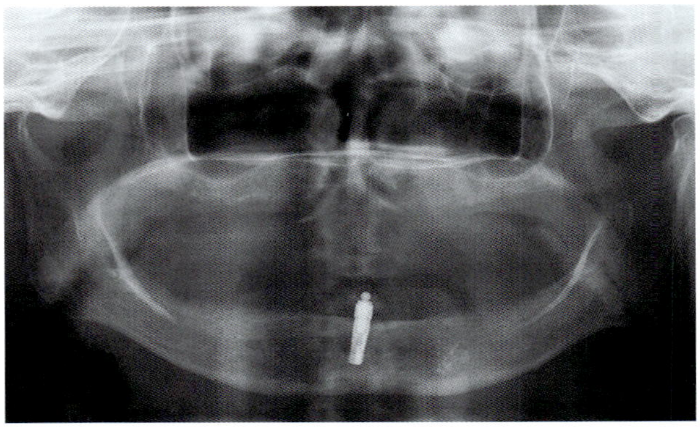

Fig 19 Panoramic radiograph after 16 years revealing no further bone loss around the midline implant as compared to the 5 year radiograph.

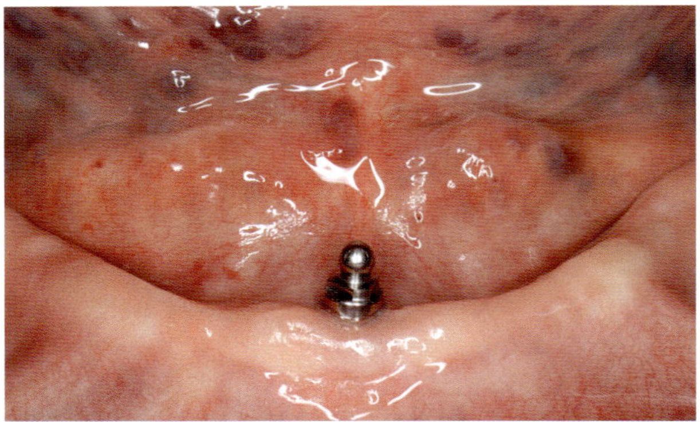

Fig 20 View of the implant at 16 years after inserting a new ball attachment (2022).

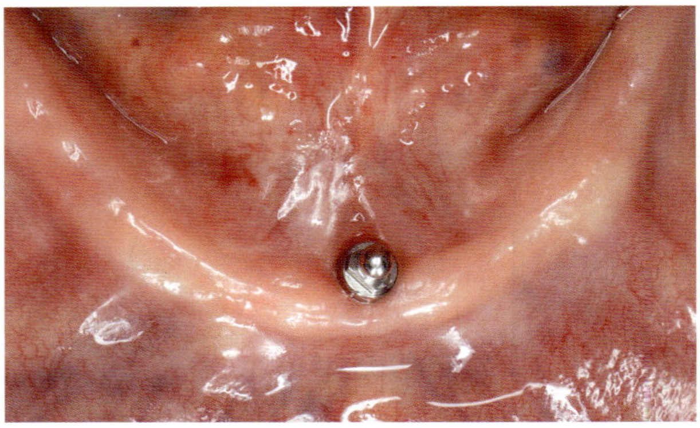

Fig 21 Occlusal view of the implant with the replaced ball attachment at 16 years (2022).

DISCUSSION

This patient's implant treatment was minimal due to a lack of financial resources. Although the patient was informed about the advantages of alternative treatments, namely either using two or more implants to better stabilize her removable prosthesis or of a fixed prosthesis with four or more implants (Goncalves and coworkers 2022; Kern and coworkers 2016), the patient chose the single-implant treatment option because the alternative would have been to continue with her unsatisfactory prosthesis without improved implant retention.

For edentulous patients with very limited financial resources, the question is usually not whether two or more implants would be a better treatment option than the single midline implant (because they cannot afford it at any rate) but whether they can afford at least one implant to improve the completely unsatisfactory retention of their complete denture (de Souza and coworkers 2022; Hartmann and coworkers 2020). Therefore, in this treatment concept developed for social reasons, the pros and cons of treatment with a complete denture without a mandibular implant and a similar treatment with a mandibular implant are usually discussed under the motto of "is one better than none?"

The documentation presented confirms that the single mandibular midline implant can retain a mandibular denture to the full satisfaction of an elderly edentulous patient over the long term. This finding is consistent with several research reports published within the last decade that demonstrated acceptable long-term function of single mandibular midline implants when implants with modern rough implant surfaces were used in a conventional delayed loading protocol (Passia and Kern 2023).

No specific risks of a single mandibular implant treatment have been identified in the available clinical studies. Although implant placement in the mandibular midline could result in injury to the supra-spinosum lingual canals, no permanent vascular or neurosensory complications were reported in any of the clinical studies (Chaar and coworkers 2022; Passia and coworkers 2020).

Conflicting results have been published on the direct comparison of the gold-standard two-implant treatment with the minimized single implant treatment in the edentulous mandible. While two clinical studies found no significant difference between the two-implant and single-implant groups in terms of chewing function and patient satisfaction (Bryant and coworkers 2015; de Resende and coworkers 2021; Walton and coworkers 2009), a different study reported higher masticatory performance in the two-implant group than in the single-implant group (Hauck and coworkers 2021). However, peri-implant aspects were not affected by the number of implants in any of the above studies.

Other disadvantages of using only one versus two implants appear to be a higher need for maintenance procedures and a higher rate of fractures (Bryant and coworkers 2015; Hauck and coworkers 2021). The use of more than two implants to improve denture stability or the ability to place a fixed prosthesis would offer additional benefits (Hartmann and coworkers 2020). However, this approach is not discussed here because the placement of multiple implants is not feasible for the target patient group due to their limited financial resources.

Therefore, the main indication for single midline implants in the edentulous mandible is a situation where the use of multiple implants is not possible for financial or other reasons. The motto of this treatment concept is therefore “one is better than none” and not “one implant is just as good as multiple implants.”

Prof Dr Matthias Kern† (1958–2025)

It is noted with sadness that the author of this chapter passed away while this book was in production.

5.2 Immediate Loading of Four Narrow-Diameter One-Piece Implants in the Edentulous Mandible

C. Raabe, N. Schenk, M. Schimmel

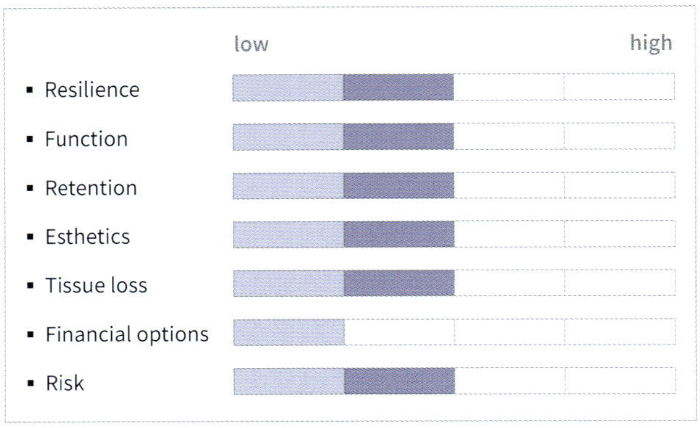

Fig 1 Patient profile.

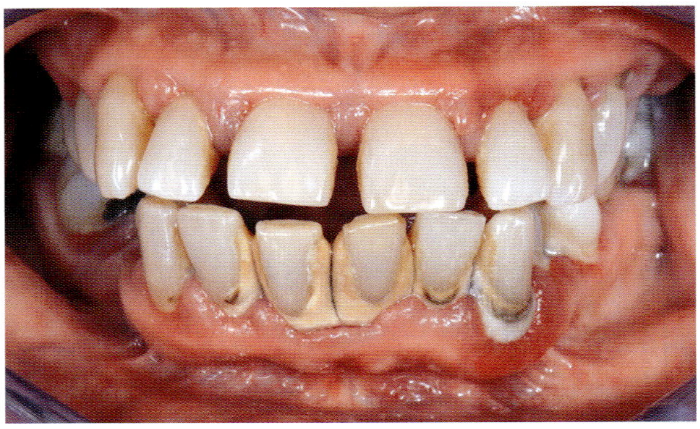

Fig 2 Baseline intraoral situation with periodontally compromised dentition.

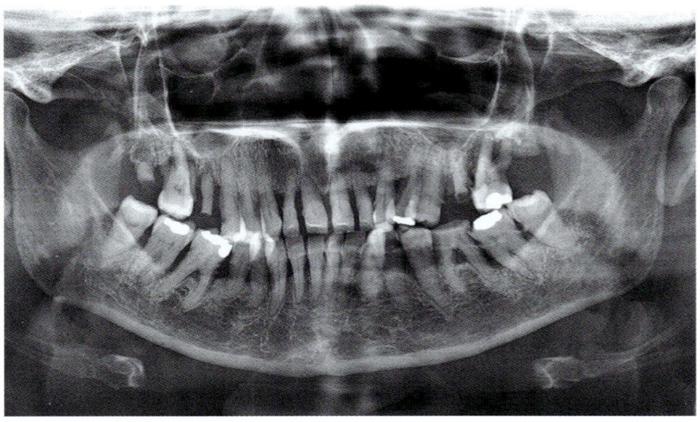

Fig 3 Baseline panoramic radiograph. The national social welfare guidelines required full-mouth clearance and the provision of immediate dentures in the present case.

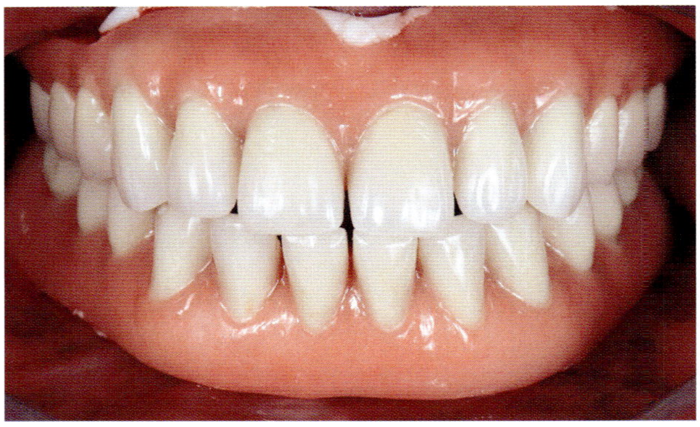

Fig 4 Complete removable dentures with relining in situ.

PATIENT CHARACTERISTICS AND PATIENT PROFILE

A 63-year-old female patient presented at the School of Dental Medicine of the University of Bern, Switzerland (zmk Bern) with the goal of improving her dental appearance and finding relief from the persistent pain and discomfort in her teeth and gums. While recognizing the need for surgical interventions, she aimed to minimize the number of surgeries required. The patient suffered from obesity and mild hypertension, treated with amlodipine and valsartan under the care of her physician. She lived independently and appeared to be active and cognitively fit. Financial limitations for dental treatment were present.

Based on this information and the clinical evaluation described below, the following patient profile (Fig 1) can be derived for this patient (for more information about patient profiles, see Chapters 2.1.3 and 3.6).

CLINICAL EVALUATION AND TREATMENT PLAN

A thorough clinical and radiological evaluation led to a diagnosis of stage IV periodontitis with a hopeless or poor prognosis for all her remaining teeth (Figs 2 and 3). Given the patient's reliance on the national social welfare system for treatment support, the treatment plan had to conform to legal regulatory guidelines, according to which full-mouth clearance was indicated in this case. Therefore, the treatment plan included the extraction of all teeth and immediate denture placement followed by relining.

According to the treatment plan, immediate dentures were prepared in the usual manner. All teeth were then extracted, and the immediate dentures were delivered during the same appointment. The dentures were relined with tissue conditioner (Kerr F.I.T.T.; Kerr, Herzogenrath, Germany) to improve fit and retention 1 week and 4 weeks after the procedure (Fig 4). After 3 months, definitive relining of both the maxillary and mandibular dentures was performed using polymethylmethacrylate (Aesthetic Blue; Candulor, Glattpark, Switzerland). The patient was satisfied with the esthetics and overall comfort but had difficulties adapting to her mandibular denture, whose lack of retention led to functional difficulties with chewing and biting, speaking, and general social interaction. Despite more than 1 year of adaptation with the denture, this functional impairment persisted. Options to improve the situation were discussed, and the patient agreed to participate in a randomized clinical trial (ITI grant 1286_2018). The study design mirrors real patient scenarios in clinical practice and aims to compare immediate loading of four new-generation narrow-diameter one-piece implants (NDI) with early loading of two standard-diameter implants.

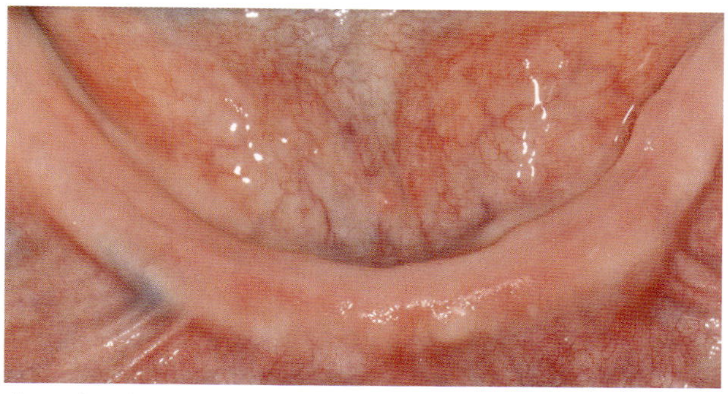

Fig 5 Edentulous mandible 2 years after extraction, frontal view. Metallic pigmentation at site 45.

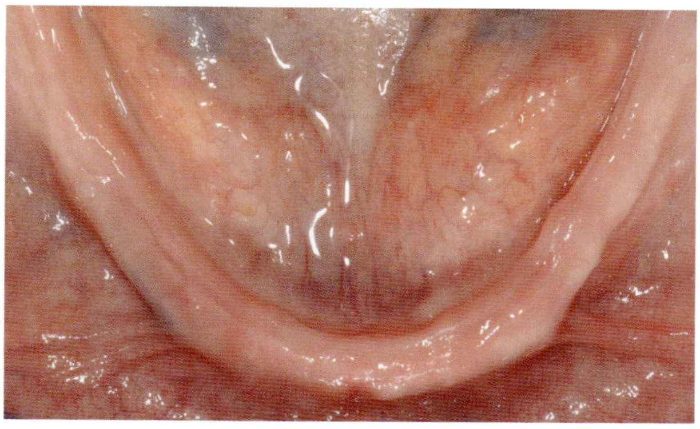

Fig 6 Edentulous mandible, occlusal view. Sufficient keratinized mucosa.

Comprehensive treatment planning included an intraoral examination that revealed edentulous jaws with moderate vertical and horizontal resorption but with sufficient keratinized mucosa. Pigmentation was noted at site 45 and suspected to be a tattoo from residual displaced restorative material (Figs 5 and 6). A cone-beam computed tomography (CBCT) scan of the mandible (Fig 7) confirmed sufficient bone dimensions for the placement of NDIs or standard-diameter dental implants (Fig 8). Evaluation of the existing dentures indicated that they could be used for the prospective integration of the attachment housings.

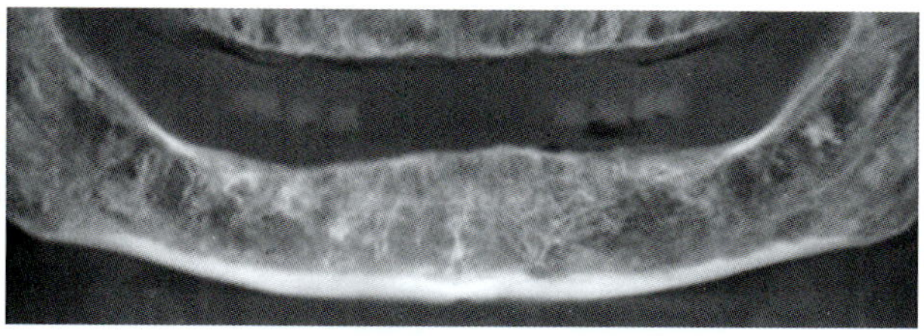

Fig 7 Reconstruction of a panoramic radiograph from the CBCT dataset.

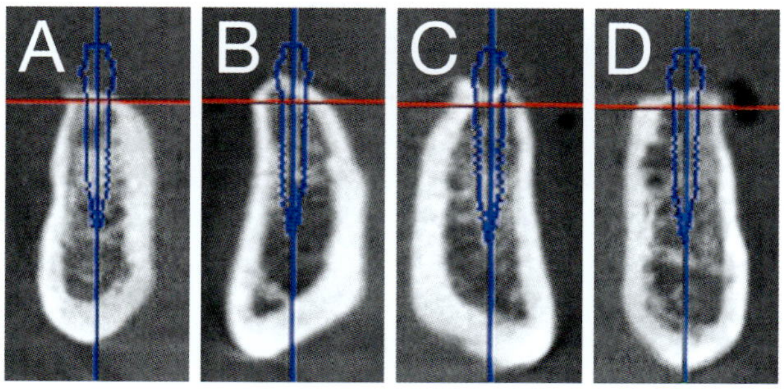

Fig 8 CBCT including virtual implant planning. Sufficient horizontal and vertical bone dimensions at the prospective implant sites 44 (A), 42 (B), 32 (C), and 34 (D).

After giving informed consent, the patient was randomized to the experimental group for NDI treatment. This treatment involved the placement of four one-piece implants with miniaturized stud attachments in the interforaminal region and the use of an immediate loading protocol (loading within 24 hours) to convert the existing denture into an implant overdenture (IOD) without metal reinforcement.

SURGICAL PROCEDURES

Surgery was performed under local anesthesia using bilateral mental blocks and lingual infiltration (articaine hydrochloride 40 mg/ml with adrenaline 10 µg/ml, Ubistesin forte; 3M ESPE, Seefeld, Germany). In such cases, a flapless approach may be considered to reduce patient morbidity. However, this approach does not allow for ridge flattening, identification of critical anatomic structures such as the mental foramen, or repositioning of the keratinized mucosa and should only be applied in the context of computer-assisted implant placement. These factors were considered necessary in this case to optimally distribute the implants without risking damage to adjacent

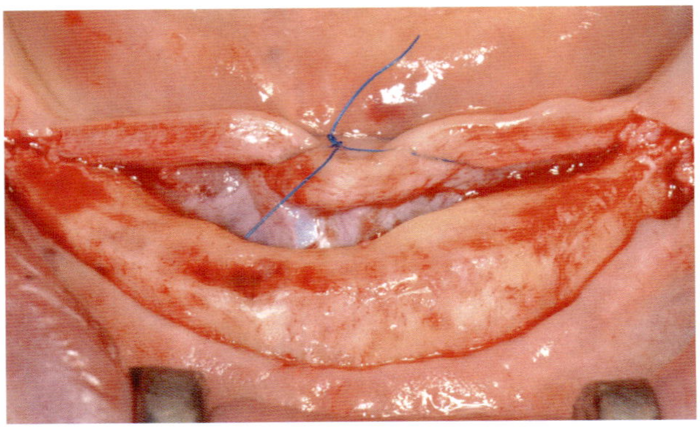

Fig 9 Mandible, frontal view. Midcrestal incision with distal vertical releasing incisions and elevation of a mucoperiosteal flap. Lingual retraction suture for better intraoperative orientation. A crestal osteotomy was performed to flatten the edentulous alveolar ridge.

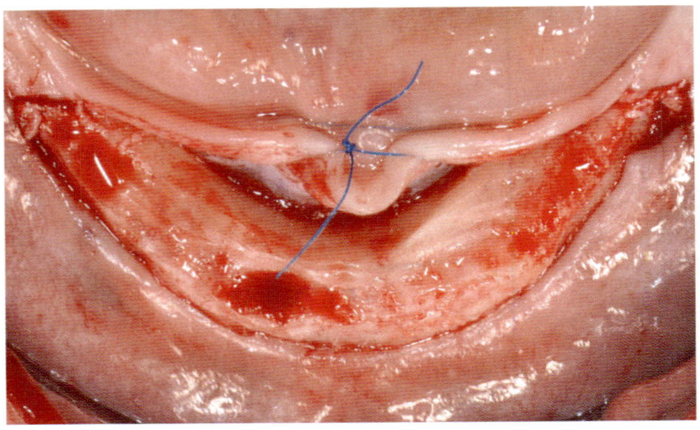

Fig 10 Mandible, occlusal view. Sufficient horizontal bone dimensions for interforaminal implant placement.

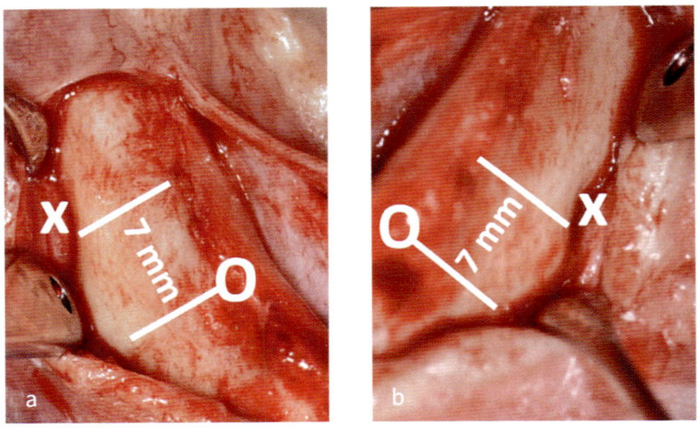

Fig 11 Bilateral visualization of the mental foramen ("X") to maintain a safety distance of 7 mm to the most posterior implant sites ("O").

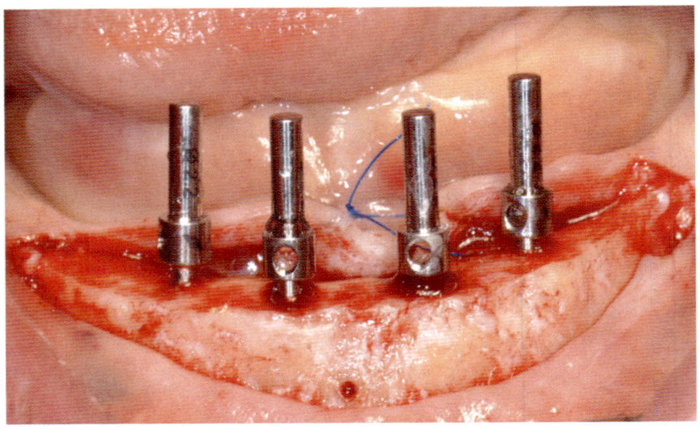

Fig 12 Mandible, frontal view. Paralleling posts in situ after initial implant bed preparation showing the orientation of the osteotomy.

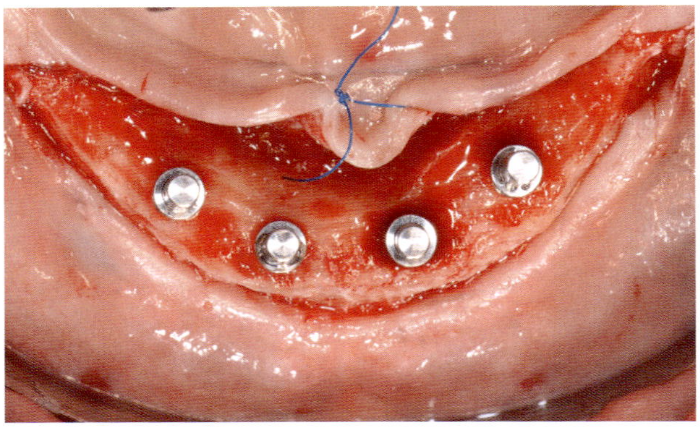

Fig 13 Mandible, occlusal view. Paralleling posts in situ.

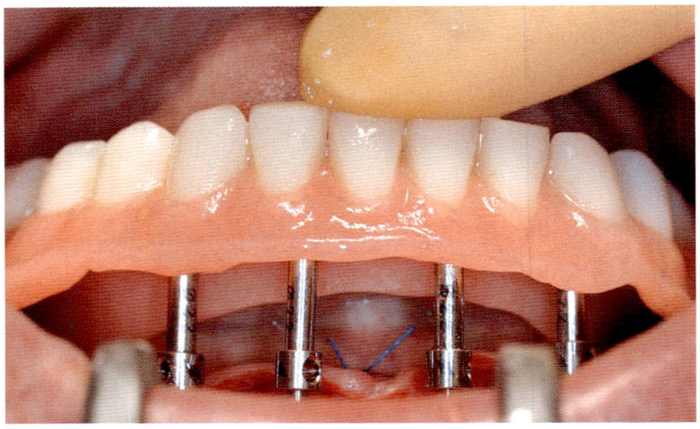

Fig 14 Visual verification of the paralleling post orientation relative to the base of the prosthesis.

structures and to preserve a wide band of peri-implant keratinized mucosa. Therefore, a conventional full-thickness flap was elevated after a mid-crestal incision respecting at least 2 mm of keratinization on both sides of the incision line and bilateral vertical releasing incisions posterior to the mental foramina. An osteotomy was then performed to flatten the crestal portion of the alveolar ridge (Figs 9 and 10).

The mental foramina were then identified to maintain a safety distance of 7 mm to the most posterior implant sites (Fig 11).

The implant positions were determined and the implant site osteotomies performed in a prosthetically oriented manner (Figs 12 to 14).

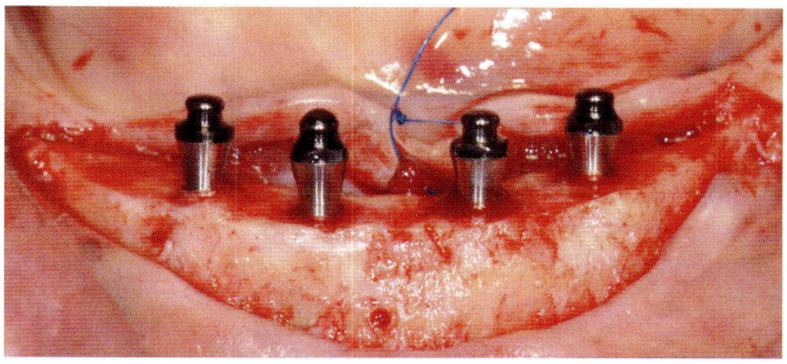

Fig 15 Mandible, frontal view. Mini-implants with the border of the machined/micro-rough implant surface positioned approximately 1 mm subcrestally.

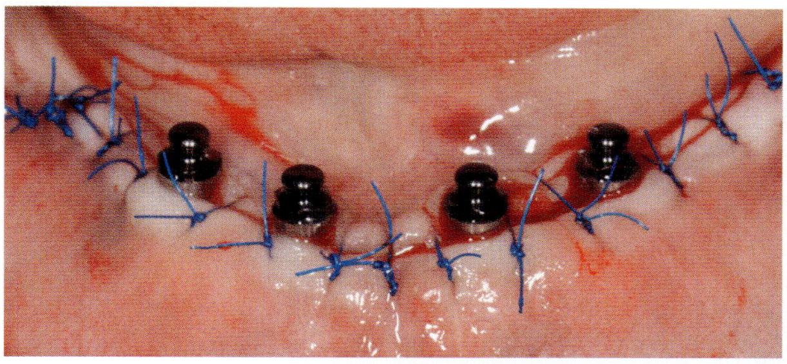

Fig 17 Mandible, frontal view. Adaptation of wound margins with single interrupted sutures (5-0 polyamide).

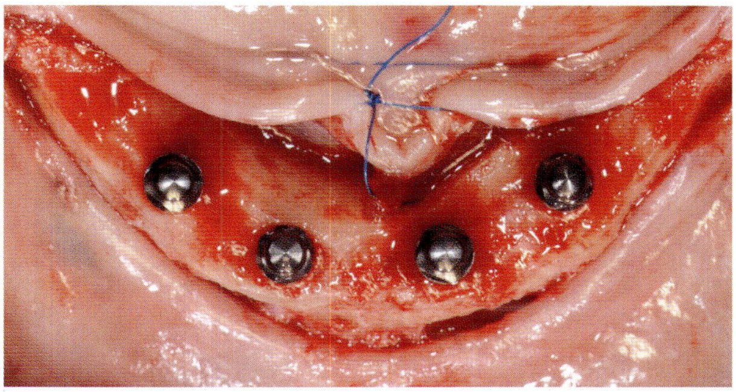

Fig 16 Mandible, occlusal view. Inserted mini-implants.

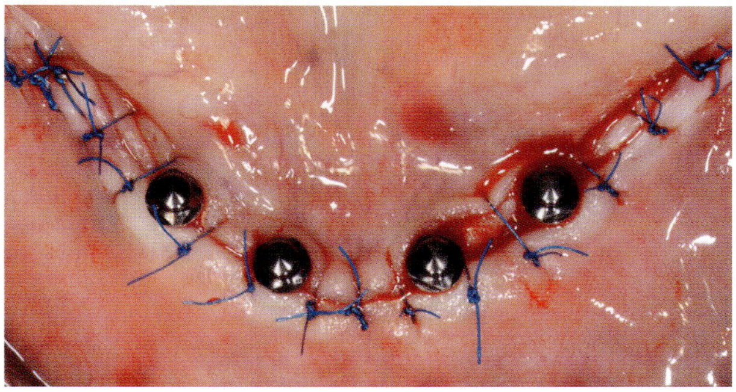

Fig 18 Mandible, occlusal view. Adaption of wound margins.

The drilling sequence of the implant system is adapted to the local bone density, which in this case presented as D2 according to Misch (2015). The implant macro-design involves an apically tapered implant body design with self-tapping threads (Fig 20), allowing for underpreparation of the implant osteotomy. Both factors are aimed at achieving high primary implant stability and facilitating immediate loading protocols. Four one-piece implants (Mini Implant GH 3.8 mm, diameter 2.4 mm, length 12 mm; Institut Straumann AG, Basel, Switzerland) were placed with an insertion torque of > 35 Ncm and the border between machined and micro-rough implant surfaces located roughly 1 mm subcrestally (Figs 15 and 16).

The mucoperiosteal flap was repositioned for transmucosal healing and adapted using non-resorbable monofilament single interrupted sutures (5-0) (Figs 17 and 18).

The postoperative panoramic radiograph shows the mini-implants in their final position (Fig 19).

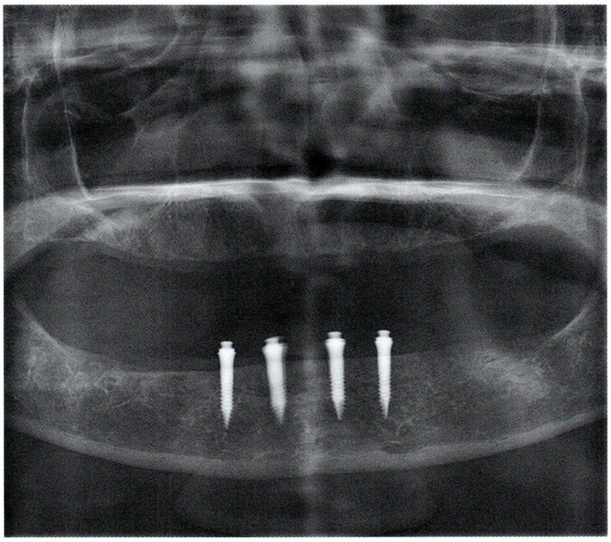

Fig 19 Postoperative panoramic radiograph.

PROSTHETIC PROCEDURES

The mini-implants include attachments as an integral part (Optiloc; Institut Straumann AG, Basel, Switzerland). The attachments are coated with black amorphous diamond-like carbon (ADLC) to reduce wear and improve their sliding properties due to a low coefficient of friction. The corresponding housings have dimensions of 4.2 mm, significantly smaller than those of other stud-type attachments (Fig 20).

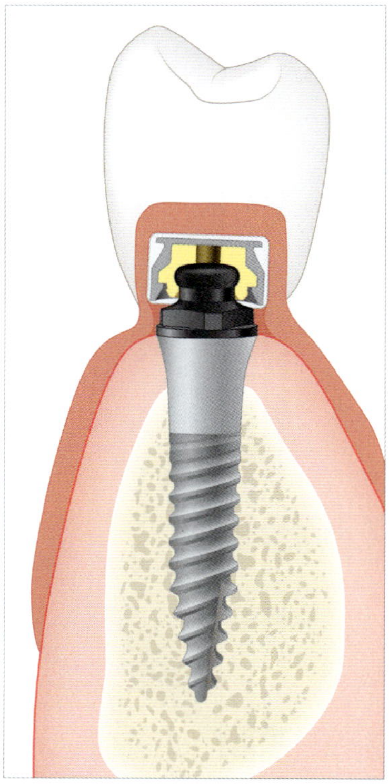

Fig 20 Schematic drawing of the Straumann Mini-Implant system with the Optiloc System in the design of a one-piece implant.

After surgery, implant housings with the lowest retention force inserts (color-coded white) were connected to the implants and the denture base was carefully relieved at the sites corresponding to these implant attachments. Care was taken to ensure that there was no contact between the housings and the denture base, even with maximum clenching. A relining impression was taken under maximum bite force effort (Fig 21). The denture was rebased in the dental laboratory (Zahrmanufaktur Bern, Bern, Switzerland), and the housings were polymerized into the denture base without reinforcement structures. The IOD was delivered on the day of surgery, and the first follow-up was scheduled for the following day.

At follow-up, the patient had experienced minimal pain and had not even taken any analgesics. The IOD was removed for the first time. At 10 days postoperatively, the wound had healed sufficiently, and the sutures were removed (Figs 22 and 23).

FOLLOW-UP AND PATIENT SATISFACTION

The patient returned for study-related assessments at 6 months (Fig 24) and 1 year (Fig 25). She continued to neglect her oral hygiene but developed only peri-implant mucositis. Radiographs showed crestal remodeling but no pathological bone loss was observed (Fig 26).

Overall, the patient was very satisfied with the treatment as the stabilization of the lower denture with four novel NDIs with miniature stud attachment led to improved masticatory performance, oral health-related quality of life, and denture satisfaction.

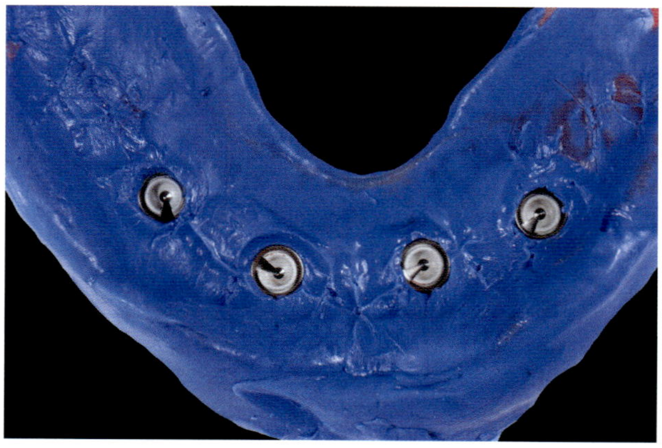

Fig 21 Relining impression immediately after surgery. The quality of the impression can be poor due to the fresh wound.

> Use this QR code to watch a highlight video with the patient reporting on her satisfaction with the treatment.

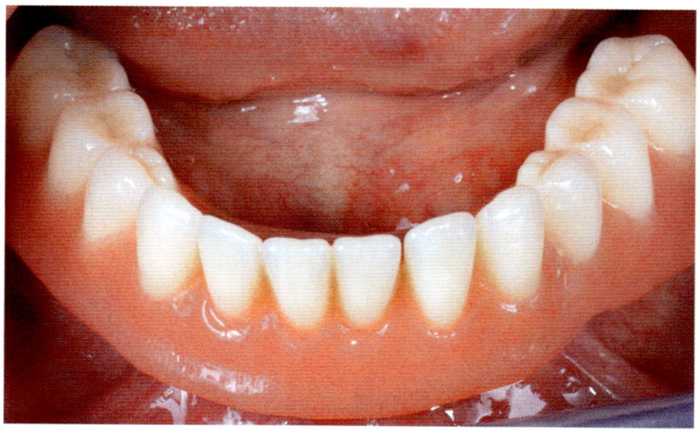

Fig 22 Delivery of the relined denture with integrated Optiloc housings and white retention inserts.

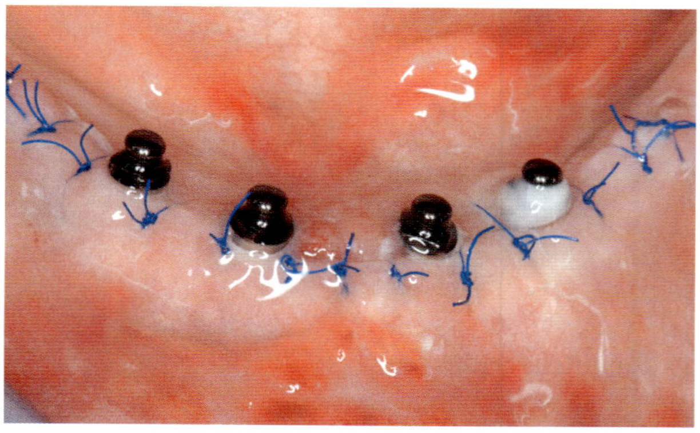

Fig 23 Mandible, frontal view. Adequate wound healing was observed 10 days postoperatively, and the sutures were removed.

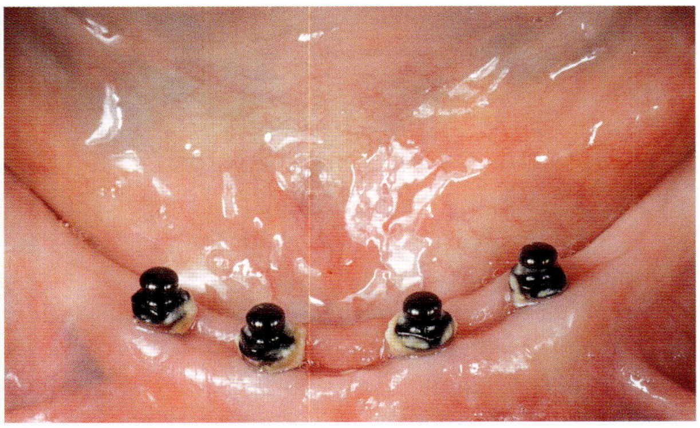

Fig 24 The patient presented with poor oral hygiene at the 6-month assessment. 80% of implant sites showed presence of plaque and 43% were associated with bleeding on probing.

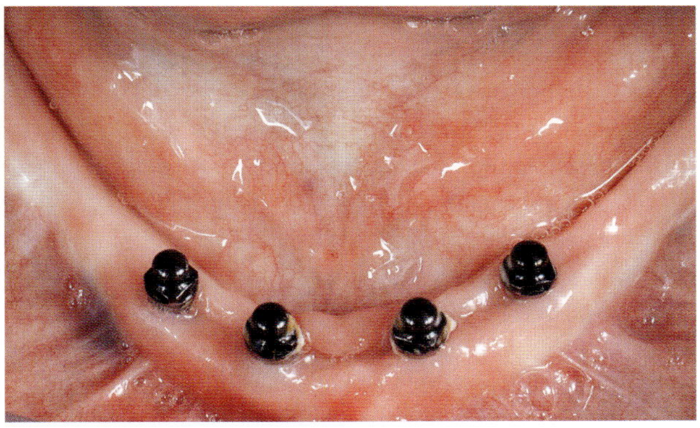

Fig 25 Oral hygiene had improved slightly as seen at the 1-year follow-up. 50% of implant sites showed presence of plaque and 31% were associated with bleeding on probing.

DISCUSSION

Mini-implants primarily include one-piece implants and represent the category of implants with the smallest diameters available on the market (Schiegnitz and Al-Nawas 2018). They are intended to provide a less invasive treatment option using standard implant placement protocols, particularly in cases of severely horizontally resorbed alveolar ridges where invasive bone augmentation procedures would be indicated for the placement of standard-diameter implants. Invasive augmentation procedures may be contraindicated in patients with general medical concerns or may not be well accepted in a geriatric patient population. Conversely, standard implant placement protocols offer advantages such as shorter treatment times, lower treatment costs and reduced morbidity compared to bone augmentation (Scherer and coworkers 2014).

Mini-implants are designed to provide a simplified prosthetic workflow by converting a complete denture to an IOD, without the need for a separate framework. The absence of a framework simplifies the prosthetic procedure and reduces the overall treatment cost for patients. However, the decision to include a metal framework from the initial conversion of a complete denture to an IOD is controversial because current evidence to support its necessity is lacking. A prospective cohort study showed that 65% of patients had no prosthesis fractures at 5 years, while 35% had single or multiple fractures in the matrix area (Enkling and coworkers 2020). Notably, the authors observed no further fractures after a small lingual metal reinforcement was incorporated into the fractured dentures. At the 10-year follow-up of the same cohort of patients, no further denture fractures were found (Schenk and coworkers 2024). However, the initial incorporation of reinforcement may not be warranted to limit costs. Instead, reinforcement could be considered as an option after the occurrence of the first fracture, serving to prevent future fractures (Enkling and coworkers 2020).

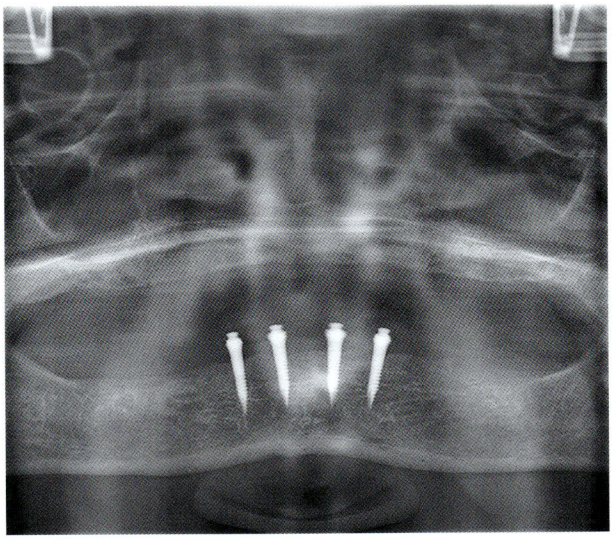

Fig 26 Panoramic radiograph at the 1-year evaluation.

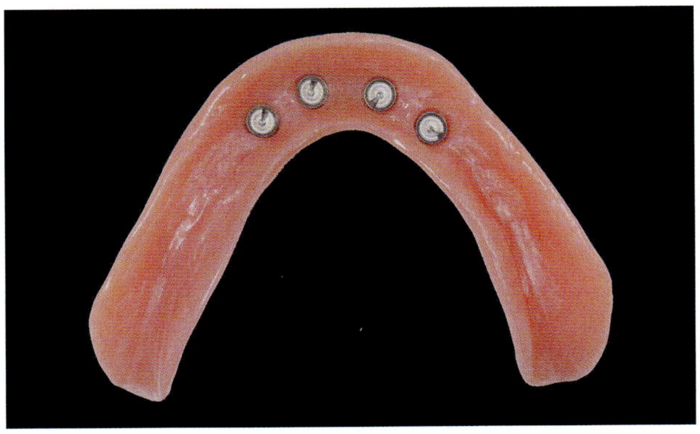

Fig 27 Denture base at the 1-year evaluation.

Immediate restoration with mini-implants involves the placement and loading of a prosthesis on the same day as implant placement, offering the advantage of immediate functional restoration (Leles and coworkers 2022). However, this approach may carry certain risks, particularly with regard to wound healing and implant survival. Postoperative wound healing involves soft-tissue swelling as a physiologic response to surgical trauma, which may conflict with the denture base, resulting in sequelae such as discomfort or mucosal ulceration. In addition, immediate loading should only be applied to implants with high primary stability in order to reduce the risk of osseointegration failure. Immediate loading has been associated with a higher incidence of implant failure compared to conventional loading (Chen and coworkers 2019). Therefore, careful patient selection, appropriate surgical techniques, and carefully controlled prosthetic designs are required to ensure successful outcomes with immediate restoration protocols.

One-piece implants may pose future risks related to mechanical wear or fracture of the implant or prosthetic components. If the retentive portion of an implant becomes severely worn or fractured, the stability and retention of the prosthesis may be compromised. In such cases, management strategies may include shortening the implant below the mucosal margin, allowing the soft tissue to heal, or removing and replacing the fractured implant. Long-term monitoring and maintenance are essential to identify and address any potential complications associated with single-piece implants and to ensure the longevity and success of the prosthetic rehabilitation.

Patients looking for greatly improved prosthesis retention

5.3 Complete Prosthetic Rehabilitation in a Fully Edentulous Patient: Palateless Maxillary CAD/CAM Implant-Supported Overdenture Using High-Performance Polymer as Framework Material and Mandibular Implant-Retained Overdenture with Stud Attachments

S. A. Sánchez

PATIENT CHARACTERISTICS AND PATIENT PROFILE

A 65-year-old female patient with a history of medically controlled type II diabetes was referred to the clinic with severe esthetic and functional problems due to complete edentulism as result of generalized stage IV periodontitis (Figs 1 to 3). Her main complaints were difficulty when chewing all types of food and poor esthetic appearance.

Clinical and CBCT analysis revealed a horizontal deficiency of the alveolar ridge caused by the extraction of the remaining teeth 4 months earlier (Figs 4 to 7).

Owing to her lifestyle, the patient had high esthetic and functional expectations. She wanted implant-supported restorations with a natural appearance, high retention and, if possible, no palatal coverage. She was compliant and motivated to follow the professional recommendations to achieve her expectations.

Based on this information and the clinical evaluation, the following patient profile (Fig 8) can be derived for this patient (for more information about patient profiles, see Chapters 2.1.3 and 3.6).

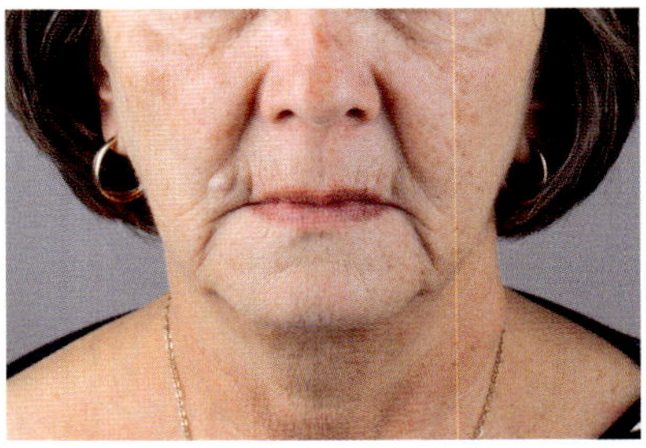

Fig 1 Initial extraoral view. Fully edentulous maxilla and mandible.

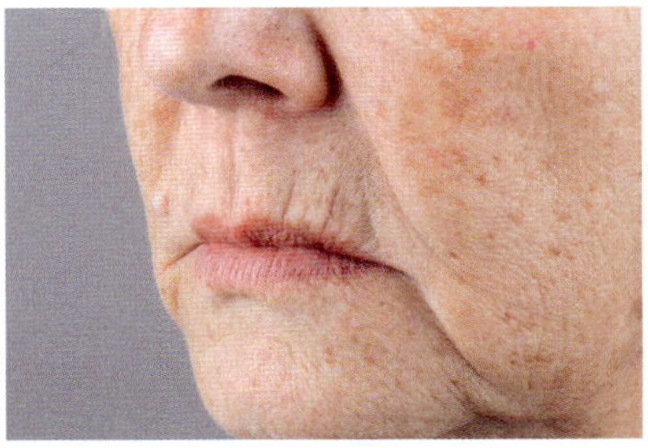

Fig 2 Preoperative extraoral view with the lower third of the face in a resting position. Lip and facial support required.

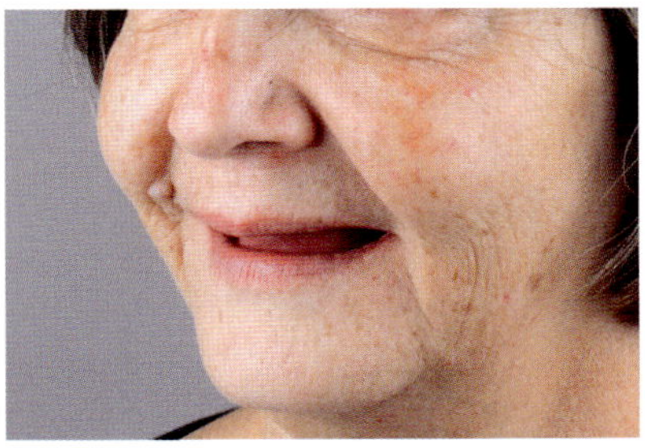

Fig 3 Moderate smile position. Lip and facial support required.

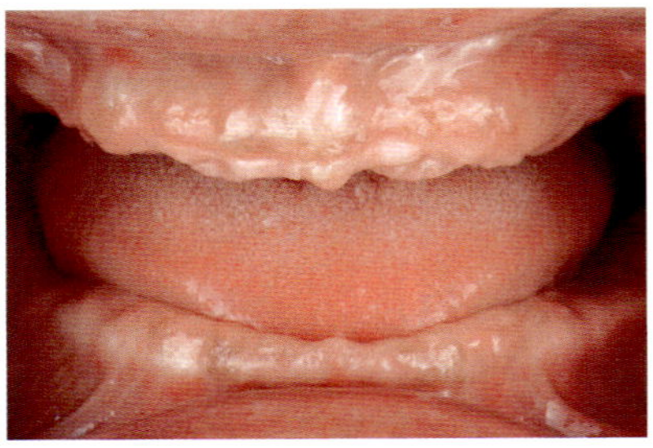 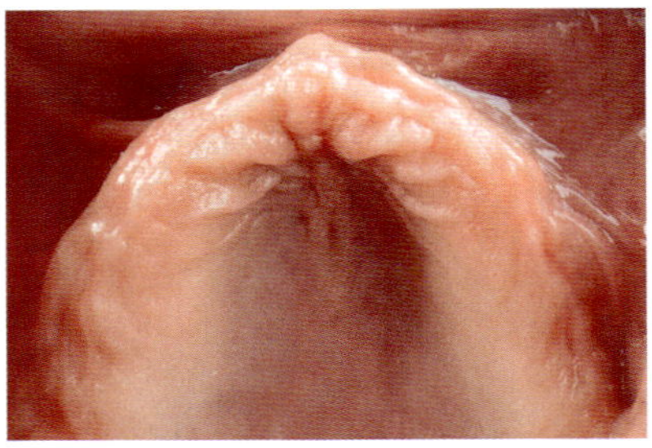 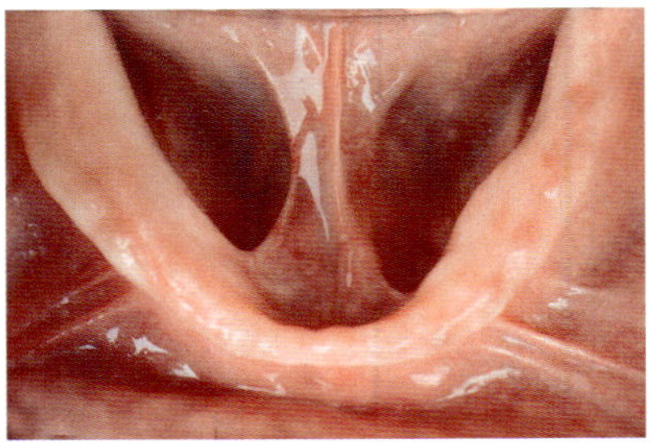

Figs 4 to 6 Preoperative views.

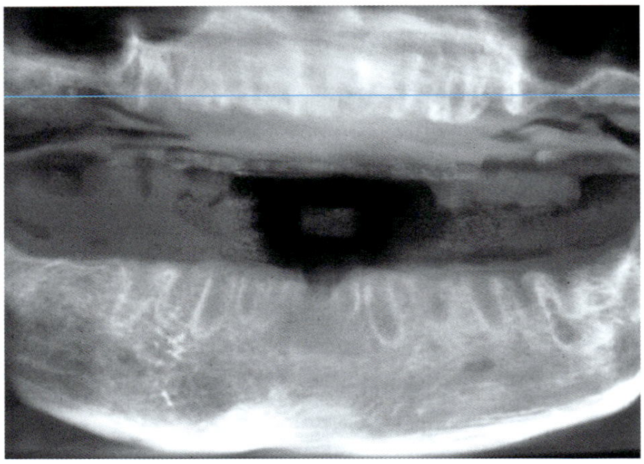

Fig 7 Preoperative panoramic view obtained from the CBCT scan.

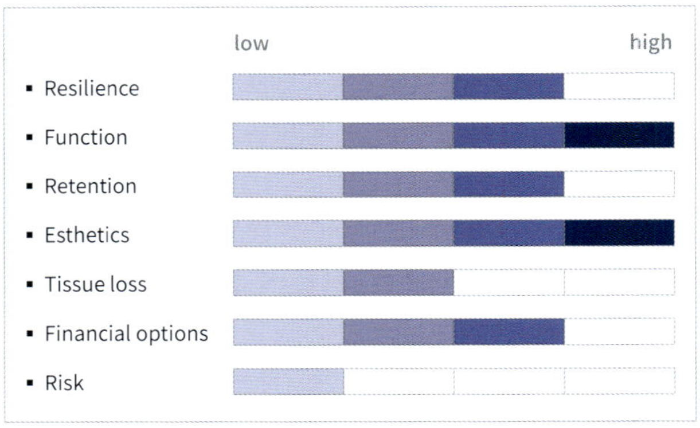

Fig 8 Patient profile. The four-point graded scale emphasizes the high expectations (esthetics, function, and retention) of the patient with regard to her future implant-supported rehabilitation. In addition, it highlights the high resilience and financial options that also played an important role in the overall treatment.

CLINICAL EVALUATION AND TREATMENT PLAN

Based on the initial intraoral and extraoral clinical assessment, CBCT analysis, a history of stage IV periodontitis (Salvi and coworkers 1998; Ravidà and coworkers 2021), a need for labial and facial support (Zitzmann and Marinello 1999), the patient's functional and esthetic demands (high esthetic expectations and rejection of palatal coverage), and financial aspects (Wolfart 2016), an individualized treatment plan was designed. It included prosthetic reconstruction of the maxilla and mandible with implant-supported prostheses that adequately supported the facial structures, could be removed by the patient, and were easy to clean, while meeting the patient's high functional and esthetic expectations.

Esthetic risk was assessed using the Edentulous Esthetic Risk Assessment (EERA) table (L. Gonzaga, W. Martin, and D. Morton), which is an important tool as part of the SAC classification. It assists clinicians in selecting the appropriate restoration type (fixed or removable) for fully edentulous patients during the diagnostic and planning phases by identifying critical risk factors that can lead to negative outcomes, especially in the maxilla, which is considered more challenging than the mandible (see Table 1).

After discussion with the patient, the following final restorations were selected:

- Maxilla: An implant-supported fixed/removable overdenture with a palateless design made of a high-performance polymer material (ceramic-reinforced polyetheretherketone, PEEK) using ceramic telescopic crowns with PEEK friction caps.
- Mandible: An implant-retained overdenture with stud attachments (Novaloc system; Institut Straumann AG, Basel, Switzerland).

The use of PEEK as a framework material for implant-supported overdentures offers important advantages, such as high biocompatibility in contact with soft tissues, low biofilm adhesion and plaque accumulation (Hahnel and coworkers 2015; Barkarmo and coworkers 2019), excellent mechanical properties (Jin and coworkers 2019; Paratelli and coworkers 2020), and a reduced volume of the final prosthesis, which improves patient acceptance and comfort.

The combination of zirconia as a prosthetic material for telescopic crowns with PEEK friction caps has proven reliable in terms of retention and wear performance (Engels and coworkers 2013; Schubert and coworkers 2018; Schimmel and coworkers 2021), biocompatibility, low biofilm formation, and superior physical properties. Additionally, these materials can be integrated into modern CAD/CAM workflows.

Table 1 EERA table underlining the risk factors inherent in this scenario if a fixed prosthesis had been considered for the maxillary arch. The need for facial and lip support provided by a buccal flange and expectation to have small buccal corridors were the main considerations that led to the suggestion of a removable solution.

Esthetic risk factors - Edentulous	Level of risk		
	Low	Medium	High
Arch	Mandible		Maxilla
Facial support (fixed)	Alveolar process provides adequate facial support	Minimal changes tolerated by the patient	Flange required for adequate facial support
Facial support (removable)	Flange provides adequate facial support	Minimal changes tolerated by the patient	Insufficient space for a flange
Labial support	Designed tooth position provides satisfactory labial support	Minimal changes tolerated by the patient	Designed tooth position causes unsatisfactory labial support
Upper lip length	Long upper lip (> 20 mm)		Short upper lip (< 20 mm)
Buccal corridor* (atrophic ridge)	Removable prosthesis		Fixed prosthesis
Smile line	No display of the ridge(s) at full smile (maxilla or mandible)		Display of the ridge(s) at full smile (maxilla or mandible)
Maxillomandibular relationship	Class I	Class II	Class III

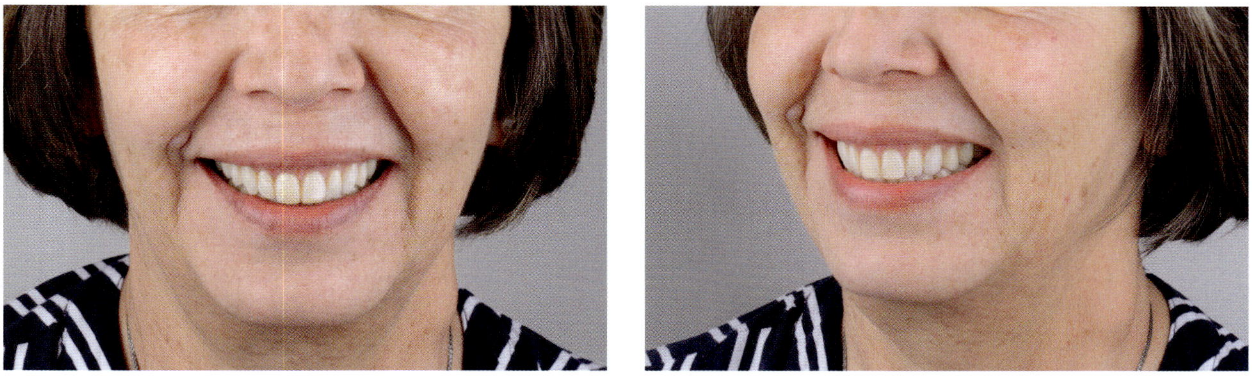

Figs 9 and 10 Transitional complete dentures. Extraoral frontal and three-quarter views. Adequate lip support provided by the buccal flange of the full prosthesis.

TRANSITIONAL PHASE

Transitional acrylic complete maxillary and mandibular prostheses (Figs 9 and 10) were fabricated with customized teeth and the proposed functional and esthetic parameters in order to establish the final tooth position prior to implant placement. This restoration-driven approach aims to optimize implant planning and placement according to the desired prosthetic reconstruction. Transitional dentures were duplicated to obtain clear radiographic guides with gutta-percha points. These were placed in the potential areas of interest and as surgical guides.

SURGICAL PROCEDURES

Following local and regional anesthesia (infiltration of articaine with epinephrine 1 : 100,000; local infiltration from premolar to premolar and a regional posterior alveolar nerve block in the posterior maxilla), as well as intravenous conscious sedation (midazolam 1.5 mg), a crestal incision was

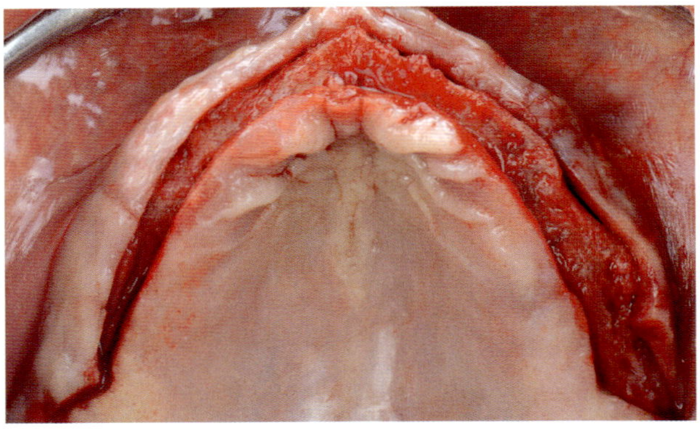

Fig 11 Maxillary implant surgery. Occlusal view of the alveolar ridge prior to implant placement.

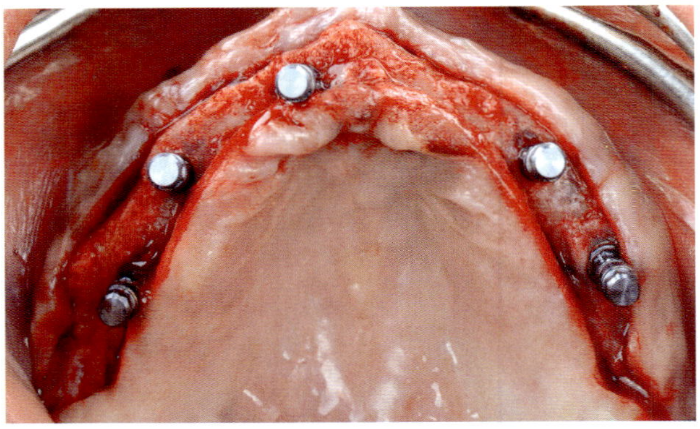

Fig 12 Maxillary implant surgery. Occlusal view of the implants placed at sites 15, 13, 11, 23, and 25.

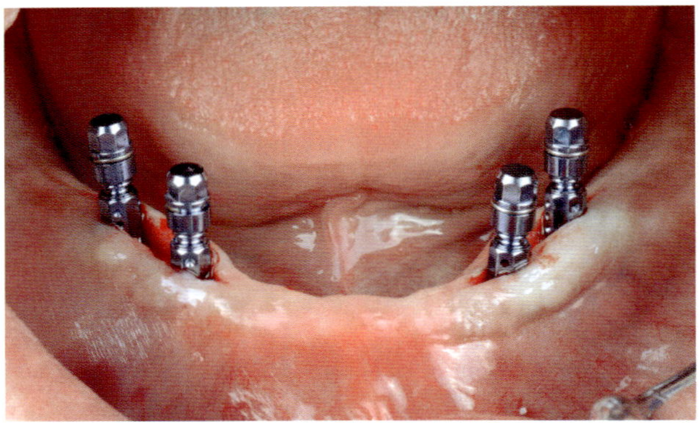

Fig 13 Mandibular implant surgery. Frontal view of the four implants.

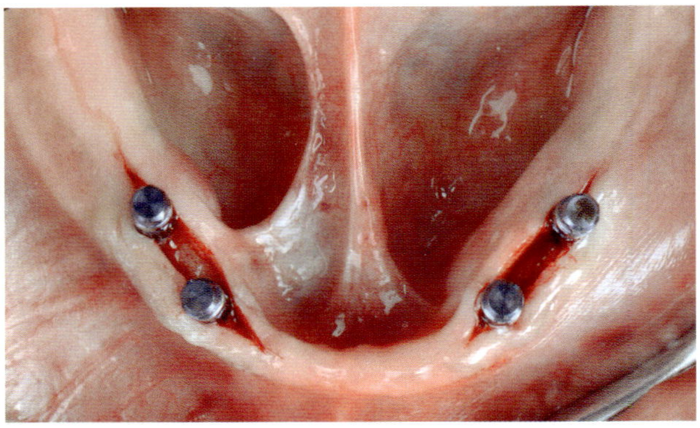

Fig 14 Occlusal view of the four implants placed in parallel alignment in the mandible.

made in the maxilla, slightly palatal to preserve the attached gingiva, and a full-thickness flap was elevated to reduce the alveolar ridge to provide an adequate platform to ensure the prosthetic volume required (Dawson and coworkers 2022) for the final prostheses (Fig 11).

Following the osteotomy, five implants (four Bone Level Tapered Roxolid SLActive, diameter 3.3 mm, length 12 mm, and one Bone Level Tapered Roxolid SLActive, diameter 4.1 mm, length 8 mm; Institut Straumann AG, Basel, Switzerland) were placed in parallel alignment (Fig 12), well distributed across the arch and with cover screws in place. Primary wound closure was achieved with a modified continuous sling suture using non-resorbable PTFE monofilament suture material.

At the second surgery (4 weeks later) – again under local anesthesia (articaine infiltration with epinephrine 1 : 100,000 and a mental nerve block in the mandible; intravenous sedation was not considered) – four narrow-diameter implants (Bone Level Tapered Roxolid SLActive, diameter 3.3 mm, length 10 mm; Institut Straumann AG, Basel, Switzerland) were placed in the mandible in an interforaminal distribution (canine and second premolar) placed in parallel alignment to avoid bone grafting in the severely resorbed anterior mandible, and important anatomical structures in the molar sites (Figs 13 and 14).

The implants were left with closure screws in place for two-phase submucosal healing (Fig 15). A conventional loading protocol was selected in both the maxilla and mandible according to the ITI Consensus Statement on loading protocols for implant-supported overdentures in edentulous jaws (Gallucci and coworkers 2009; Gallucci and coworkers 2014; Schimmel and coworkers 2014).

After 8 weeks of healing, a second surgical procedure was performed to uncover the implants and to place healing abutments that preserved the attached gingiva (Figs 16 and 17).

PROSTHETIC PROCEDURES

The first step was to accurately transfer the 3D position of the implants and soft tissue to the laboratory using conventional impressions taken with an open-tray technique using polyvinyl siloxane in custom trays. Cast models with implant analogs were fabricated, scanned, and digitized; from this point, a complete digital workflow was used to fabricate the final restoration.

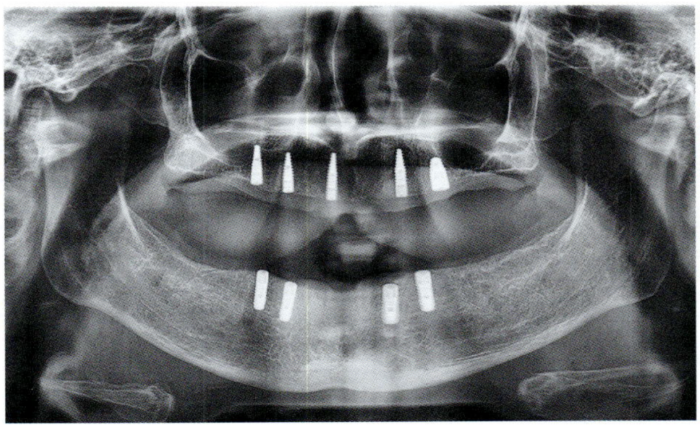

Fig 15 Panoramic radiograph after 8 weeks of healing.

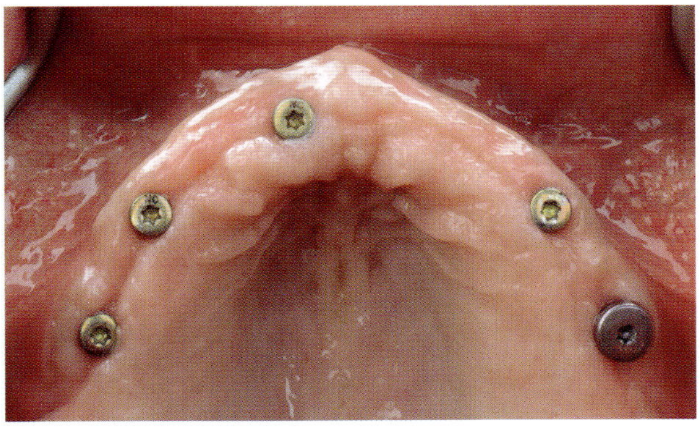

Fig 16 Occlusal view of the five uncovered maxillary implants.

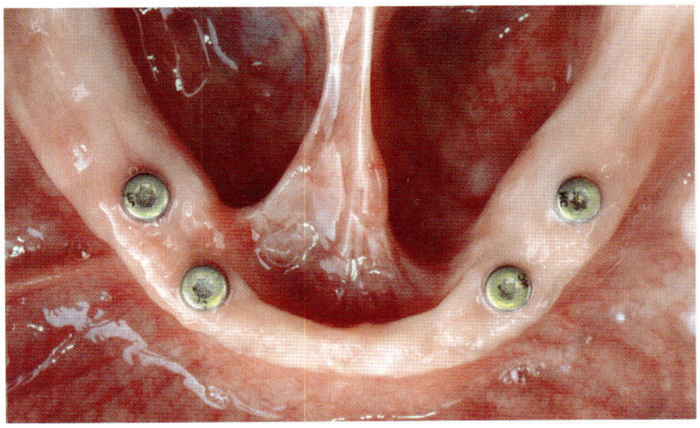

Fig 17 Occlusal view of the four uncovered mandibular implants.

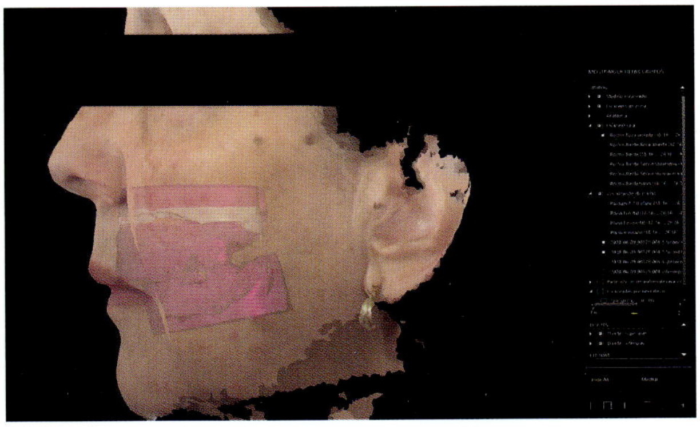

Fig 18 3D digitization of the patient's face in the natural head position with upper and lower baseplates and wax rims with correct intermaxillary parameters.

Posteriorly, the craniomandibular relationship was registered using Udo Plaster's PlaneSystem (Zirkonzahn, Gais, Italy), which is an innovative digital approach to acquiring specific occlusal information such as the three-dimensional position of the maxilla, inclination of the occlusal plane, bite registration, and mandibular function analysis (Plane Analyzer). This system integrates a virtual articulator (PS1 Articulator) with facebow transfer at the reproducible natural head position (Plane Finder) in an upright posture and a three-dimensional facial scanner (Face Hunter; all Zirkonzahn) using a triangulated structured light technique to perform a surface scan of the patient's face for a facially driven prosthetic design (Att and coworkers 2019; Okawa and coworkers 2019).

The patient's facial 3D dataset was obtained using the optical 3D facial scanner with a bite plate for image fusion (Transfer Fork; Zirkonzahn) and 3D patient analysis. The 3D facial scan provides the clinician and laboratory with valuable patient information and facilitates communication with the patient.

Once the necessary clinical information (three-dimensional positions of implants, soft tissues, and craniomandibular registration plus facial scanning) were acquired and merged in the CAD software, the digital design process of the final restorations was initiated. The CAD software allows full control of the prosthesis with 3D data of the esthetic and functional parameters verifying occlusal contacts and excursion movements in the virtual articulator (Figs 18 to 21).

For the maxillary arch, five telescopic crowns were designed and milled in 3Y-TZP monolithic zirconia (Prettau 2 Dispersive; Zirkonzahn) according to the previous digital set-up (Figs 22 to 25) and cemented on the abutments (four Variobase NC abutments, diameter 3.8 mm, abutment height 3.5 mm, gingival height 1 mm, and one RC abutment, diameter 4.5 mm, abutment height 3.5 mm, gingival height 1 mm; all Institut Straumann AG, Basel, Switzerland).

The final prosthesis consisted of a CAD/CAM framework milled in ceramically reinforced PEEK (Tecno Med Mineral; Zirkonzahn) with no palatal coverage and anatomical reduction to receive customized monolithic ceramic prosthetic teeth (IPS e.max CAD; Ivoclar Vivadent, Schaan, Liechtenstein) (Figs 26 to 32).

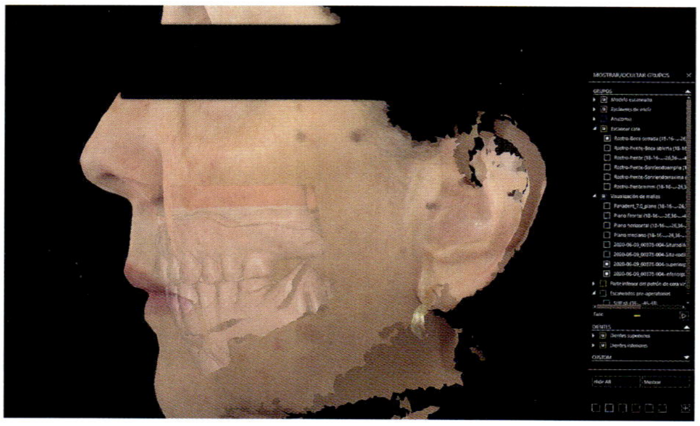

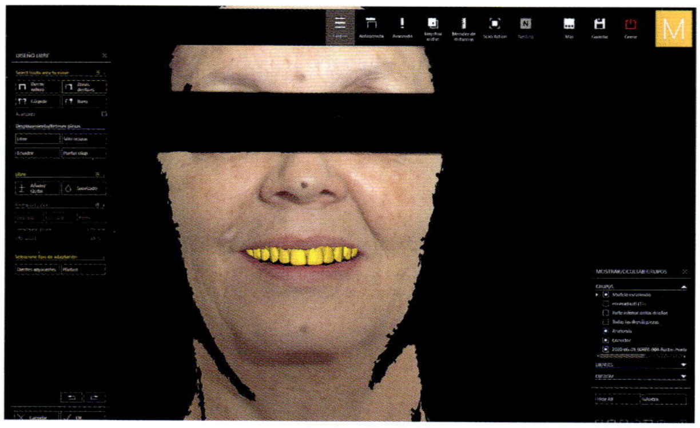

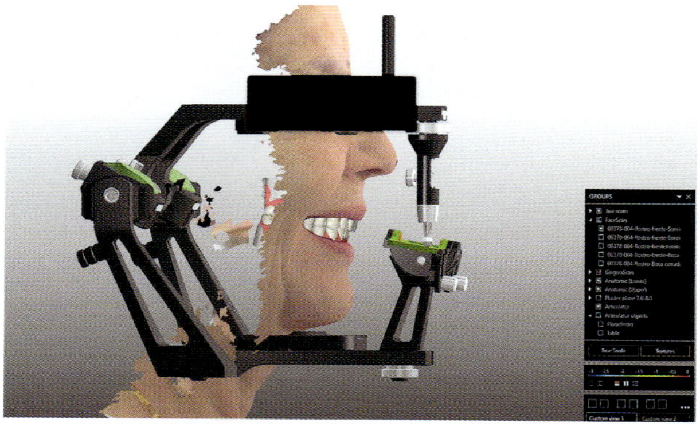

Figs 19 to 21 Facial data integrated into the virtual articulator with final virtual design of the restorations.

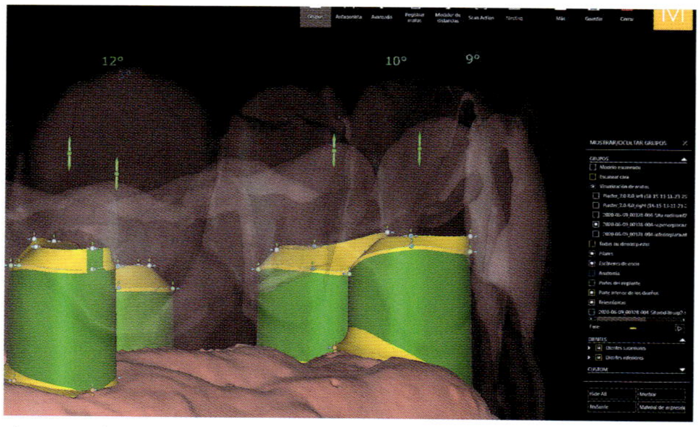

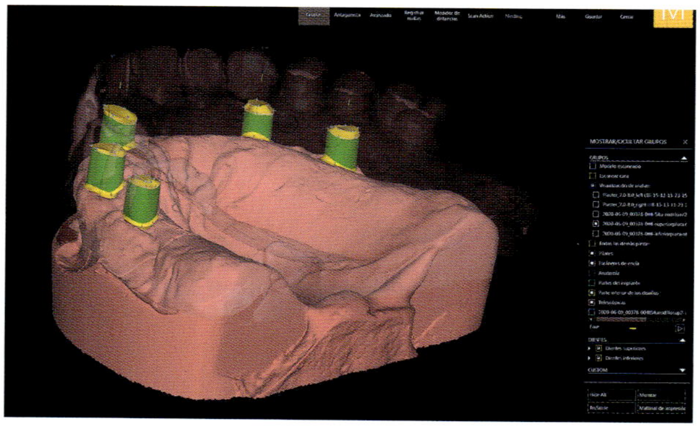

Figs 22 and 23 Virtual designs of the maxillary telescopic crowns.

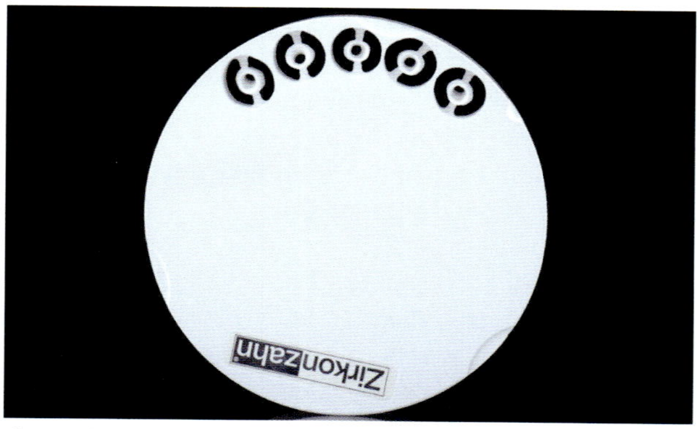

Fig 24 Telescopic crowns milled from 3Y-TZP zirconia.

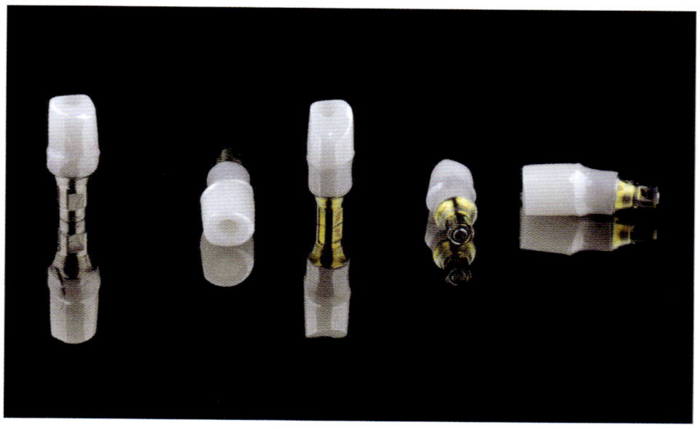

Fig 25 Polished maxillary telescopic zirconia crowns cemented on Variobase abutments.

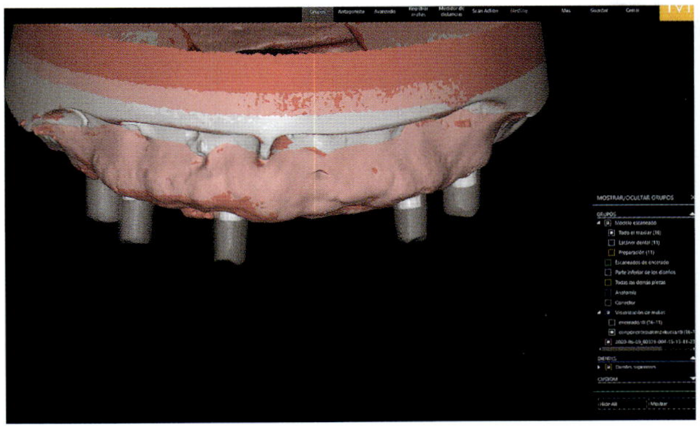

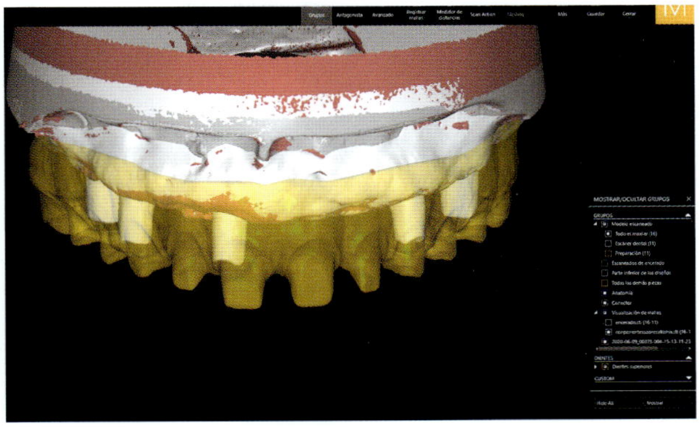

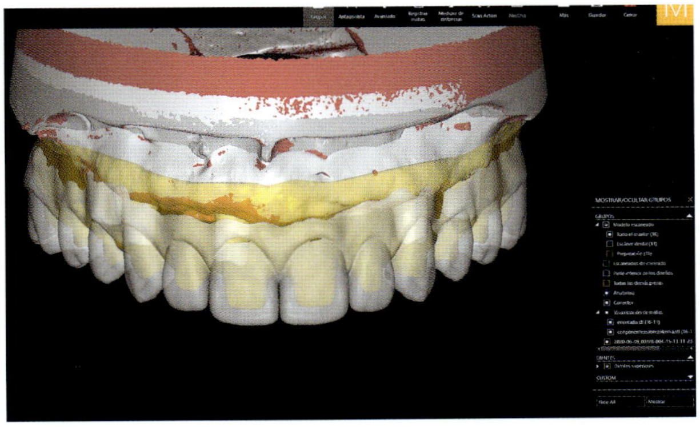

Figs 26 to 28 Final virtual design of the maxillary overdenture in the CAD software before fabrication.

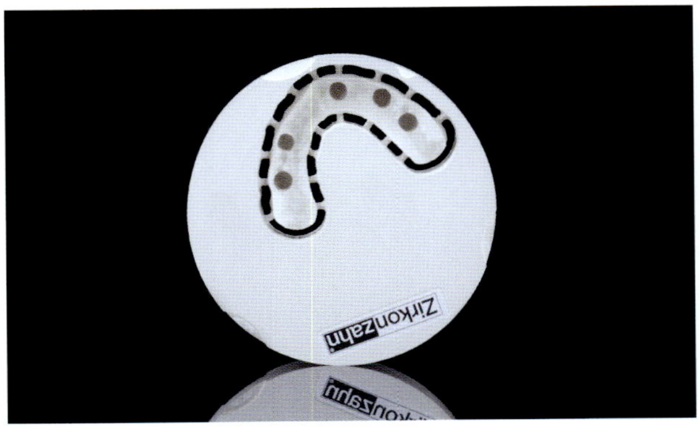

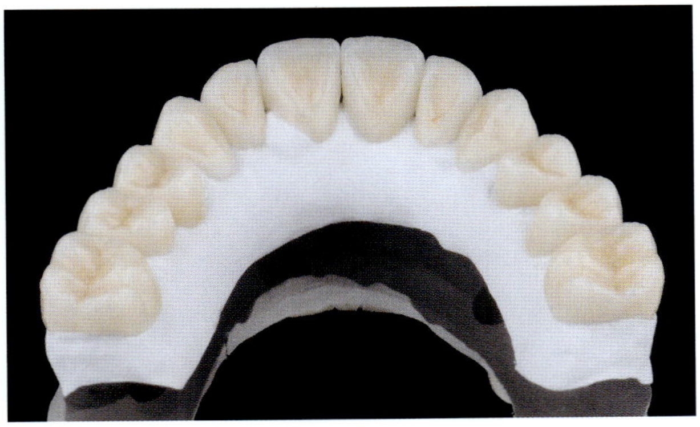

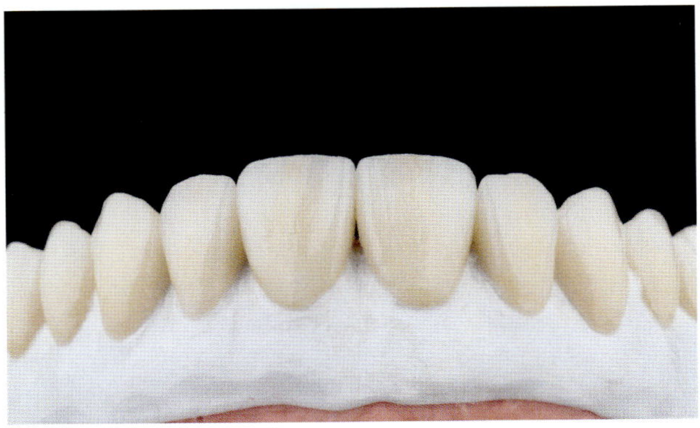

Figs 29 to 31 Maxillary framework milled from reinforced PEEK. The customized ceramic teeth were milled from lithium disilicate glass ceramic and cemented to the reinforced denture base.

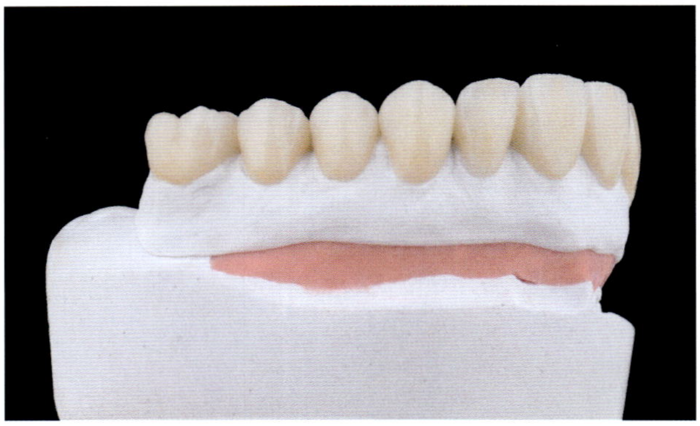

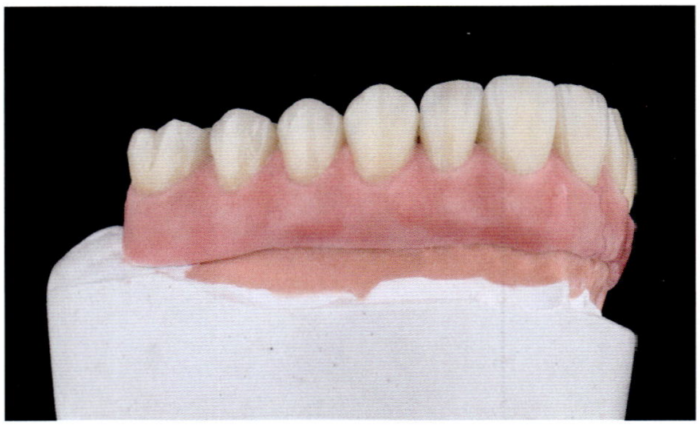

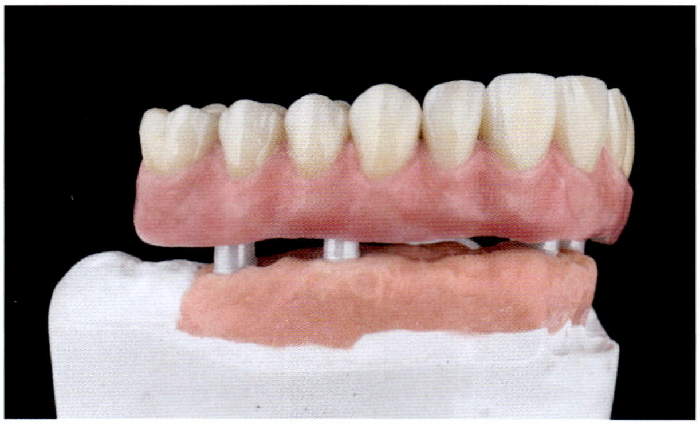

Figs 32 to 34 Final characterization with pink veneering composite.

The custom-designed ceramic teeth were prepared for bonding using 5% hydrofluoric acid (IPS Ceramic Etching gel; Ivoclar Vivadent) for 20 seconds, rinsing of the etched surface with air-water spray for 30 seconds followed by the application of a silane coupling agent (Clearfil Ceramic Primer Plus; Kuraray America, NY, USA) (Saavedra and coworkers 2009; Guarda and coworkers 2013; Menees and coworkers 2014).

The PEEK framework was sandblasted with 50-µm alumina particles at 2 bar of pressure, cleaned with oil-free compressed air, followed by the application and polymerization of a laboratory dental adhesive (Visio.link; Bredent medical, Senden, Germany) (Rosentritt and coworkers 2015). The ceramic teeth were loaded with dual curing resin cement (Panavia V5; Kuraray America, NY, USA), seated and excess cement was removed with floss and brush. The material was polymerized with a light-curing unit with multi-wavelength LED (bre.Lux Power Unit; Bredent Medical, Senden, Germany) for 90 seconds.

Finally, indirect pink veneering composite (Crea.Lign; Bredent medical) was used to reproduce the gingival anatomy according to the described bonding protocol (Figs 33 and 34).

The telescopic crowns were screwed in and tightened to 35 Ncm; the access holes were blocked with PTFE and the final prosthesis was delivered (Figs 37 and 38).

The final mandibular restoration was an implant-retained overdenture in pink PMMA base material with dense, highly crosslinked polymer prosthetic teeth. Four straight abutments (Narrow Crossfit Novaloc, diameter 3.8 mm, height 3 mm; Institut Straumann AG, Basel, Switzerland) were selected as the retention system for the final prosthesis (Figs 35 and 36). These abutments have the advantage of requiring minimal interocclusal space (8–11 mm from the edentulous ridge to the opposing occlusal table) (Dawson and coworkers 2022), avoiding additional surgical bone re-

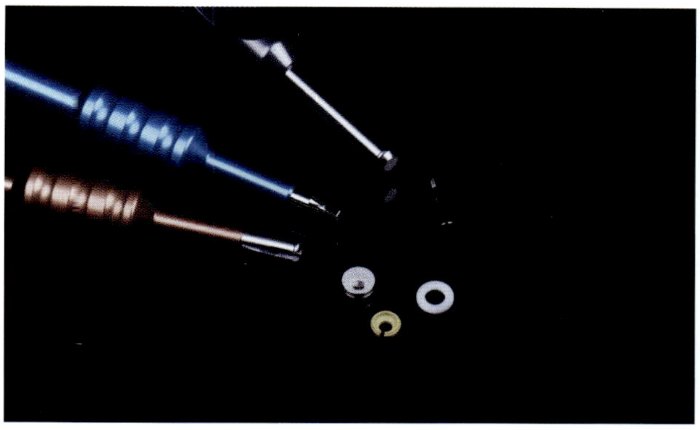

Fig 35 Novaloc retention system.

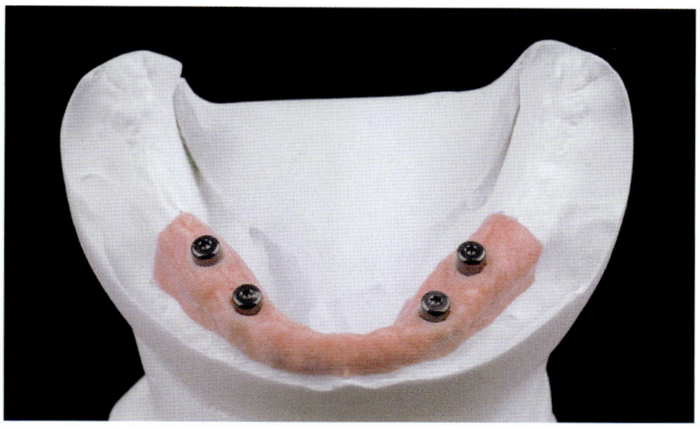

Fig 36 Novaloc abutments presented in the model with artificial soft tissue showing the correct gingival height.

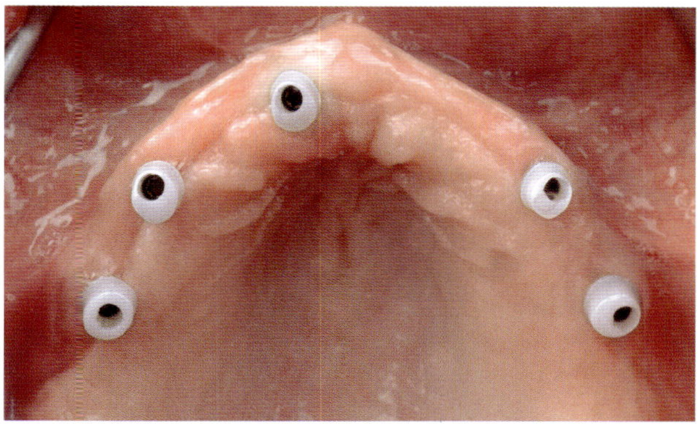

Fig 37 Occlusal view of the five telescopic abutments tightened to 35 Ncm.

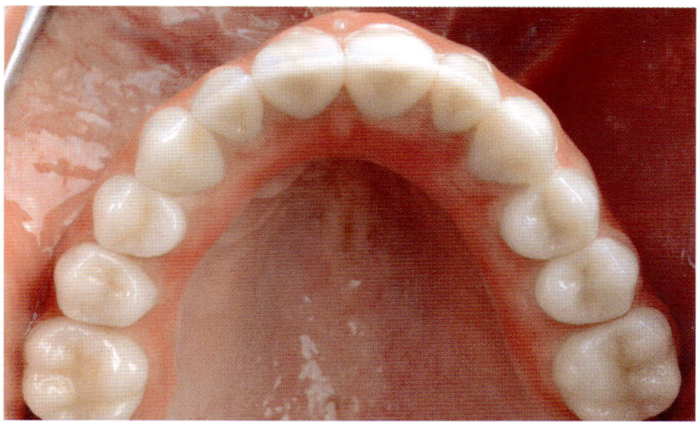

Fig 38 Occlusal view of the maxillary implant-supported overdenture.

duction to accommodate other types of more space-consuming retention systems and still offering long-lasting retention and high wear resistance (Friedrichsen and coworkers 2024).

The intraoral abutment pick-up process was performed using dual-cure self-adhesive pink composite (Attachment Processing Material; Zest Dental Solutions, CA, USA) (Figs 39a-d). After finishing and polishing, light-retention PEEK Novaloc retention inserts (white color) were placed.

FOLLOW-UP AND PATIENT SATISFACTION

The final intraoral and extraoral views 2 weeks postoperatively illustrate the very pleasing and natural result achieved (Figs 40 to 43). The patient was very satisfied with the esthetic and, more importantly, the functional outcome. She reported being able to eat and chew different types of food, something she described as a life-changing experience.

Given her history of stage IV periodontitis, the patient was scheduled for a stringent maintenance regime and professional oral hygiene every 4 months, and radiographic controls once a year (Figs 44a-b).

During the maintenance visits, the implant-supported prostheses were subjected to an ultrasonic bath with cleaning solution (Tartar and Stain Remover; Henry Schein Dental, NY, USA) for 25 minutes, followed by removal of small stains and possible calculus remnants by air-polishing (Airflow Max) with 14-µm erythritol powder (Airflow Plus Powder; both EMS Dental, Nyon, Switzerland) on the prosthesis and finally surface polishing with goat-hair brushes with composite polishing paste.

At the 3-year follow-up visit, the peri-implant soft tissues showed no signs of inflammation or recession. There was no significan bone resorption around the implants and no prosthetic complications were present (Figs 45 and 46).

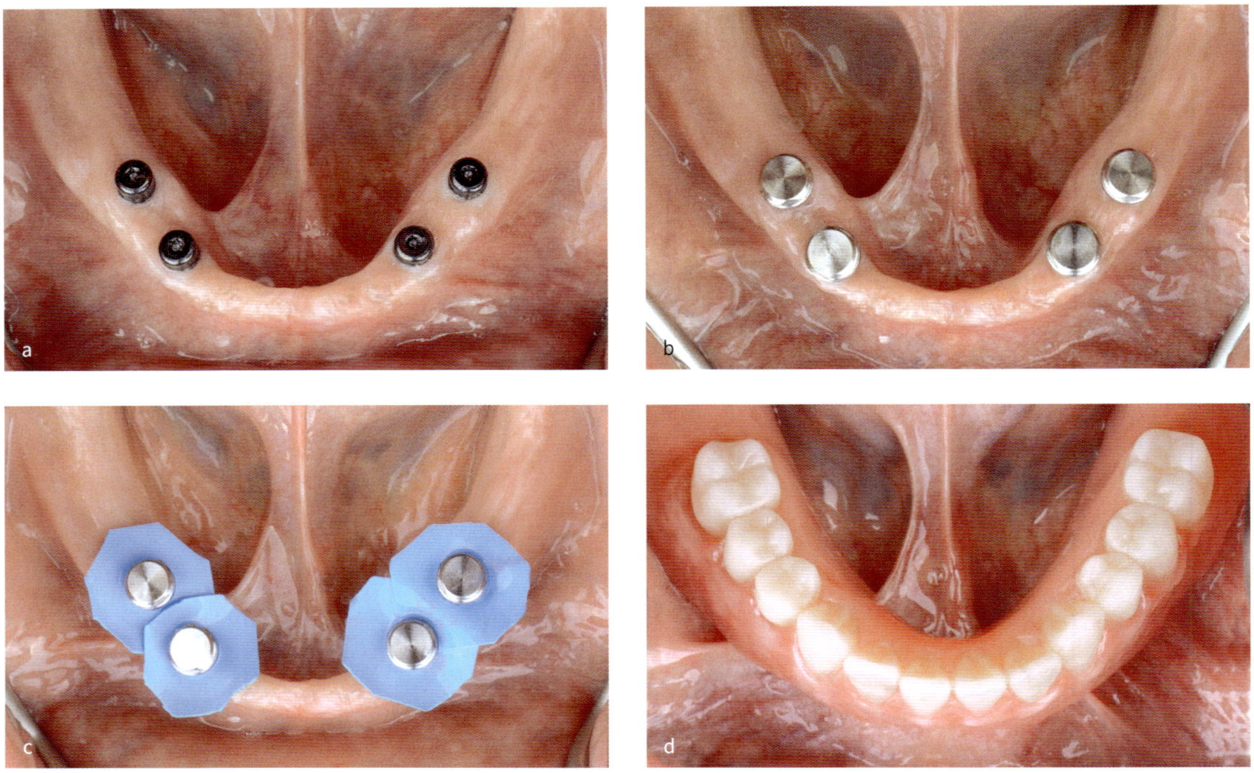

Figs 39a-d Intraoral direct pick-up procedure. Intraoral occlusal view of Novaloc abutments tightened to 35 Ncm (a). Titanium matrix housings in situ (b). Block-out rings placed over the abutments to prevent excess dual-cure resin below the matrix housings (c). After verifying adequate passive seating of the final prosthesis, the final pick-up was performed with finger pressure using dual-cure self-adhesive resin.

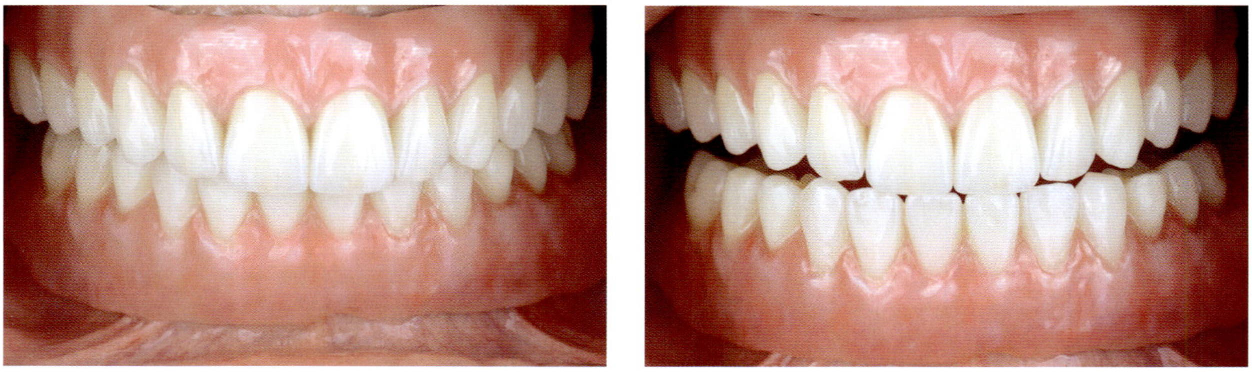

Figs 40 and 41 After 2 weeks in function. A mutually protected occlusion with lateral progressive group function was designed as the occlusal scheme in this rehabilitation.

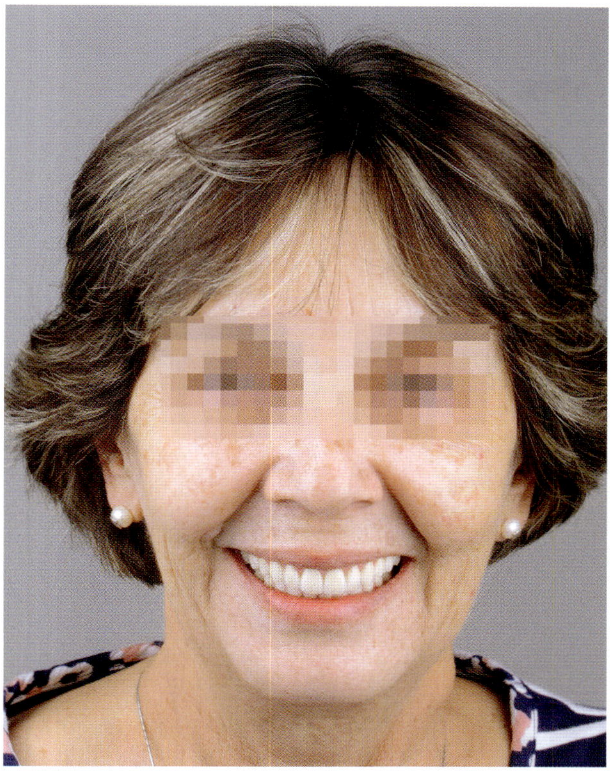

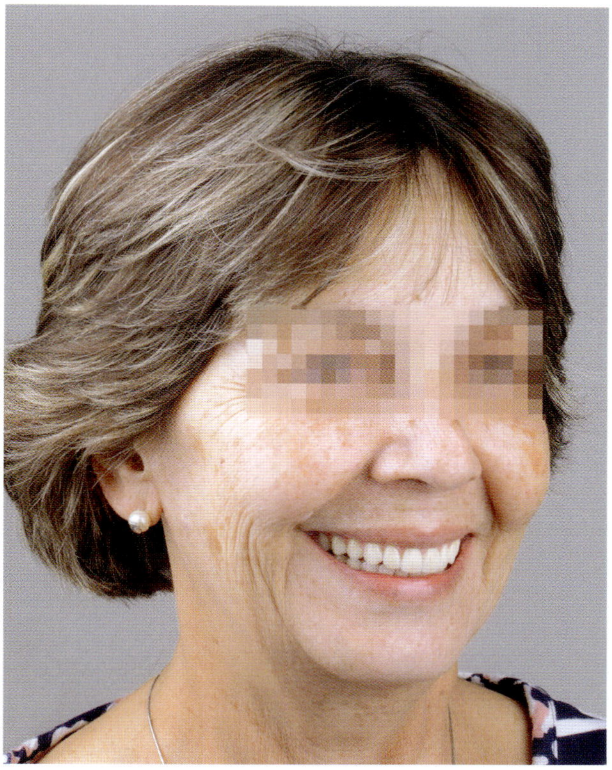

Figs 42 and 43 Final extraoral view of the bimaxillary implant-supported rehabilitation.

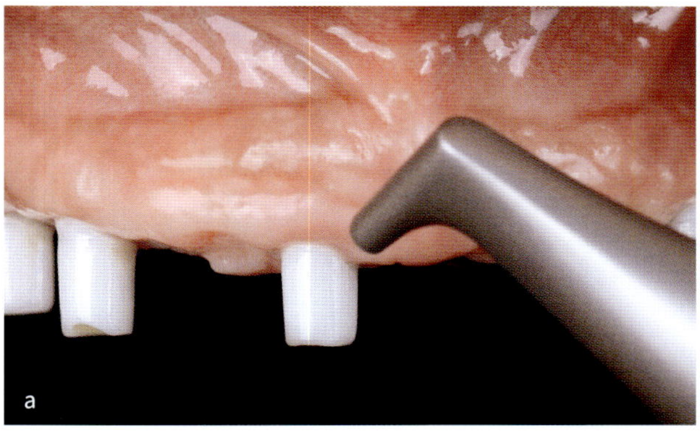

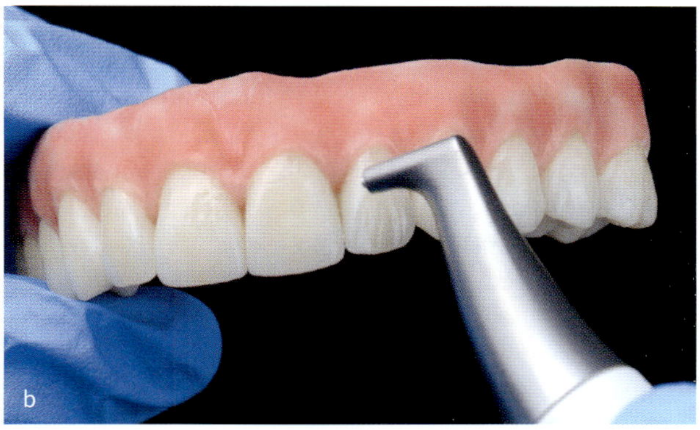

Figs 44a-b At the 3-year maintenance visit, using an air-polishing system with 14-µm erythritol powder on the abutments and prosthesis.

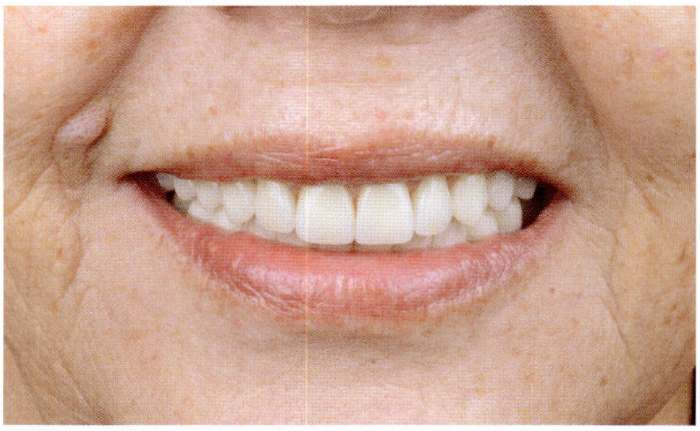

Fig 45 Patient's smile after 3 years of function.

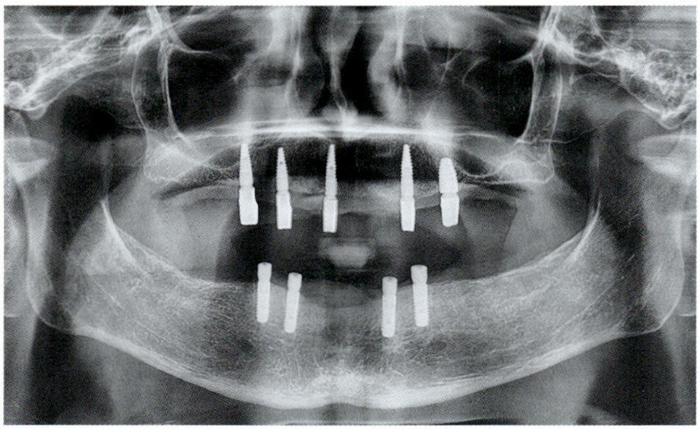

Fig 46 Panoramic radiograph at 3 years.

DISCUSSION

Initially, the patient presented with important risk factors identified by the interdisciplinary team, such as a history of stage IV periodontitis, the need for facial tissue support, the desire for a fixed and palateless maxillary prosthesis (if possible), and high esthetic and functional expectations. During the initial phase with transitional removable complete dentures, an attempt was made to educate the patient about the advantages, disadvantages, and possible limitations of different types of prostheses (fixed or removable) in light of the existing risk factors.

In the maxilla, a fixed-removable overdenture made of a high-performance polymer material (ceramically reinforced PEEK), with zirconia telescopic crowns and friction caps as the prosthetic solution allowed an optimized esthetic result by supporting the facial structures with a buccal flange, avoiding palatal coverage and providing a mechanical behavior similar to that of a fixed restoration (which was an important requirement), with the advantage of being easy to remove, clean, and maintain even at the patient's advancing age.

In the mandible, an implant-retained overdenture on four narrow-diameter implants with stud attachments with PEEK matrix inserts (Novaloc) was considered an effective solution. It provided long-term retention and was cost-effective.

Because the mandibular interocclusal space was limited (8 mm measured from the edentulous ridge to the opposing occlusal table) (Dawson and coworkers 2022), a mandibular implant-supported overdenture with frictional retention such as telescopic crowns, as in the maxilla, would have required adjunctive surgery (reduction of the alveolar bone) at the same time as implant placement (an option rejected by the patient). It would have required more interocclusal space for the prosthetic components and materials (prosthetic screw, abutment, friction cap, framework, and prosthetic teeth) for an esthetic and durable restoration, increasing morbidity and treatment complexity.

Another challenge in this clinical scenario was the limited alveolar bone available (mainly due to horizontal deficiencies of both anterior alveolar ridges) to place the optimal number of implants with a favorable distribution according to the maxillary and mandibular prostheses. The use of narrow-diameter implants allowed us to place an adequate number of implants anteroposteriorly while avoiding bone augmentation. This resulted in reduced cost, morbidity, time savings and less complexity in the overall treatment process.

Use this code to watch a highlight video with the patient reporting on her satisfaction with the treatment.

CONCLUSION

The patient scenario included a full-mouth reconstruction (with a 3-year follow-up) to replace the missing teeth and to provide ridge and facial-tissue support in a completely edentulous elderly patient, restoring esthetics and chewing efficiency with implant-supported overdentures designed and fabricated utilizing digital technology with contemporary high-performance polymeric and ceramic materials.

Undoubtedly, a careful diagnosis, risk assessment, and treatment plan incorporating the patient profile analysis were fundamental to providing the patient with an individualized solution using dental implants to improve her initial condition.

ACKNOWLEDGMENTS

Surgical procedures
Dr Said A. Sánchez and Dr Elena Balcázar – León, Mexico

Prosthodontic procedures
Dr Said A. Sánchez – León, Mexico

Laboratory procedures
MDT Eric Sánchez Alonso – Aguascalientes, Mexico

Patients who wish for the prosthesis to be as stable as natural teeth

5.4 Conventional Loading of Four Implants in the Edentulous Maxilla and Restoration with a Bar-Supported Overdenture

H. J. A. Meijer, J. W. A. Slot, G. M. Raghoebar

PATIENT CHARACTERISTICS AND PATIENT PROFILE

A 64-year-old male patient was referred to the University Medical Center Groningen, The Netherlands, for dental implant treatment. The patient had been edentulous in both the maxilla and mandible for 25 years. During these 25 years, three conventional dentures had been fabricated, the most recent one being 2 years old. The patient complained of inadequate retention and stability of his maxillary and mandibular dentures. The esthetic aspect was of medium importance to the patient. His medical history was unremarkable.

Intraoral examination revealed extreme resorption of the maxillary ridge and moderate resorption of the mandibular ridge. Retention and stability of both dentures were low, and the occlusion was balanced without anterior contact. Radiographic analysis included a panoramic rotational radiograph, a lateral cephalometric radiograph, and a posteroanterior oblique radiograph. The radiographs were also evaluated for sinus pathology (Figs 1a-c).

Based on this information and the clinical evaluation described below, the following patient profile (Fig 2) can be derived for this patient (for more information about patient profiles, see Chapters 2.1.3 and 3.6).

CLINICAL EVALUATION AND TREATMENT PLAN

A diagnostic set-up helped determine the available space for a removable bar-supported implant overdenture or a fixed full-arch dental prosthesis (FDP) on implants. The choice between a fixed full-arch FDP and an implant-supported overdenture is influenced by the patient's preference, possibility of lip support, degree of bone resorption, ease of cleaning, available prosthetic space, phonetics, esthetics, general satisfaction, and economic situation (Heydecke and coworkers 2003; Boven and coworkers 2015).

Financial considerations (reimbursement by the health insurance company) were the main reason for the patient's choice of a removable implant-supported overdenture, but also a desire for better retention and stability. If there is sufficient bone in the anterior region and enough space for the restoration, it is advantageous to place implants in the anterior region, as this reduces morbidity and shortens the treatment time (Slot and coworkers 2013).

However, this patient had been edentulous for a long time, so there was not enough bone for reliable placement of the implants. Therefore, sinus floor augmentation and ridge width reconstruction with iliac crest bone grafts was planned prior to implant placement (Raghoebar and coworkers 2019). After a 3-month healing period, four tissue-level implants were to be placed in the posterior maxilla in a single-stage procedure.

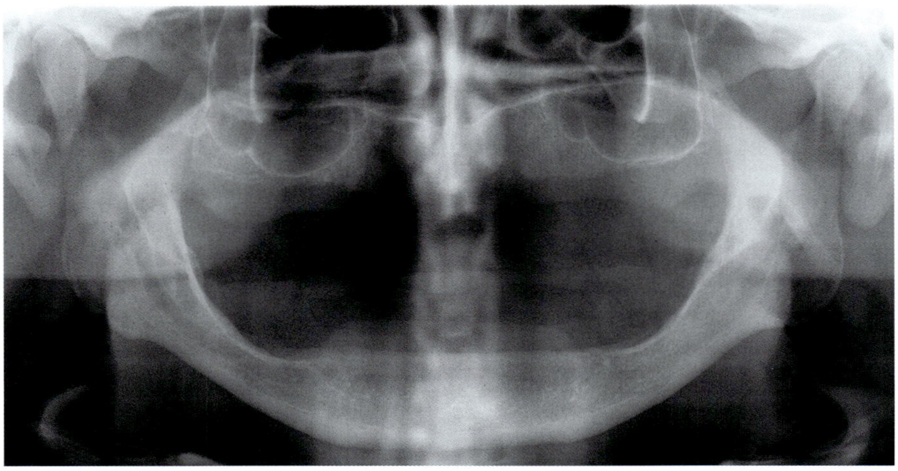

Fig 1a Baseline panoramic rotational radiograph.

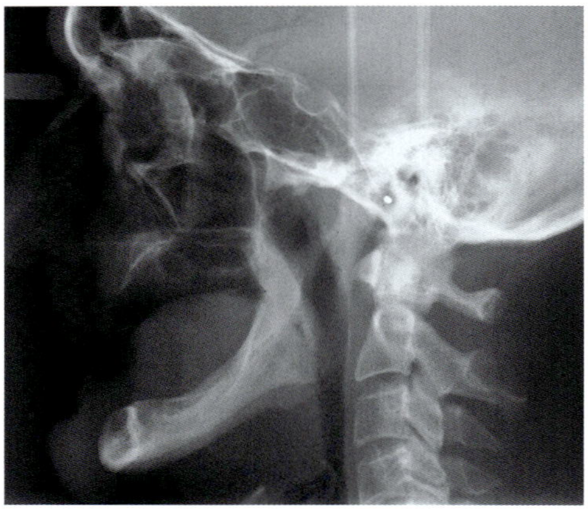

Fig 1b Baseline lateral cephalometric radiograph.

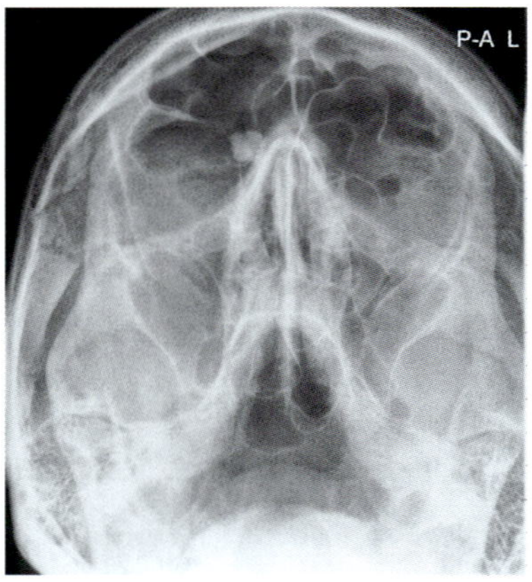

Fig 1c Baseline posteroanterior oblique radiograph.

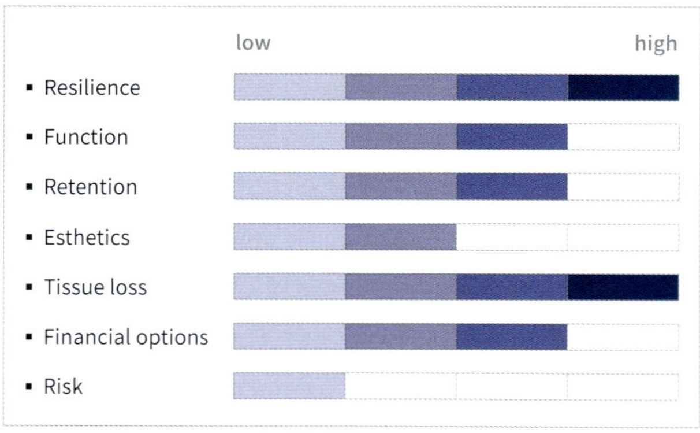

Fig 2 Patient profile.

Four implants and a bar attachment provide adequate retention and stability for a maxillary overdenture (Roccuzzo and coworkers 2014; Slot and coworkers 2022). In addition, four implants were proposed in the interforaminal regions of the mandible. Two implants in the mandible are now considered more than sufficient for overdenture support, but at the time of this treatment proposal, it was thought that with an opposing natural (partial) dentition or an implant-supported maxillary overdenture, four mandibular implants would be preferable. After 3 months of osseointegration in both jaws, an overdenture supported by a bar attachment was to be fabricated.

The patient was informed of the potential risks and gave his informed consent.

SURGICAL PROCEDURES

The surgical procedure was performed under general anesthesia. A bone graft was harvested from the medial surface of the anterior ilium. After harvesting the bone grafts, the maxillary surgical sites were infiltrated with a local anesthetic containing epinephrine (Ultracaine D-S forte; Sanofi-Aventis Netherlands, Gouda, The Netherlands) as a vasoconstrictor. The palatal mucosa was incised just below and parallel to the top of the alveolar crest.

After vertical releasing incisions were made in the buccal mucosa, a mucoperiosteal flap was elevated to expose the alveolar crest and the lateral wall of the maxilla. When necessary, the mobility of the reflected flap was improved by a relieving incision in the periosteum at the base of the buccal flap.

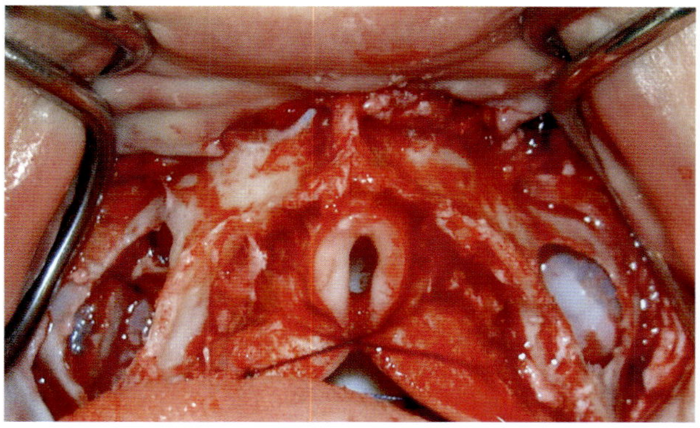

Fig 3 Bilateral sinus elevation. The membrane was raised and the mobilized part of the lateral sinus wall was rotated medially and upward together with the raised membranes.

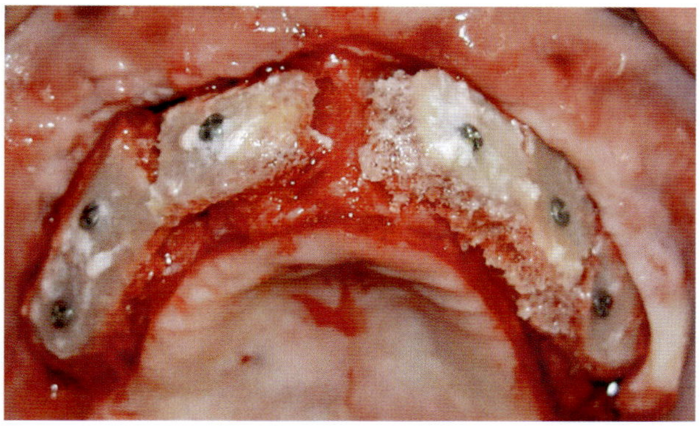

Fig 4 The cancellous portion of the graft was repositioned toward the maxilla. The grafts were fixed with 1.5 mm osteosynthesis screws.

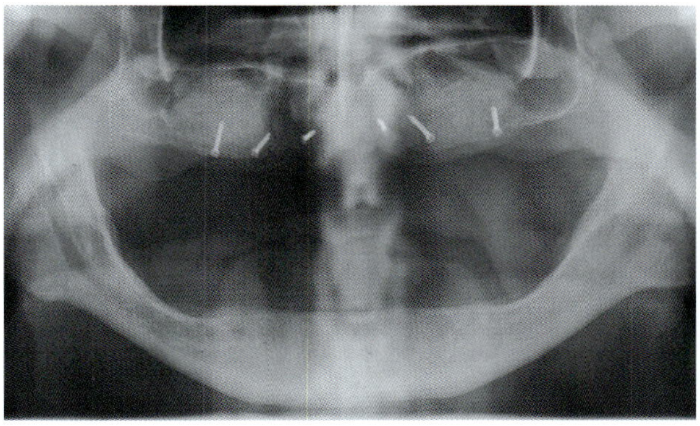

Fig 5 Panoramic radiograph 6 weeks after maxillary sinus floor augmentation and lateral bone augmentation.

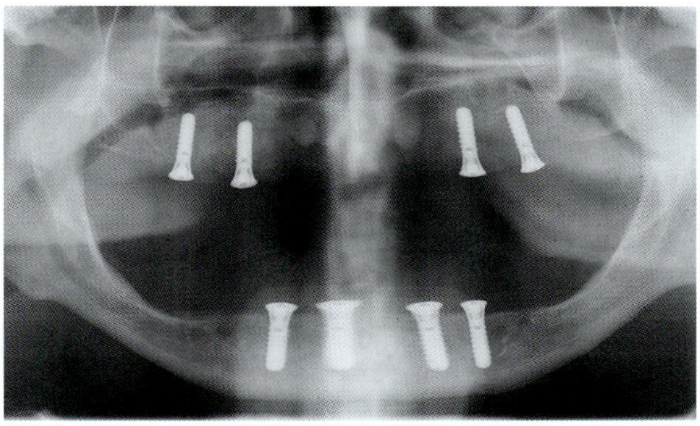

Fig 6 Panoramic radiograph 6 weeks after placement of the tissue-level implants.

The lateral wall of the maxillary sinus was fenestrated with a round bur at high speed and adequately cooled with sterile saline. Care was taken to preserve the mucosa. The Schneiderian membrane was elevated and the mobilized portion of the lateral sinus wall was rotated medially and upward together with the elevated membrane (Fig 3). The space created between the residual maxillary ridge and the membrane was filled with graft material.

The cortical bone grafts to reconstruct the bone width were placed on the exposed maxillary alveolar process as buccal onlay grafts. The cancellous portion of the graft was repositioned toward the maxilla. The grafts were fixed with 1.5 mm osteosynthesis screws (Fig 4). No membranes were used to cover the lateral wall defect after bone graft placement because the bone grafts completely covered the fenestration in the lateral wall of the sinus (Raghoebar and coworkers 1997). The target maxillary bone height after grafting was at least 13 mm (Fig 5).

The patient was not allowed to wear his denture for 2 weeks after surgery. Subsequently, the acrylic base was relieved in areas where it could have contacted the graft sites, and the denture was relined with an elastic liner (GC Reline II Extra Soft; GC, Tokyo, Japan).

After 3 months of healing, four tissue-level dental implants (Straumann Standard SLA implants RN, diameter 4.1 mm, length 12 mm; Institut Straumann AG, Basel, Switzerland) were placed in the maxilla in a single-stage procedure. The implants were placed semi-guided with a surgical guide in predetermined positions within the grafted sites (16, 13, 23, 26). Thanks to the bone augmentation performed in a separate session, there was enough bone volume to place the implants. At the same time, four implants for an overdenture were placed in the mandible (Fig 6).

Directly after implant placement, the patient was allowed to wear the dentures again after relieving the space around the implants and relining with an elastic liner. The patient was given oral hygiene instructions for cleaning the healing abutments.

The patient received amoxicillin for the sinus floor elevation and implant placement, starting with 3 g Clamoxyl p.o. (GlaxoSmithKline, Utrecht, The Netherlands) 1 hour before surgery and continuing at 3 × 500 mg/d for 7 days after surgery.

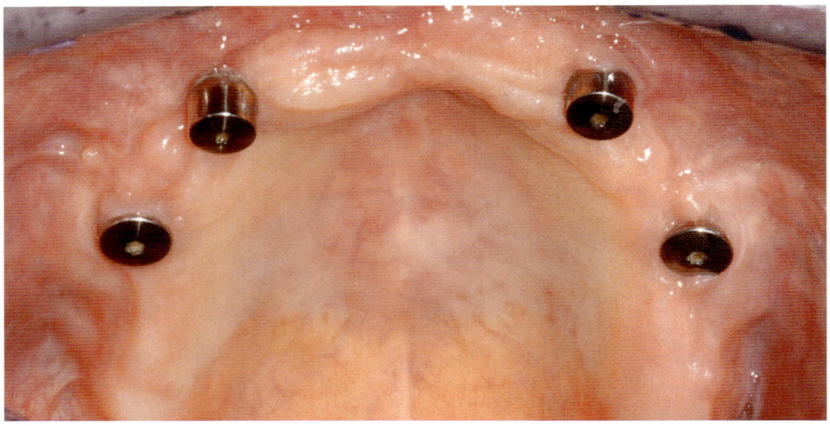

Fig 7 Four tissue-level implants with healing abutments at the end of the 3 month osseointegration period.

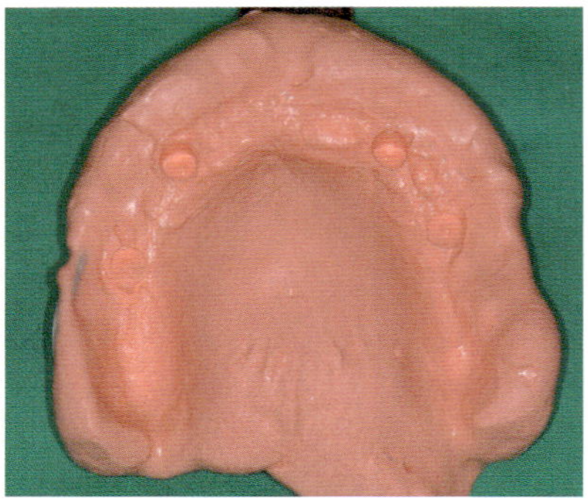

Fig 8 Preliminary impression for fabrication of a custom impression tray.

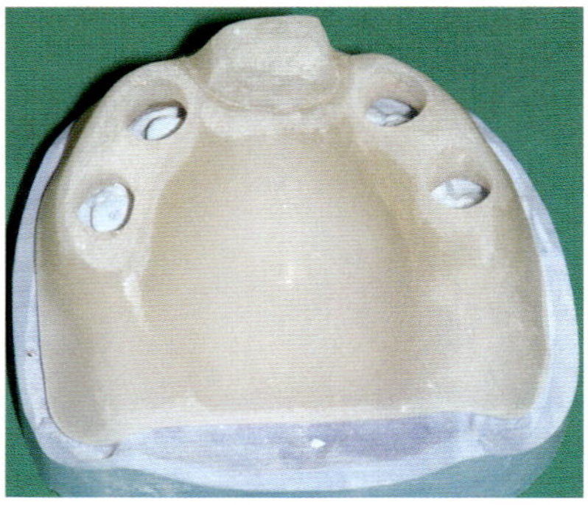

Fig 9 Preliminary cast with custom impression tray.

Postoperatively, the patient was prescribed a 0.2% chlorhexidine mouthrinse (Corsodyl; GlaxoSmithKline) to be applied for 2 × 1 min/d for 2 weeks.

PROSTHETIC PROCEDURES

After 3 months of osseointegration (Fig 7), prosthetic procedures were initiated. A preliminary impression was taken with stock metal trays and irreversible hydrocolloid (Cavex CA 37; Cavex Holland, Haarlem, The Netherlands) (Fig 8).

A preliminary cast was fabricated using type IV dental stone (GC Fujirock EP; GC Europe, Leuven, Belgium). A custom acrylic impression tray (Lightplast base plates; Dreve Dentamid, Unna, Germany) was fabricated with openings for screw-retained impression copings (Fig 9). The impression copings were fixed to the implants with the integrated positioning screws (Fig 10). The tray was placed over the impression copings and any contact between the copings and the tray was eliminated to allow the tray to rest firmly on the denture-bearing mucosa, with the positioning screws exiting through an opening in the tray. The tray margins were molded with a thermoplastic resin material (ISO Functional; GC Europe).

The final full-arch impression was taken with polyether (Impregum F; 3M ESPE, St. Paul, MN, USA). A syringe was used to inject impression material around the copings. The tray was filled with more impression material and placed on the alveolar process. During polymerization, the positioning screws of the copings were exposed to facilitate removal of the impression (Figs 11 to 13).

After removal of the tray, implant analogs (RT Implant Analog; Institut Straumann AG, Basel, Switzerland) were connected to the impression posts and a master cast was poured in type IV stone (GC Fujirock EP; GC Europe). This reproduced the implant sites and the denture-bearing area (Fig 13). Composite-resin record bases (Lightplast base plates; Dreve Dentamid) with an occlusal wax rim were fabricated to determine the vertical dimension of the occlusion and to record the maxillomandibular relationship (Figs 14 to 16).

The bite rims in the patient's mouth were stabilized with addition-cured silicone (Futar D; Kettenbach, Eschenburg, Germany) (Figs 17 and 18) and transferred to an articulator (Artex; Girrbach Dental, Pforzheim, Germany).

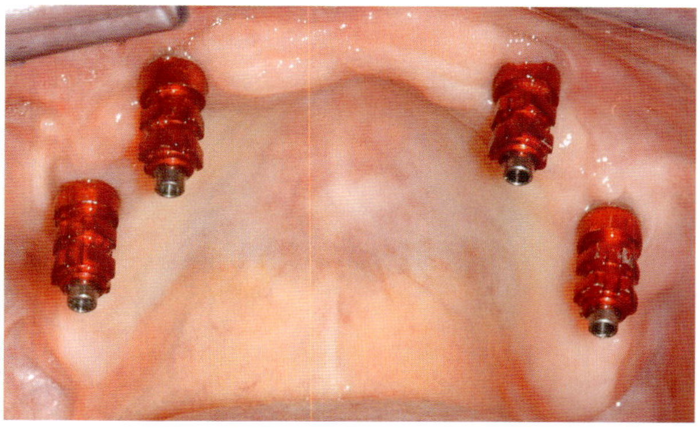

Fig 10 Impression posts on the implants.

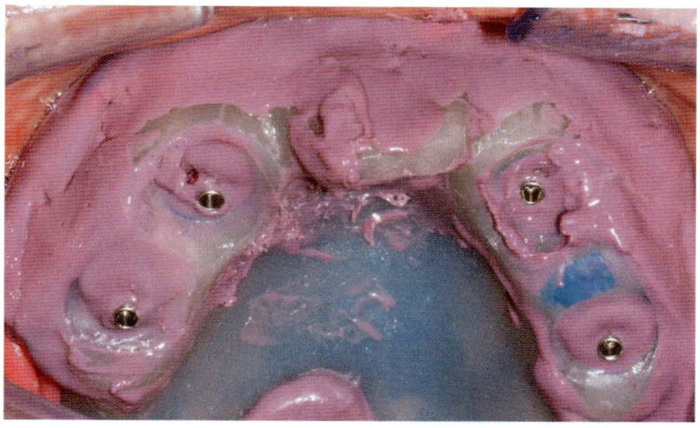

Fig 11 Final impression taken with a rigid polyether material. The screws of the impression posts are visible.

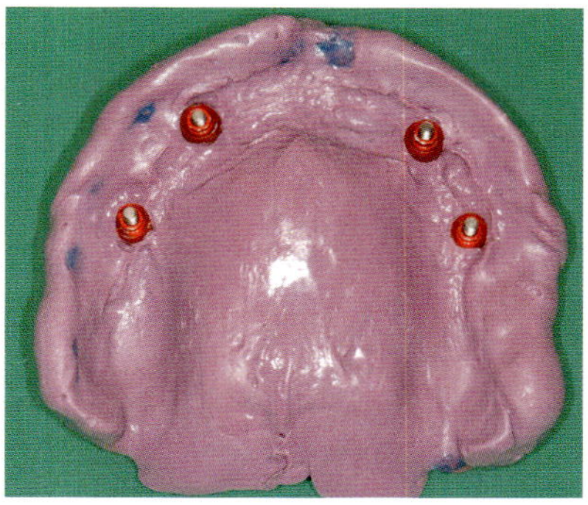

Fig 12 Basal side of the final impression.

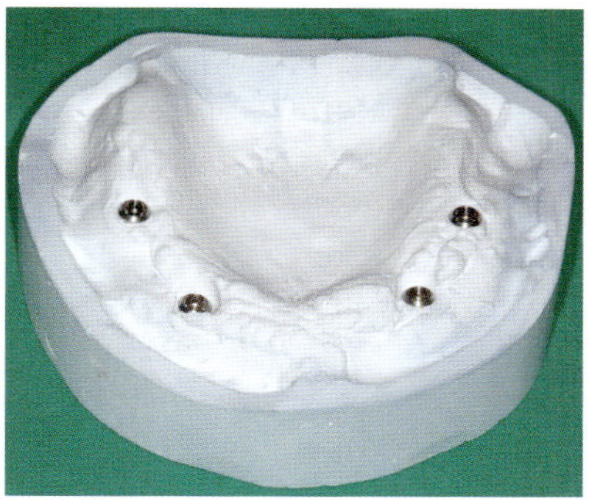

Fig 13 Final stone cast with implant analogs.

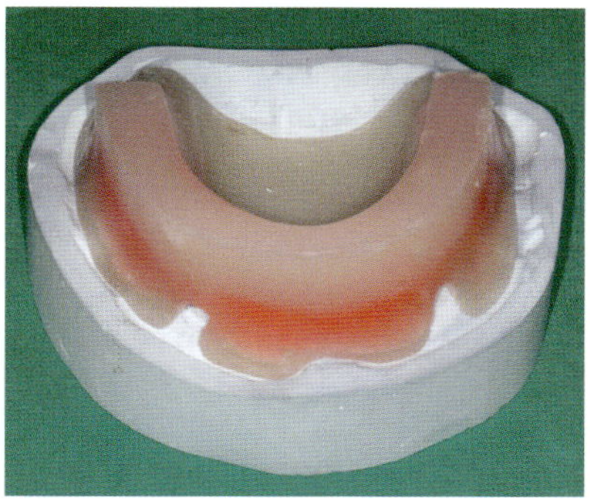

Fig 14 Occlusal wax rim on a composite-resin record base.

Fig 15 Maxillary bite rim base with two bite registration aids.

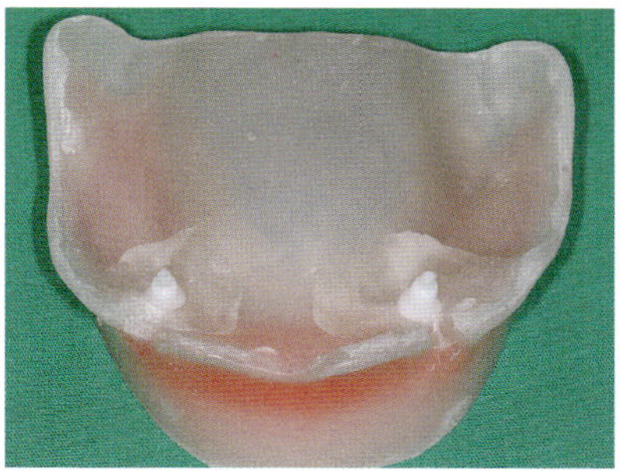

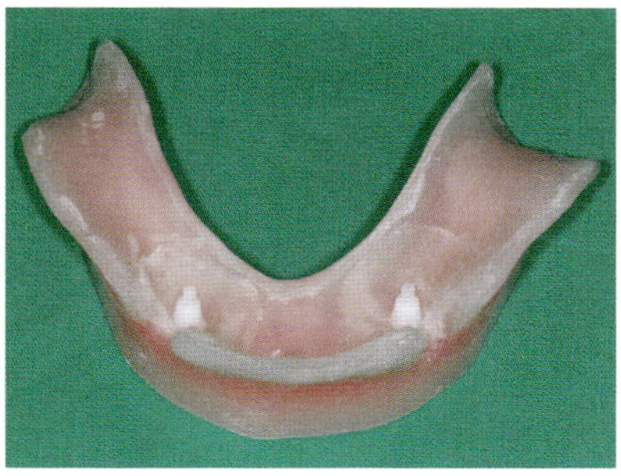

Fig 16 Mandibular bite rim base with two bite registration aids.

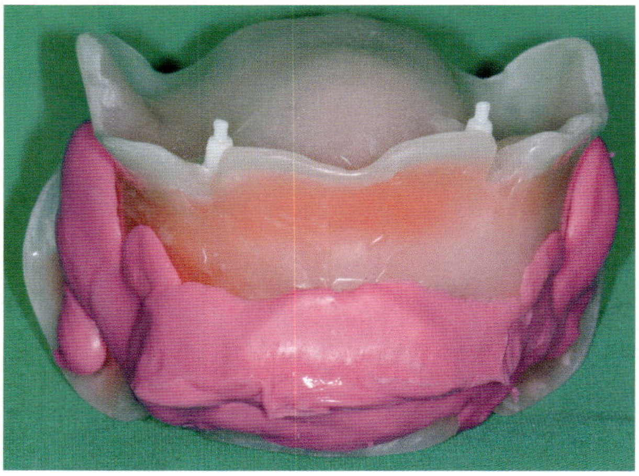

Fig 17 Maxillomandibular relationship stabilized with addition silicone (frontal view).

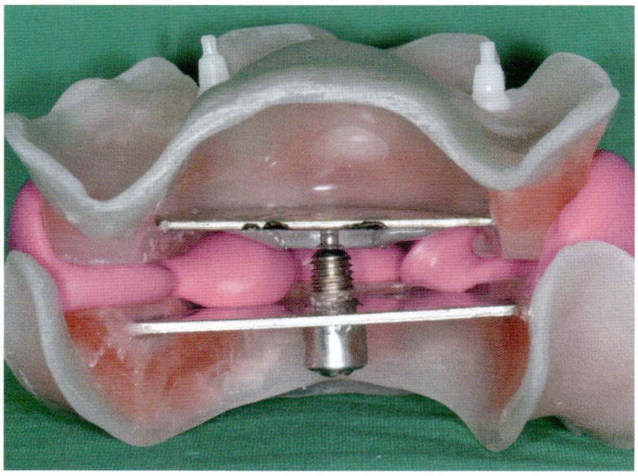

Fig 18 Maxillomandibular relationship stabilized with addition silicone (dorsal view).

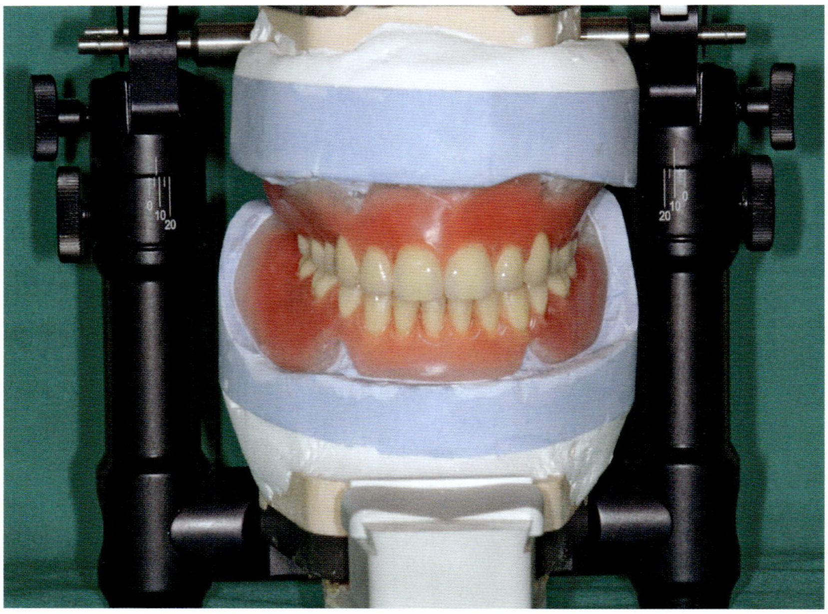

Fig 19 Tooth set-up in the articulator.

Acrylic denture teeth (Vivodent S PE; Ivoclar Vivadent, Schaan, Liechtenstein) were selected and placed on the base (Fig 19). The resulting trial denture was evaluated and adjusted as necessary to develop a balanced occlusion. Esthetics, phonetics, centric relation, occlusion, and vertical dimension were verified. The final result was approved by the patient.

The dental laboratory digitized the casts and arrangement and designed an ovoid bar, clips, and reinforcement on the implant analogs (Exocad, Darmstadt, Germany). It appeared that there was sufficient restorative space to accommodate the bar, clips, and reinforcement, confirming that the option of a bar/clip attachment, including a reinforcing structure, was indeed available (Figs 20 and 21).

The file was sent to a milling service (ES Healthcare, Hasselt, Belgium) where the maxillary and mandibular bars were milled from titanium. The resulting bars were placed on the original cast (Fig 22). Gold retentive clips (Cendres + Métaux, Biel/Bienne, Switzerland) were selected to fit the bars (Fig 23).

A refractory duplicate cast was fabricated with a silicone duplicating material (Elite Double 22; Zhermack, Badio Polesine, Italy). A framework pattern for the reinforcement structure was waxed onto the refractory cast. The modeled framework was cast in cobalt-chromium (Vitalium PH2; Elephant-Dental BV, Hoorn, The Netherlands) (Fig 24). The retention clips were laser-welded to the reinforcement structure under direct vision (Fig 25).

The reinforcement was integrated into the acrylic resin (Mega CRYL N; Megadental, Büdingen, Germany) of the overdenture. The advantage of this type of attachment is improved attachment performance with fewer fractures and less loosening of the clips (Slot and coworkers 2012).

The overdenture was processed and finished (Figs 26 and 27). The milled bars were placed on the implants, the attachment screws were tightened to 35 Ncm using a torque controller (Straumann Torque Control Device; Institut Straumann AG, Basel, Switzerland), and the overdenture was delivered (Figs 28 and 29).

After placement, the adaptation of the clips to the bar was checked with a silicone-based disclosing material (Fit Checker; GC, Tokyo, Japan), and the occlusion and articulation were examined. The patient was instructed on how to remove and insert the overdenture and how to clean it and the bar. If necessary, the retention force of the clips could be adjusted at this time.

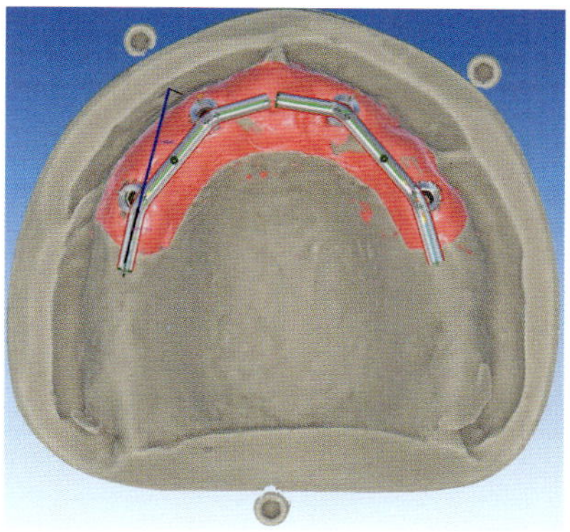

Fig 20 3D model with bar design on four implants (different patient).

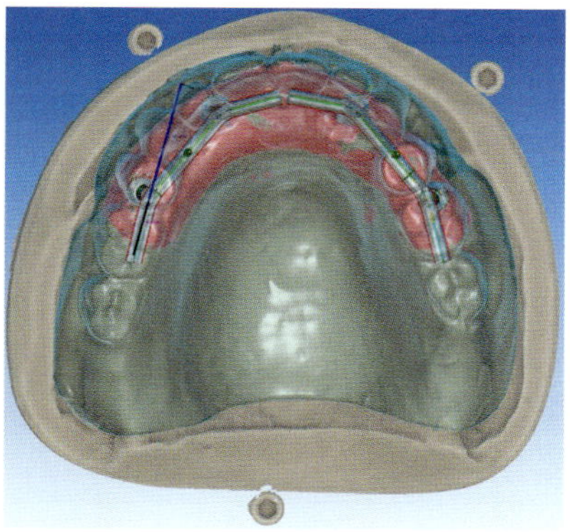

Fig 21 3D model with bar design in relation to tooth set-up (different patient).

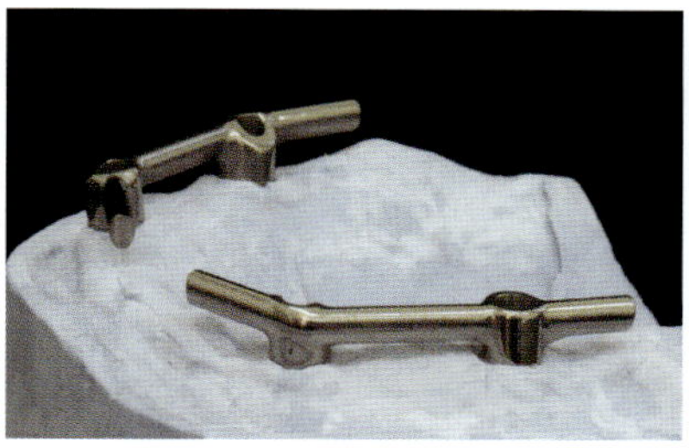

Fig 22 Titanium bars on final cast (different patient).

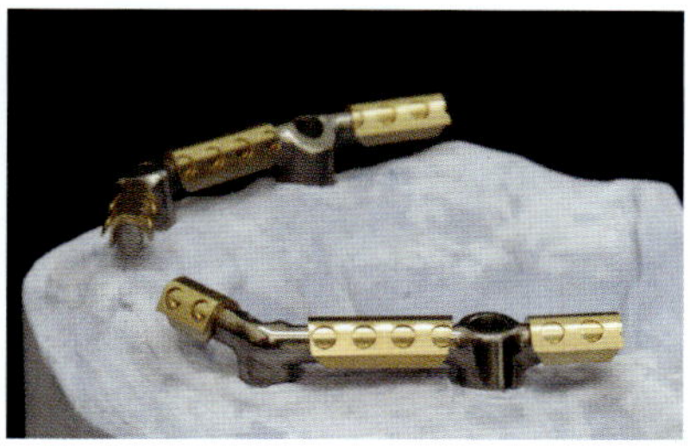

Fig 23 Titanium bars with gold clips (different patient).

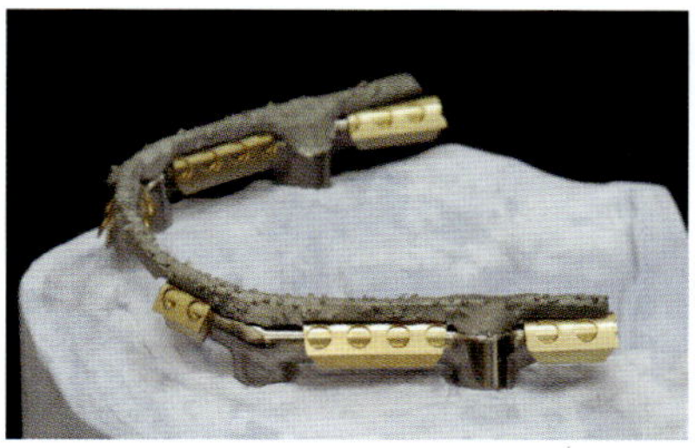

Fig 24 Titanium bars, gold clips. and cobalt-chromium reinforcement (different patient).

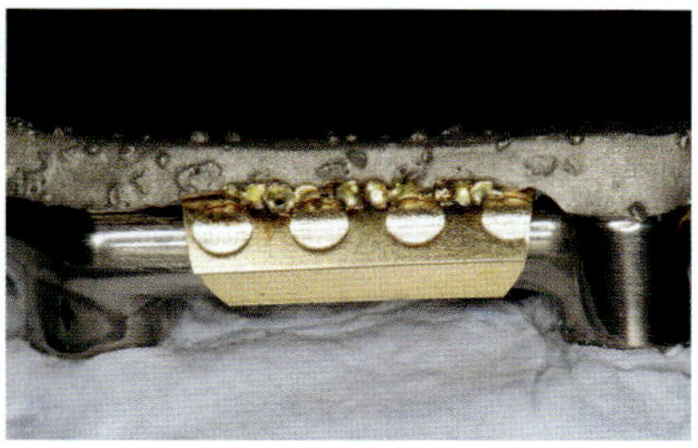

Fig 25 Clips laser-welded to cobalt-chromium reinforcement (different patient).

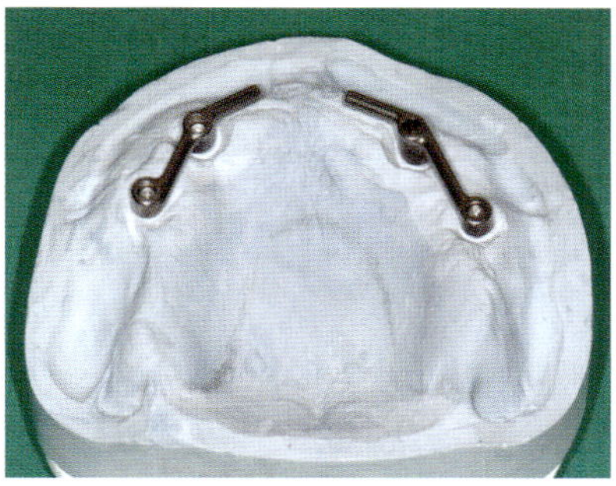

Fig 26 Titanium bars with anterior cantilevers on the master cast.

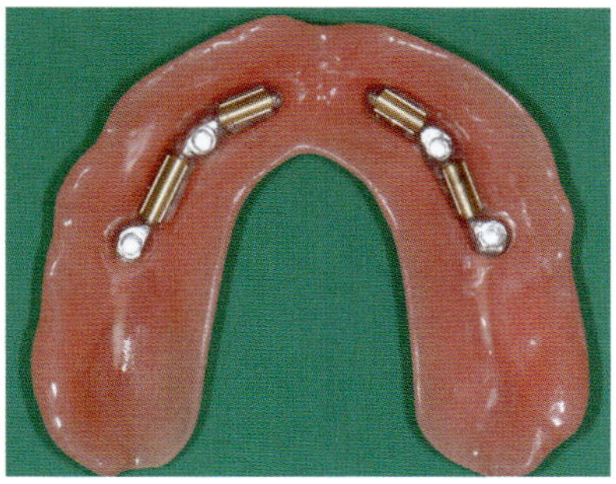

Fig 27 Basal side of the overdenture with gold clips attached to the reinforcement.

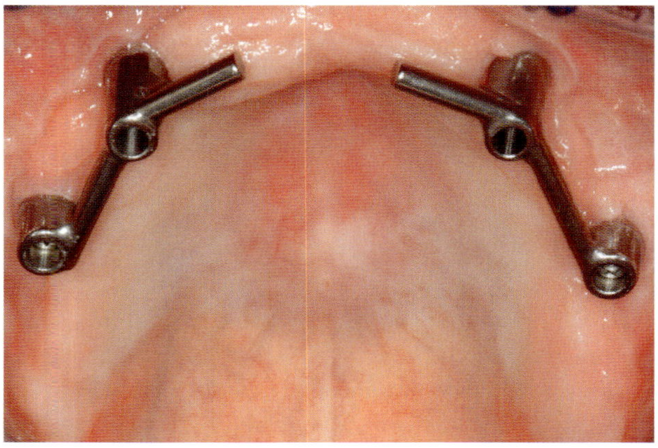

Fig 28 Titanium bars attached to the implants.

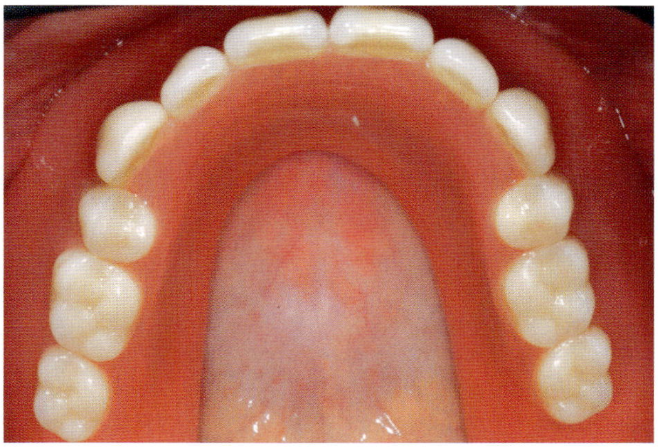

Fig 29 Intraoral view of the bar-supported overdenture.

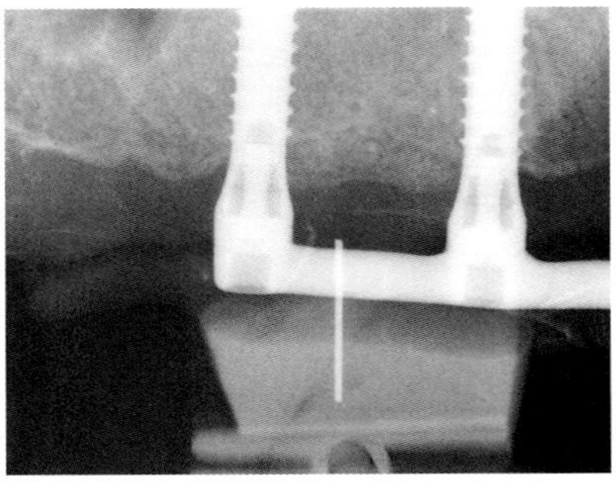

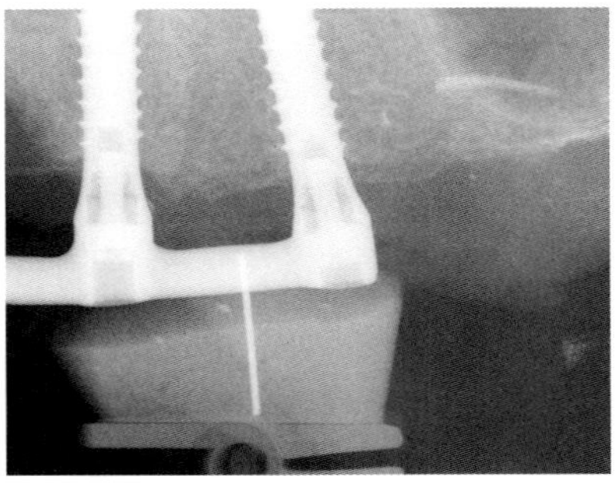

Fig 30 Intraoral radiograph 1 week after delivery of the overdenture (right part of the maxilla).

Fig 31 Intraoral radiograph 1 week after delivery of the overdenture (left part of the maxilla).

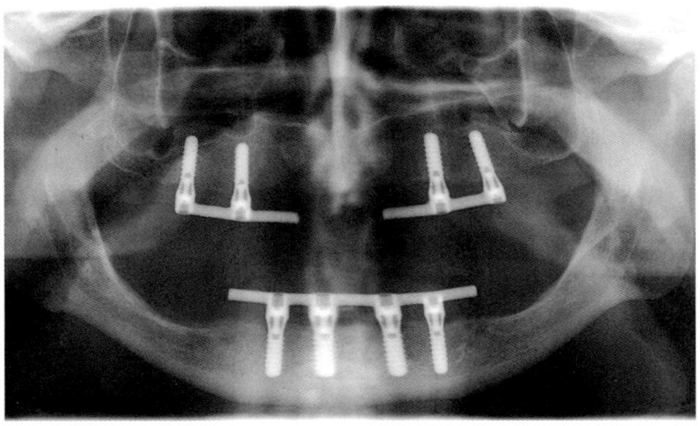

Fig 32 Panoramic rotational radiograph after 1 year in function.

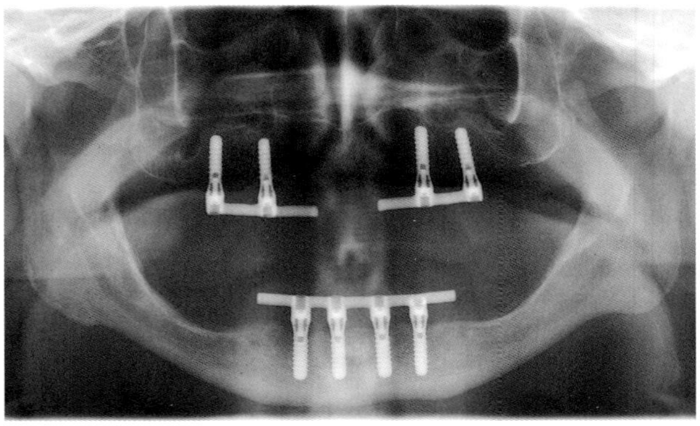

Fig 33 Panoramic rotational radiograph after 5 years in function.

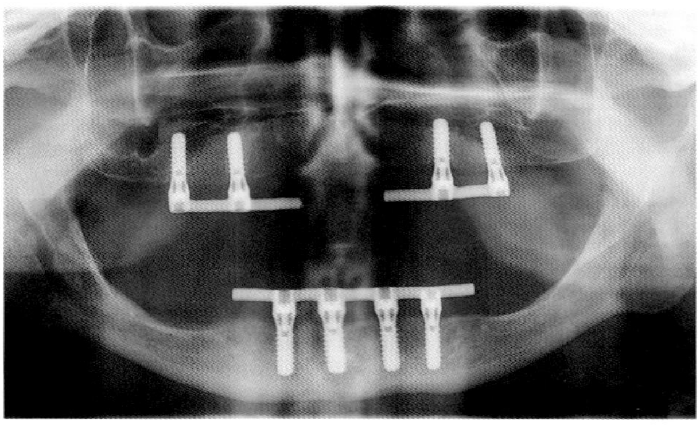

Fig 34 Panoramic rotational radiograph after 10 years in function.

The first follow-up examination was performed 1 week after delivery of the overdenture. Peri-implant radiographs were taken to record peri-implant bone levels at the beginning of the functional period (Figs 30 and 31).

FOLLOW-UP AND PATIENT SATISFACTION

A regular annual recall program was established. The status of the alveolar process was evaluated intraorally along with the peri-implant status (at that point: no plaque and no calculus, no infection of the peri-implant mucosa, sulcus depth not exceeding 3 mm, no bleeding on probing). The prosthesis was evaluated for fit, occlusion and articulation, denture base or tooth fracture, and clip loosening or fracture. At the 1-year, 5-year and 10-year follow-ups, the patient presented with a satisfactory clinical situation with healthy soft tissue, stable probing depths, and favorable peri-implant bone levels (Figs 32 to 34).

There were no complications during the 10 years and the patient was still very satisfied with the improved function of his maxillary denture.

DISCUSSION

The case presented here is an example case from a randomized controlled trial comparing a bar-supported maxillary overdenture on four implants with a bar-supported maxillary overdenture on six implants. The overall conclusion of the randomized controlled trial after 1, 5 and 10 years was that bar-supported overdentures on four implants in the posterior region of an augmented maxilla resulted in high implant survival, limited peri-implant marginal bone loss, healthy peri-implant soft tissue, and high patient satisfaction (Slot and coworkers 2013, 2019, 2022). No significant differences were found between the four-implant overdenture group and the six-implant overdenture group. For economic reasons, the treatment with four bar-connected implants to support a maxillary overdenture should be preferred. This number of implants was also confirmed in a systematic review with meta-analysis by Di Francesco and coworkers (2019).

Due to the extremely resorbed maxillary alveolar process, there was insufficient bone height and width to place the implants without bone augmentation. This type of augmentation requires more bone than is available intraorally. Therefore, it was decided to augment the sinus floor and reconstruct the alveolar ridge width with iliac-crest bone grafts. Although it has been reported that implant survival rates in jaws augmented with iliac-crest grafts were lower than in jaws augmented with intraoral bone grafts, and although more donor-site complications were reported, implant survival rates were high at 5 and 10 years (McKenna and coworkers 2022).

Overdentures with bar attachments offer many advantages in patients with severely resorbed edentulous ridges. Bars provide good retention, have low maintenance costs, provide the correct dimensions, and facilitate the insertion and removal of the denture (Bueno-Samper and coworkers 2010). Bar design is individualized. Digital planning software can be a helpful tool to gain insight into available space. Ideally, the workflow should be driven by backward planning, starting with the ideal positions of the future prosthetic teeth. There must be sufficient restorative space to accommodate the bar, clips, and reinforcement structure. Preferably, the bar and clips should not be positioned in the anterior region because the metal could compromise esthetics by shading the acrylic resin. A split-bar design with separate bars on two implants in the posterior region is preferred. Another rationale for a split-bar design is that implants should be more or less parallel to make it possible to allow the bar to conform to the implant for greater stability and to reduce the forces acting on the screws. In the edentulous maxilla, this is often not possible with four implants for anatomical reasons.

The advantage of CAD/CAM bars is that parallel-walled ovoid bars can be designed with an optimal insertion path of the overdenture. The gold clips can be easily adjusted for more or less friction, depending on the patient's preference and manual dexterity. The gold clips are laser-welded to the reinforcement structure, resulting in much less loosening than when embedded in acrylic resin. However, in the rare event of clip fracture or loosening, it is not possible to reattach the clips to the supporting structure. The retentive portions of the clip must be positioned conventionally in acrylic resin (Slot and coworkers 2012).

ACKNOWLEDGMENTS

Laboratory procedures

Gerrit van Dijk – Groningen, The Netherlands

5.5 Mandibular Implant-Retained Overdenture on a CAD/CAM-Milled, Parallel-Walled CrCoMo Bar

A. Boeckler, D. Morton

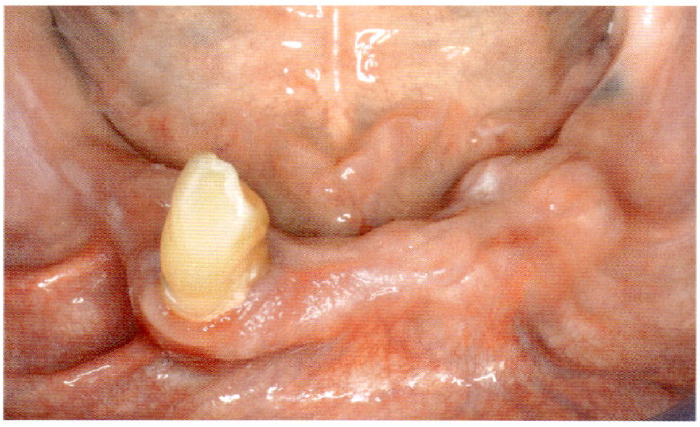

Fig 1 Baseline situation. Partially dentate patient.

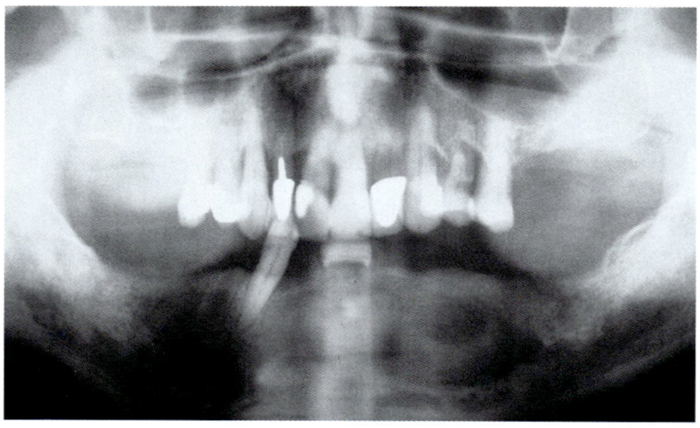

Fig 2 Baseline panoramic radiograph.

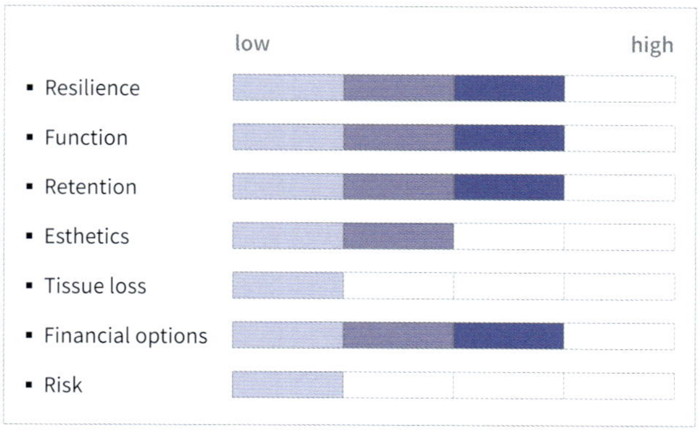

Fig 3 Patient profile.

PATIENT CHARACTERISTICS AND PATIENT PROFILE

A 72-year-old male patient, partially dentate, presented with a request for a more functional and esthetic solution for his mandibular arch. He had lost his mandibular teeth over a period of more than twenty years due to a combination of periodontal disease and dental caries. He was not satisfied with his existing mandibular prosthesis, which was stabilized by his single remaining tooth 43 (Fig 1). A pretreatment panoramic radiograph confirmed the absence of pathology (Fig 2). The patient was ambulatory, alert, and philosophical, and denied any health problems that would affect the dental treatment.

The patient had indicated that the esthetic appearance of his teeth was of moderate importance to him. His focus was on functional improvement. The patient had initially rejected the proposed treatment, but after detailed explanations of the procedures and their likely outcome, as well as alternative treatment options such as implant-supported fixed prostheses or a conventional denture, he felt more confident with the proposed treatment and believed it provided good value for money.

Based on this information and the clinical evaluation described below, the following patient profile (Fig 3) can be derived for this patient (for more Information about patient profiles, see Chapters 2.1.3 and 3.6).

CLINICAL EVALUATION AND TREATMENT PLAN

Intraoral evaluation found tooth 43 to be associated with gingivitis and probing depths of 5–6 mm. Additionally, the tooth demonstrated class II mobility according to Miller (1938). The mandibular mucosa appeared healthy with a mostly adequate band of keratinized tissue. As a result of tooth loss occurring over an extended period, the residual ridge was inconsistent in volume, with the anterior more robust than the posterior regions.

The remaining maxillary teeth were considered stable despite increased mobility (class II) subsequent to periodontal treatment as a result of horizontal and vertical bone loss.

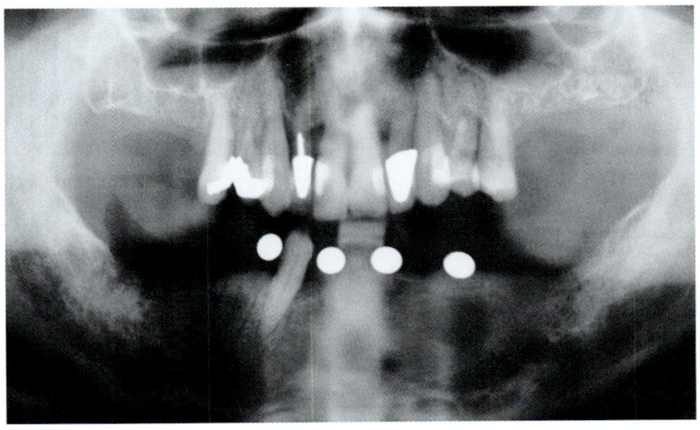

Fig 4 Panoramic radiograph with stainless-steel reference balls.

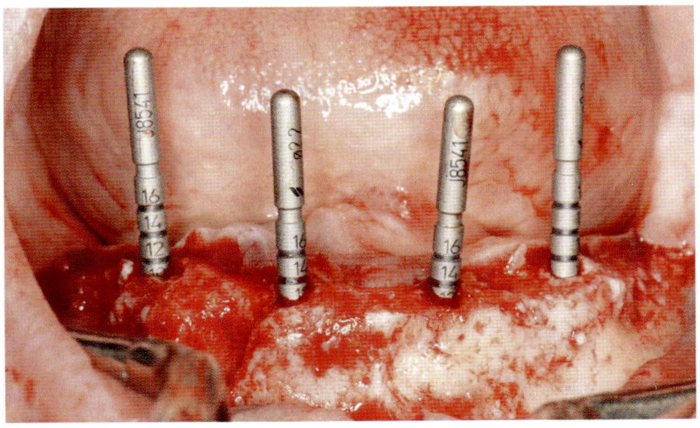

Fig 5 Guide pins to confirm the proper inclination of the implant bed after each size of twist drill.

Probing depths ranged between 3 and 5 mm. The existing prosthesis replacing the molars was stabilized by clasps on the premolars.

To facilitate implant planning, a panoramic radiograph was obtained using a duplicate of his existing removable partial prosthesis (Fig 4). Stainless-steel reference balls were incorporated into the duplicate denture to facilitate assessment of the vertical bone height in the mandible and to relate the mental foramen to the markers. The radiograph indicated adequate height for the placement of four dental implants while providing for an appropriate safety zone around the mental nerve.

Several treatment alternatives were proposed for the mandibular arch. Each option included the extraction of tooth 43 and delivery of an immediate mandibular complete denture, to be followed by one of:

- A definitive conventional complete denture
- An attachment-supported definitive complete denture on two or four implants
- A definitive complete denture supported by a digitally designed milled bar attachments
- A complete implant-supported fixed mandibular prosthesis

The patient explained that until recently he had been satisfied with the functional and esthetic characteristics of his removable partial prosthesis. He was therefore more comfortable with the idea of a new removable treatment option assisted by dental implants. Risks associated with the proposed treatment options were presented, including compromised healing subsequent to the extraction of tooth 43, and failure of one or more of the implants. The difficulty associated with domestic oral hygiene, the risk of biofilm-associated failure resulting from plaque adhesion to the bar and denture base, the loss of retention associated with the attachments, and the biomechanical failure of the bar or the metal/acrylic prosthesis were also discussed.

Once all questions had been answered to the patient's satisfaction, the patient consented to the following treatment plan:

Extraction of tooth 43, immediate placement of four dental implants and delivery of an immediate mandibular complete denture. After healing of the implants, surgical reentry (second-stage surgery) with concurrent grafting to improve the width of the keratinized mucosa around the healed implants. After healing of the soft-tissue grafts, fabrication of an implant-supported bar-retained complete mandibular denture.

SURGICAL PROCEDURES

The radiographic template was converted into a surgical template by removing the stainless-steel markers and modifying the space to provide mesiodistal and orofacial guidance during the preparation of the osteotomies.

After anesthesia was provided with articaine and epinephrine 1 : 100,000 (articaine hydrochloride 40 mg/ml with adrenaline 0,012mg/ml), a full-thickness mucoperiosteal flap was elevated with distal vertical releasing incisions. Tooth 43 was extracted, exposing a moderate defect of the buccal alveolar bone. The osteotomies for the implants were prepared with twist drills according to the manufacturer's guidelines. The osteotomies were reviewed using guide pins after each twist drill diameter to confirm their proper inclination (Fig 5). Four dental implants (Bone Level SLActive, diameter 4.1 mm, length 10 mm; Institute Straumann AG, Basel, Switzerland) were placed and cover screws were positioned without incident. A panoramic radiograph was obtained immediately after the surgery (Fig 6).

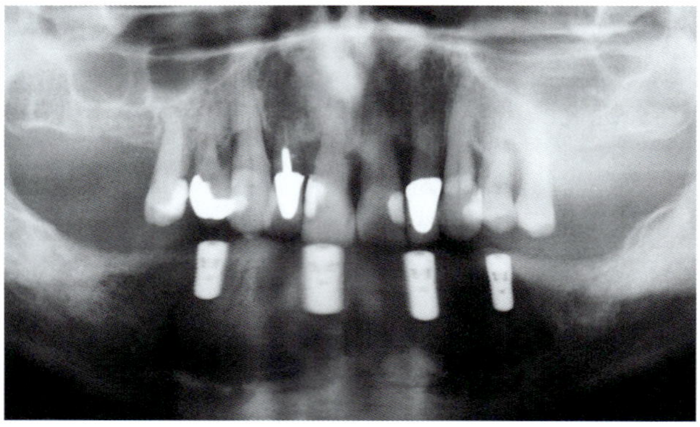

Fig 6 Panoramic radiograph with implants in place.

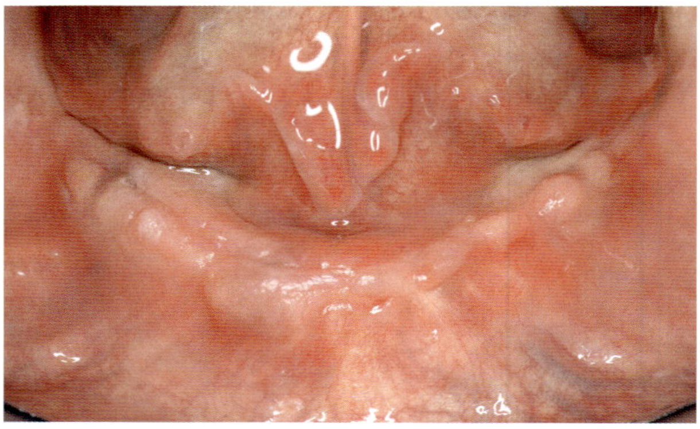

Fig 7 Healed mandible with osseointegrated implants.

The immediate denture was relieved in the regions of the four implants and relined with tissue conditioner. After minor occlusal adjustments, the patient was discharged with postoperative instructions. The implants healed without complications within 3 months.

The implants were surgically uncovered under local anesthesia and their stability was confirmed. The band of keratinized mucosa around the implants was increased with apical repositioning of the flap (Fig 7). Healing abutments (4 mm in height) were connected (Fig 8).

The patient's immediate denture was modified to provide space above the healing abutments and relined with tissue conditioner. After 8 weeks, the peri-implant tissues were evaluated and considered stable and healthy.

PROSTHETIC PROCEDURES

The healing abutments were removed and screw-retained abutments (SRA) were connected at the appropriate torque. Open-tray impression copings were positioned on each abutment (Fig 9), and a polyvinyl siloxane (PVS) impression was made. Implant analogs were positioned in the impression and verified for adaptation (Fig 10). Healing caps were placed on each SRA. The patient's immediate denture was relieved to provide space and relined with tissue conditioner.

The master cast was poured in type IV dental stone. A matrix was fabricated on the master cast; passive seating was confirmed clinically to verify the accuracy of the cast. Stabilized baseplates and wax rims were fabricated and used to record the patient's centric relation position and vertical dimension of occlusion. A facebow registration was also obtained and the casts were transferred to a semi-adjustable articulator. The trial denture was prepared and the records confirmed during clinical try-in. The patient approved the esthetic tooth set-up and gave his consent to proceed (Fig 11).

The trial denture and master cast were scanned and the data transferred to a software program. Using the approved denture as a guide, the bar and the abutment/attachment complex were digitally designed on four screw-retained abutments (SRA; Institute Straumann AG, Basel, Switzerland) (Fig 12). The design maintained adequate space for the attachments, framework, base resin, and denture teeth.

The metal bar was milled in cobalt-chromium-molybdenum (CoCrMo) alloy, finished and tapped to facilitate the placement of five Locator abutments (Locator Implant Attachment System; Zest Dental Solutions, Carlsbad, CA, USA). The passivity of the bar was evaluated on the verified master cast, and the contours and available space for oral hygiene were evaluated and confirmed (Figs 13 and 14). The finished bar was then evaluated intraorally. A passive fit and appropriate contour were confirmed.

A putty matrix fabricated from the wax trial denture was used to reposition the denture teeth and relate the definitive overdenture to the bar (Fig 12). A framework was designed to adapt accurately to the milled bar and cast in cobalt-chromium (CoCr) alloy. The framework was designed to maintain space for each Locator attachment to be picked up in acrylic resin. The definitive denture base was then waxed up over the supporting framework, and final contours were established. The denture was invested, processed in polymethyl methacrylate (PMMA), and finished (Fig 15).

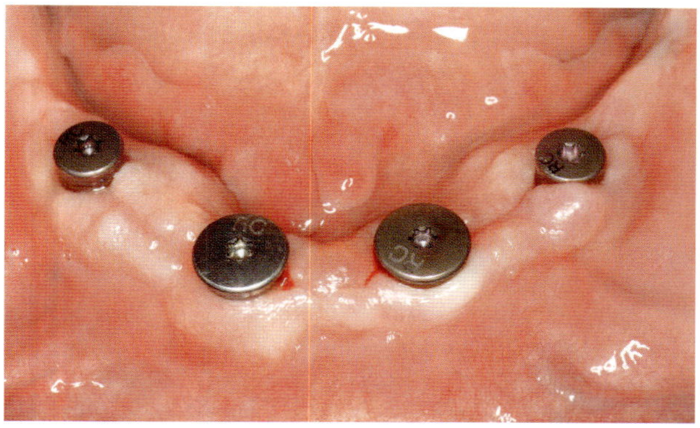

Fig 8 Healing abutments.

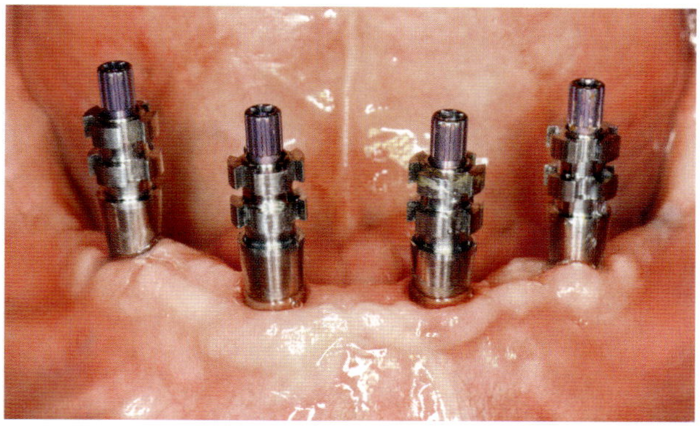

Fig 9 Impression copings.

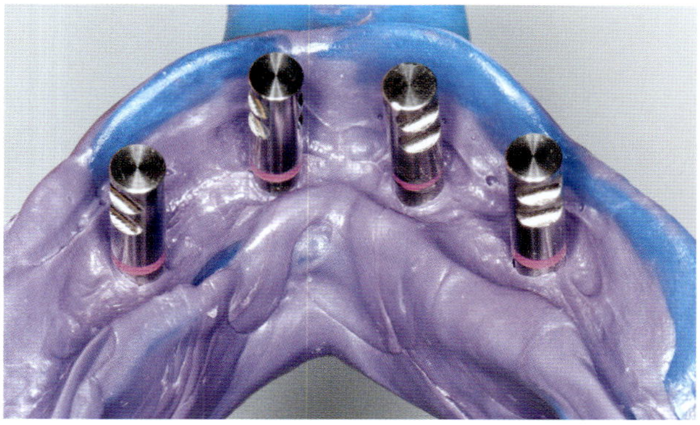

Fig 10 Impression with implant analogs.

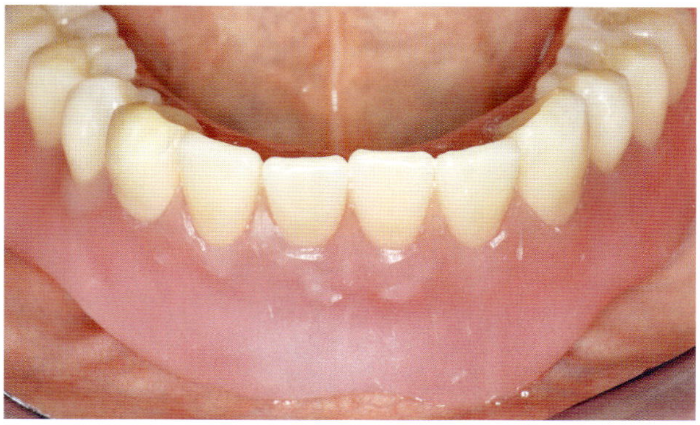

Fig 11 Trial denture.

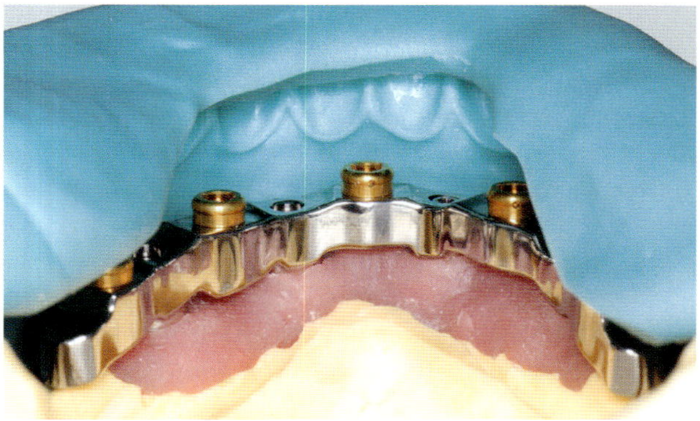

Fig 12 Putty matrix fabricated from the trial denture.

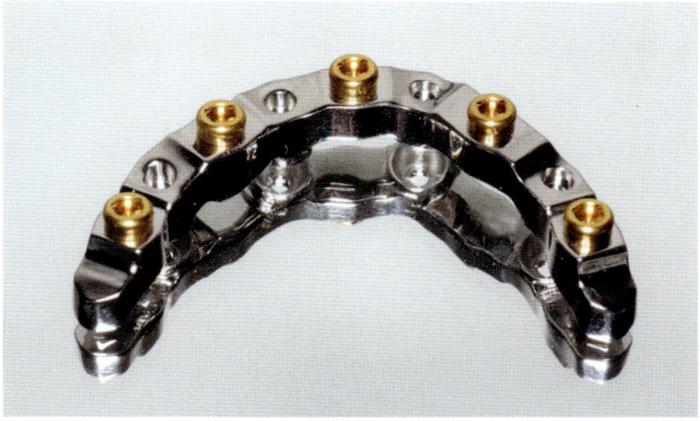

Fig 13 Milled metal bar with Locator attachments.

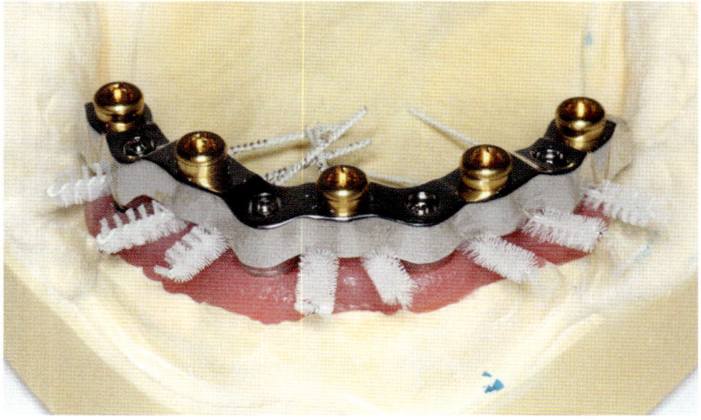

Fig 14 Evaluation of contour and space for oral hygiene.

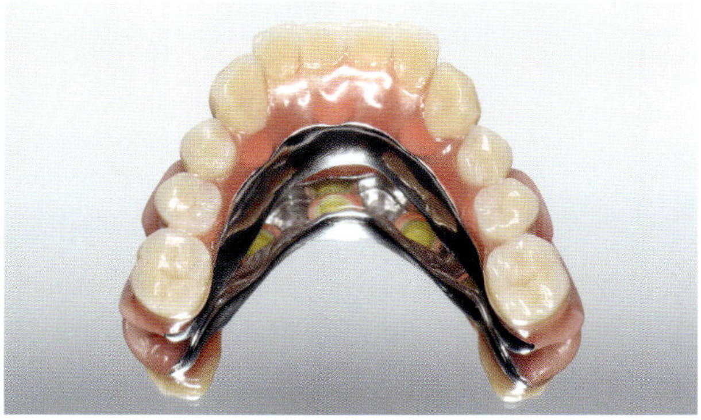

Fig 15 The finished denture.

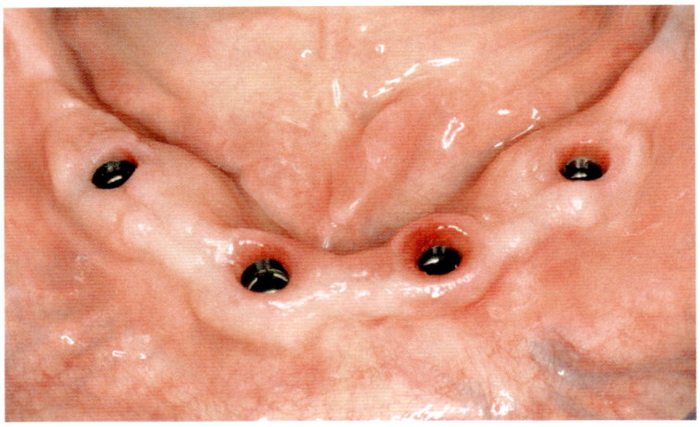

Fig 16 Mandible with matured gingiva.

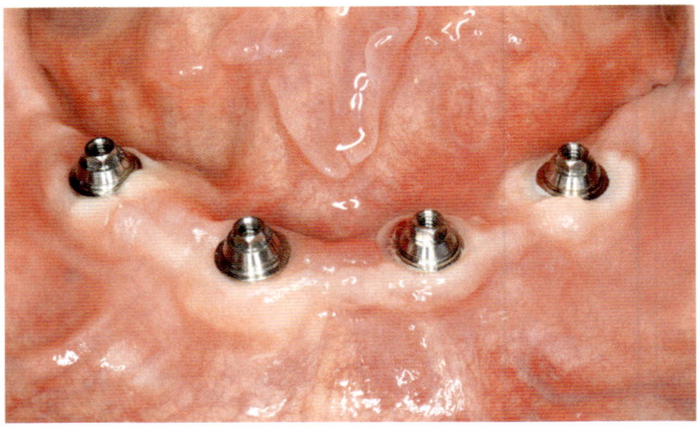

Fig 17 Screw-retained abutments.

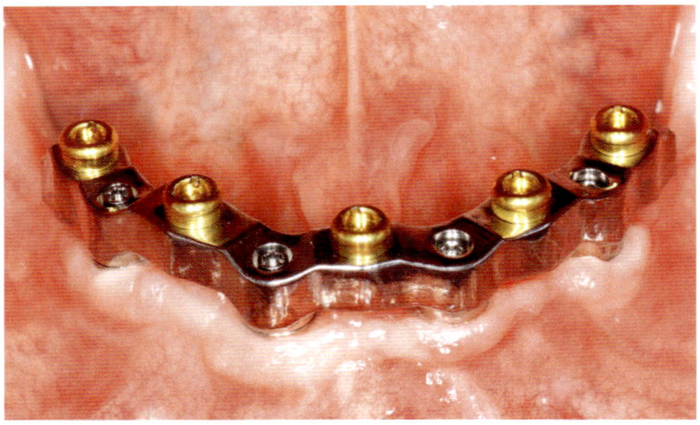

Fig 18 Finished metal bar with passive fit.

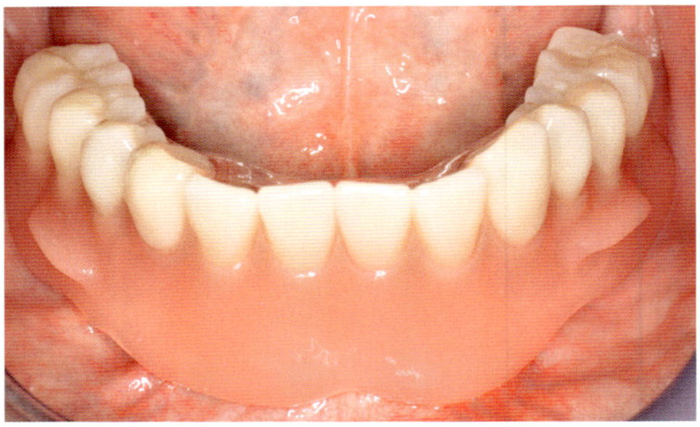

Fig 19 The denture was evaluated for tissue adaptation.

Prior to picking up the Locator attachments, the denture was evaluated for adaptation to the tissues and adjusted as required. A clinical remount was performed and the occlusion carefully adjusted. The Locator attachments were picked up individually.

The benefit of single attachments in combination with a solid milled bar is, that the retentive components of the attachment system—such as Locator—are manufactured in an industrial process. Compared to alternative attachment systems for bars (e.g., galvanic matrices, spark-eroded friction pins, ovate-shaped retentions according to Dolder, etc.) the maintenance is comparable easy to manage and the financial costs are low.

The torque of each SR abutment (35 Ncm) and retaining screw (15 Ncm) was confirmed (Figs 16 to 19) and the prosthesis was delivered to the patient.

It was confirmed that the patient could remove and insert the prosthesis without complications. He was given detailed instructions for home care and advised to return for evaluation after 1 week, 1 month, and 3 months to confirm effective maintenance, occlusion, and esthetic satisfaction.

The patient returned for evaluation as recommended. At the 1-week appointment, he described some difficulty removing the prosthesis. The five standard-range nylon retentive inserts initially provided were replaced with three extended-range inserts with medium retentive capacity and two retentive inserts with zero retention to add stability while enabling removal with greater ease (Figs 20 and 21). The patient expressed complete satisfaction with the retentive capacity of the new inserts and was able to remove and replace the prosthesis without difficulty. The passive fit of the bar structure was confirmed clinically and by panoramic radiograph (Fig 22).

FOLLOW-UP AND PATIENT SATISFACTION

According to the Implant Disease Risk Assessment (IDRA), the design of the screw-retained milled bar structure provides optimal access for oral hygiene procedures.

The patient was placed on a customized supportive periodontal care (SPC) program and referred to a dental hygienist for professional plaque removal every 4 months. The patient has been diligent with the recommended follow-up protocol and continues to maintain excellent oral hygiene.

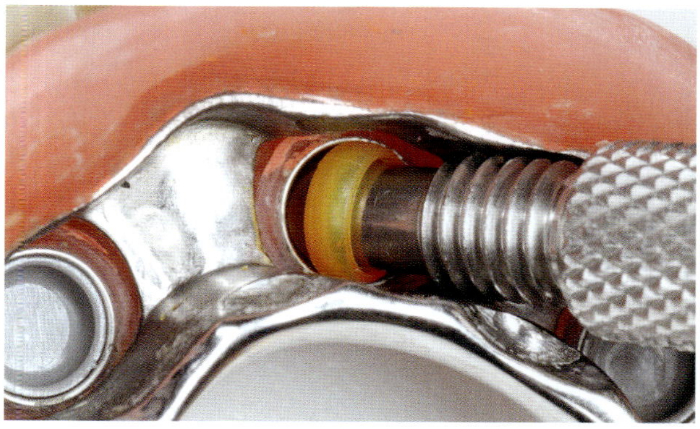

F g 20 Replacement of nylon inserts.

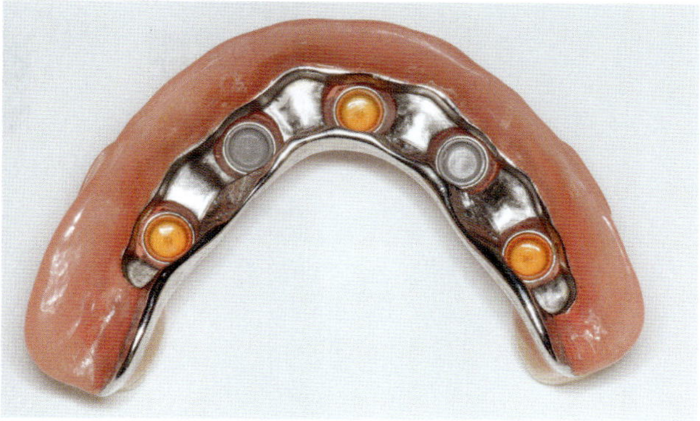

Fig 21 Extended-range inserts.

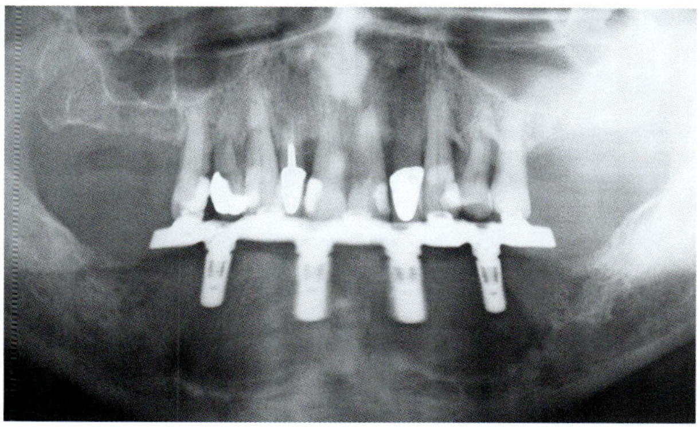

Fig 22 Panoramic radiograph with screw-retained bar.

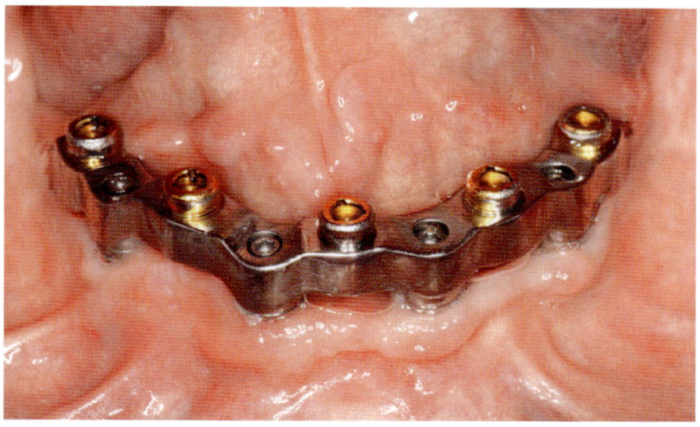

Fig 23 Clinical follow-up of metal bar.

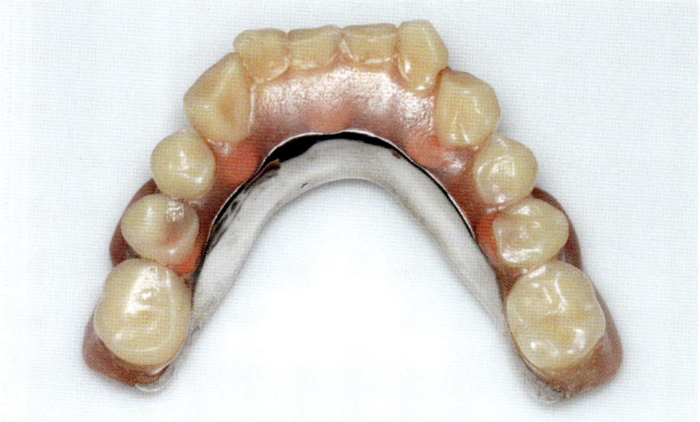

Fig 24 Denture with abraded acrylic teeth.

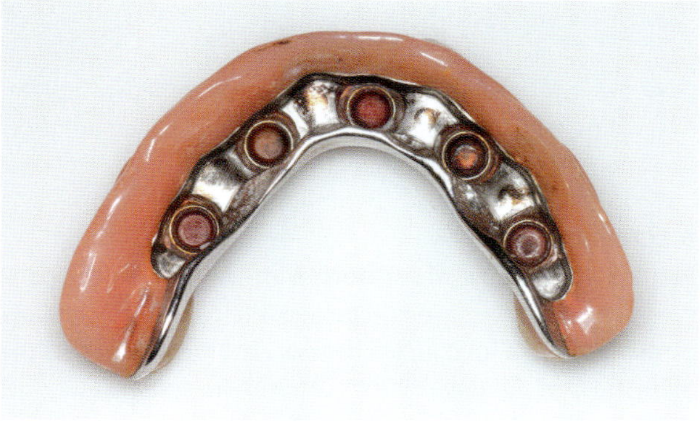

Fig 25 Worn extended-range nylon inserts.

Over 11 years of follow-ups, only minor adjustments and repairing were needed (Figs 23 to 25). The Locator attachments were changed due to retention loss after 4 years and again after another 5 years of service.

This relatively long period of function of Locator inserts can be explained by the stability of the denture on the bar structure. The control of movement, in particular bending moments, between the bar and prosthesis seems to be beneficial in the long term. Nevertheless, the Locator attachments showed mechanical wear, manifested as loss of retention over time (Fig 23). To address this problem, five light-retention extended-range inserts were integrated (Fig 25). Alternatively, the worn Locator abutments can easily be replaced in combination with new inserts in the future.

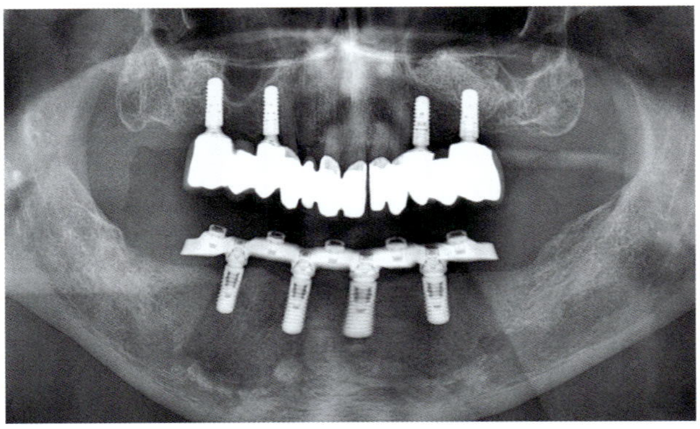

Fig 26 Panoramic radiograph of the metal bar after 11 years in function.

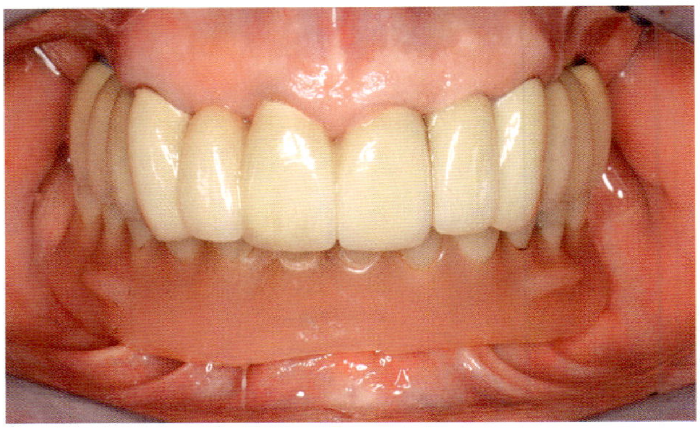

Fig 27 Intraoral situation with denture in place.

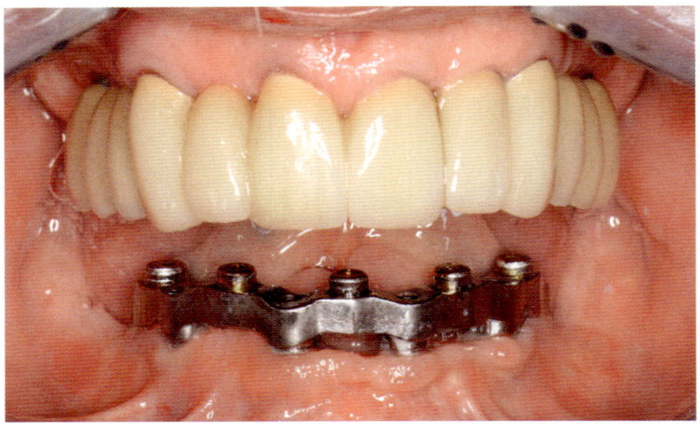

Fig 28 Intraoral situation presenting the bar structure with worn Locator abutments.

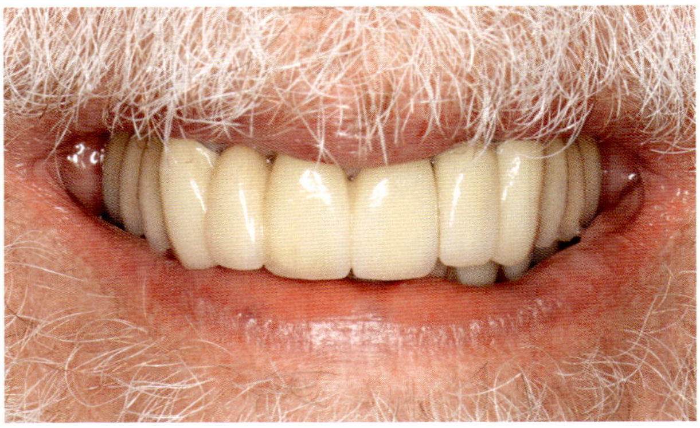

Fig 29 The patient's smile.

Over the last 11 years, the patient has remained completely satisfied with the functional and esthetic outcome of his treatment (Figs 26 to 29).

DISCUSSION

Rationale for the use of Locators: With CAD/CAM-milled bars, the friction elements are freely selectable. Single attachments combined with a solid milled bar have the advantage that the retentive components of the attachment system—such as the Locator system—are industrially manufactured. Maintenance is relatively easy and inexpensive compared to alternative bar attachment systems (such as electroplated matrices, spark-eroded friction pins, or ovoid Dolder retentions). The milled bar is effective in providing stability (resistance to movement in all directions other than the path of insertion and removal) and uses friction to provide retention. While Locator attachments can assist with stability, the milled bar is the primary stabilizing factor. However, while Locators provide direct retention (resistance to movement away from the tissue), the bar does not.

Rationale for using five (rather than three or four) Locators: During treatment planning, the patient expressed a desire for a stable prosthesis with superior retention, so it was decided to place five Locators to be on the safe side. After the first few weeks of training, the patient became very comfortable with handling the restoration and noticed an excessive retention force. Had this been recognized earlier, the number of the attachments could have been safely limited to the standard three or at most four Locators.

Locators provide retention along the path of insertion and removal. They are most effective when widely distributed (in the anterior and posterior regions) and reasonably symmetrical (right and left side). A greater number of attachments will usually enhance this distribution, while the amount of retention achieved will still vary depending on the choice of inserts.

Advantages of parallel bars over round bars: The advantage of single attachments combined with a solid milled bar is that the retentive components are industrially manufactured. A classic round bar on implants (four in this case) that were positioned to form a polygon has almost no effective degrees of freedom. There is no biomechanical advantage of a round bar design on four implants over the milled design. Furthermore, a parallel bar resists torquing forces. For example, when chewing forces are applied to the front of a round bar, the restoration can pivot and lift at the back. Parallel bars resist this torque and improve the stability of the restoration.

Incorporation of natural teeth into the restoration: An alternative solution would have been a mixed tooth/implant-supported restoration on telescopic crowns, in this case a telescopic crown on tooth 43 and three implants in the edentulous regions, also with telescopic crowns. If the last remaining canine in this case had exhibited only low mobility (grade I) and no need for periodontal treatment, the mixed concept could have been considered. But here the remaining natural tooth was in no condition to remain in place for 10 years or more in a telescopic restoration; the risk of early loss was significant. In addition, the telescopic tooth/implant design—which appears to be more popular in Europe than in the Americas or Asia—is expensive.

Rationale for analog impressions: Analog impressions are still the most reliable. And even with an optical impression, we make a try-in with a screw-retained mock-up before milling. However, optical impressions are improving, but both options still require verification casts and an intraoral evaluation of fit—any errors will usually be costly.

5.6 Fully Guided and Minimally Invasive Implant Placement as the Basis for Effective Digital Fabrication of a Tapered-Crown Full-Arch Prosthesis

P. Gutmann, T. Peter, P. Parvini, P. Weigl

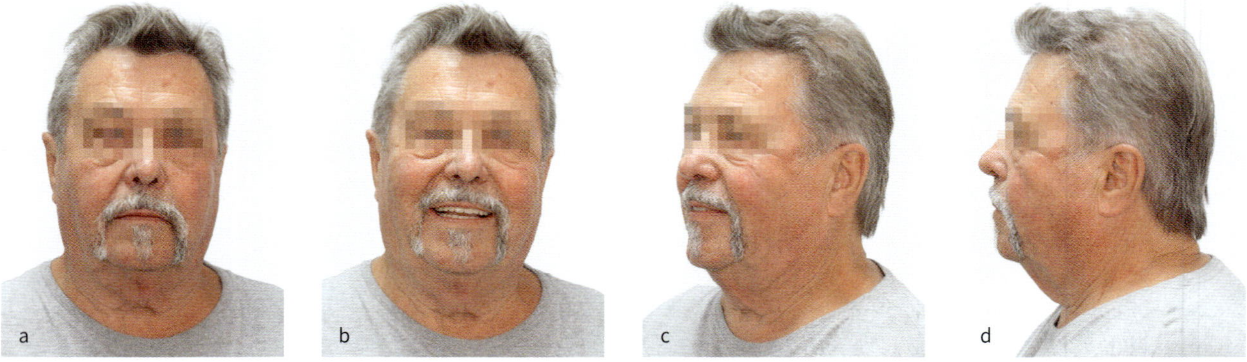

Figs 1a-d Initial extraoral situation.

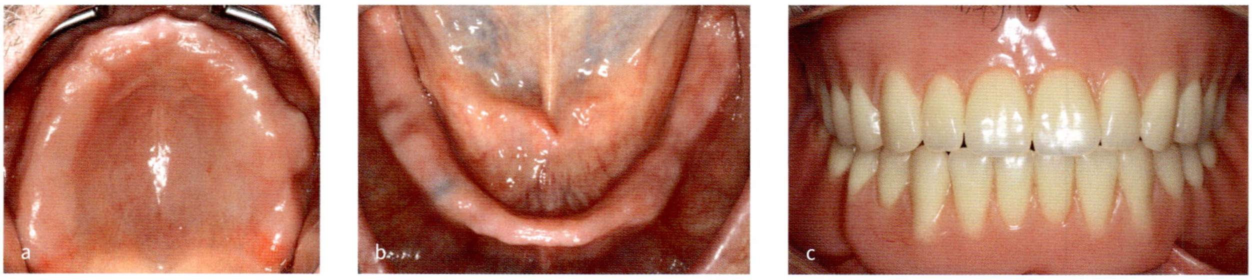

Figs 2a-c Initial intraoral situation.

A 74-year-old male patient presented to the Department of Oral Medicine at the Goethe University in Frankfurt, Germany. The patient had been edentulous for 15 months and had been treated with a complete denture by students in the undergraduate program.

During a recall appointment, the patient complained of poor retention of his maxillary complete denture (Figs 1a-d and 2a-c). The prosthetic site consisted of a rigid and thick maxillary ridge with an undercut in the left posterior region. The prosthesis covered the entire palate and was dislodged by biting on solid foods such as apples. The patient did not have high esthetic expectations, but he did want improved chewing comfort and "fixed teeth." He was particularly interested in a palate-free maxillary restoration that would require little long-term maintenance and allow him to bite firmly and enjoy the taste experience. As a former chef, he really missed the latter.

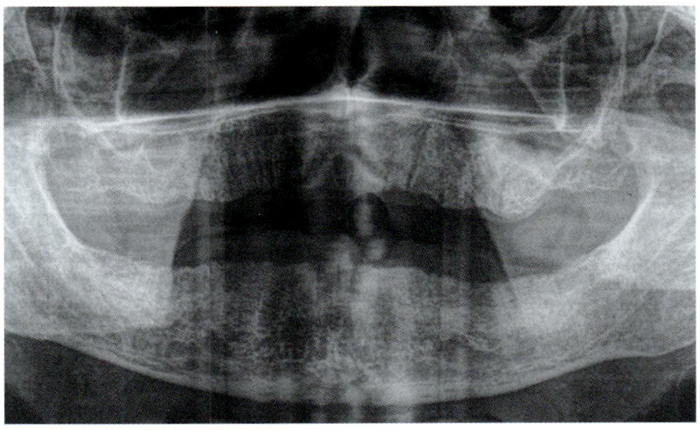

Fig 3 Initial radiograph.

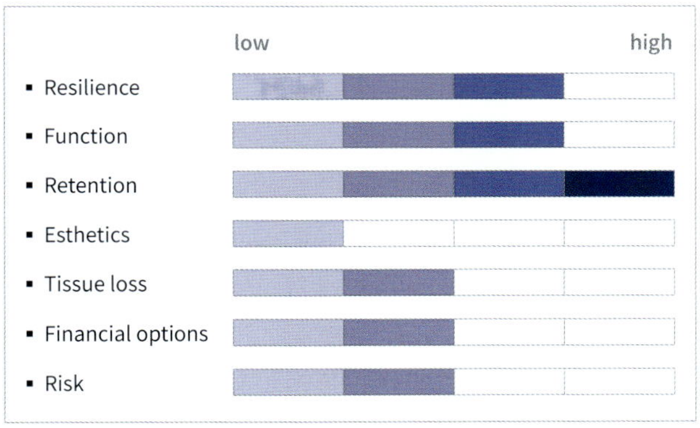

Fig 4 Patient profile.

The patient had been retired for several years, lived with his wife, and was physically and mentally fit. With a busy family life and a long commute, he wanted quick and painless implant-based therapy in as few sessions as possible. With his savings, the patient was able to afford high-quality treatment.

The patient was on direct oral anticoagulants (apixaban 5 mg/d) as a preventive medication due to atrial fibrillation. The patient had previously undergone surgical resection for gastric MALT lymphoma and was treated with chemotherapy and rituximab (no radiation). Due to his medical history, the patient wanted a less painful and minimally invasive form of treatment. There were no general medical conditions that would have increased the risk of implant loss. The patient regularly attended recall appointments and took excellent care of his prostheses. He did not smoke, did not have diabetes, and did not have a history of head and neck radiation.

The following patient profile was determined according to Wolfart et al. (2023) (Fig 4).

Patient wishes and expectations

- **Resilience:** The patient was physically fit and very resilient. He would have liked a little downtime to help his family at home (level 3).
- **Function:** The patient tolerated removable dentures well and would have continued to tolerate removable dentures (level 3).
- **Retention:** The patient's main concern was a palate-free denture that was as stable as possible (level 4).
- **Esthetics:** Esthetics and appearance of the denture were of secondary importance to the patient (level 1).

Patient-related baseline factors

- **Tissue loss:** Due to the vertical loss of the anterior alveolar ridge and the ease of cleaning, a telescopic prosthesis seemed a suitable solution (level 2).
- **Financial options:** The patient had public health insurance and wanted to invest his savings in a new prosthetic rehabilitation. Because of the priority of an uncovered palate to improve taste and the poor retention of the complete maxillary denture, the patient initially financed a new implant-supported restoration in the maxilla (Srinivasan and coworkers 2023) (level 2).
- **Risk:** After evaluation of the existing orthopantomogram (Fig 3) in combination with the clinical assessment of the oral-vestibular width of the maxillary ridge (Fig 2), it was determined that the available bone volume was sufficient for the placement of four to eight implants. This would satisfy the patient's desire for a palate-free prosthetic rehabilitation with a full-arch bridge or an overdenture (level 2).

Because of the previous oncologic treatment—resection of a gastric MALT lymphoma combined with chemotherapy—the next step was to evaluate the risk of implant placement. The patient's oncologists found no contraindication to the placement of oral implants, nor did they assert an increased risk of late complications due to compromised peri-implant soft-tissue attachment. Concerns were expressed, however, in the event of a massively traumatic surgical procedure, which would occur with extensive soft-tissue flap formation and/or bone augmentation. Patient compliance was good due to the perceived oncologic follow-up every 6 months.

Based on this information and the clinical evaluation described below, the following patient profile (Fig 4) can be derived for this patient (for more Information about patient profiles, see Chapters 2.1.3 and 3.6) (Wolfart 2023).

CLINICAL EVALUATION AND TREATMENT PLAN

The clinical evaluation and patient profile (Fig 4) did not argue against implant-supported prosthetics. Due to the patient's history of oncologic disease, fully guided implant placement was preferred, which can be performed without the formation of a mucosal flap and then in a minimally invasive manner.

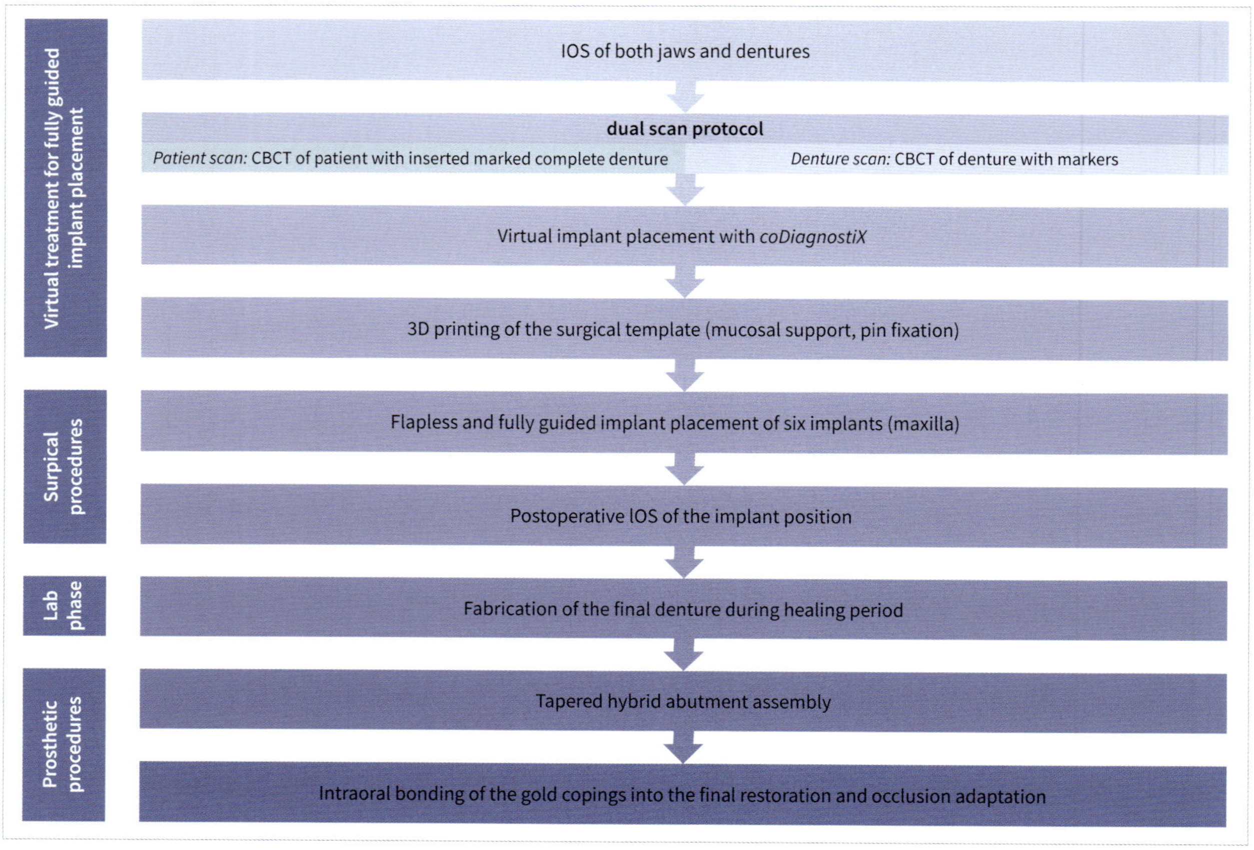

Fig 5 Treatment protocol.

In the financial options parameter, the patient profile (Fig 4) indicated a minimum number of implants—four in total—for a full-mouth restoration (Slot and coworkers 2023; Payne and coworkers 2018). However, six implants were recommended for the patient (Slot and coworkers 2023) to counteract the risk of slowed metabolism due to chemotherapy. Immediate loading of the implants was not considered.

The patient found the daily hygiene of a screw-retained fixed bridge to be very time-consuming. In addition, the esthetically unattractive vertical atrophy of the anterior alveolar ridge can be resolved with a removable overdenture without tissue augmentation (Srinavasan and coworkers 2023). The Locator attachment (Zest Dental Solutions, Carlsbad, CA, USA) was not favored as an anchoring element because of the high maintenance required. A bar connecting the six implants requires a similar level of hygiene as a screw-retained full arch bridge (Park and coworkers 2019; Boven and coworkers 2020). A double-crown attachment consisting of a tapered zirconia male and a corresponding electroformed fine gold female was chosen because of the low aftercare requirements and easy hygiene measures for the patient (Rinke and coworkers 2015; Schwindling and coworkers 2017a; Schwindling and coworkers 2017b; Brandt and coworkers 2019). This attachment provides an absolutely rigid and micromovement free anchorage of the overdenture (Weigl and Lauer 2000).

The following treatment plan (Fig 5) as derived from the patient profile was agreed upon:

- Dual-scan procedure: CBCT of patient, prosthesis, and radiopaque markers and prosthesis scan
- Virtual implant placement (coDiagnostiX; Dental Wings, Chemnitz, Germany) for residual bone volume and prosthetic requirements
- 3D-printed surgical template for fully guided mucosa punch and implant placement
- CAD file representing the tapered-crown denture (conical zirconia hybrid abutment; electroplated gold coping; resin-veneered framework with prosthetic teeth)
- Flapless fully guided implant placement (Chmielewski and coworkers 2019; La Monaca and coworkers 2022; Poli and coworkers 2023)
- IOS of real clinical implant position
- Delivery of the final restoration after a healing period of at least 3 months (intraoral bonding of the gold copings to the final restoration)

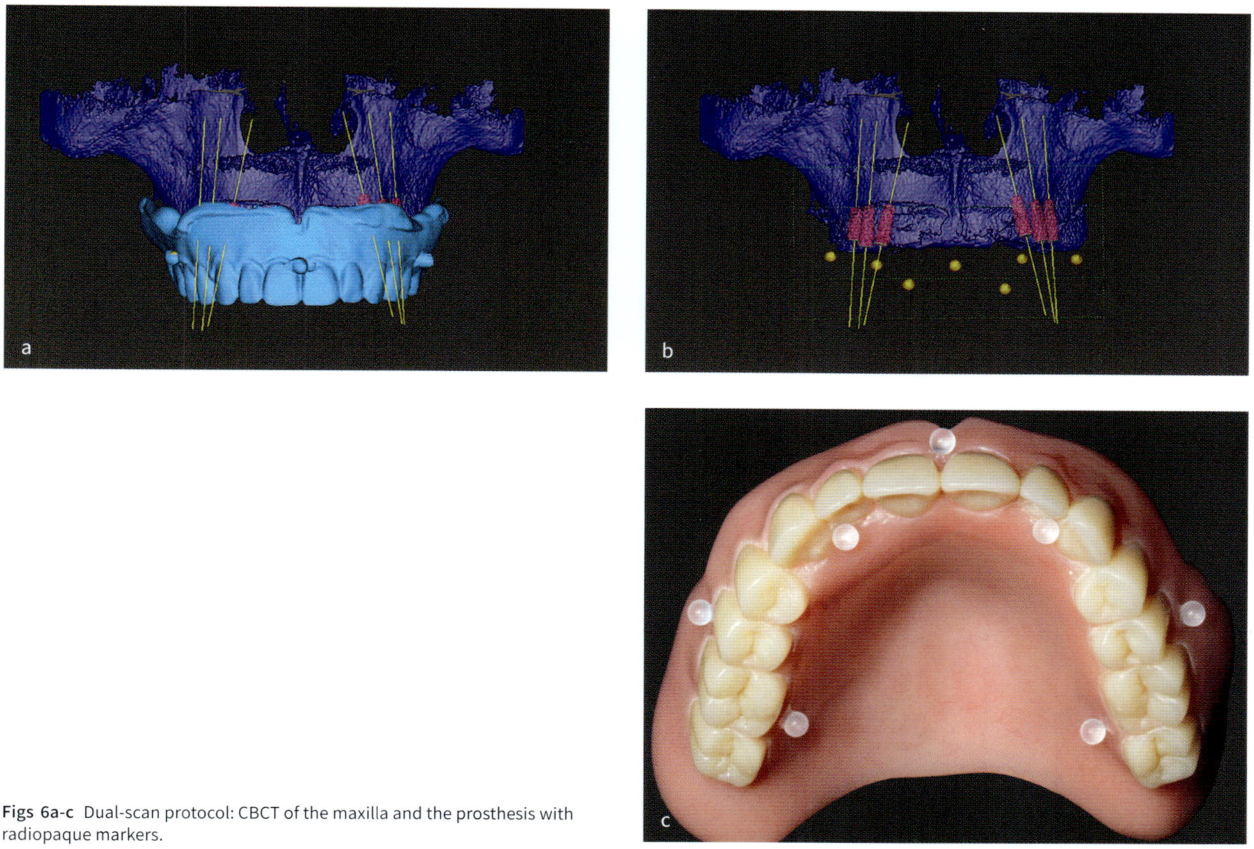

Figs 6a-c Dual-scan protocol: CBCT of the maxilla and the prosthesis with radiopaque markers.

After the intraoral examination, an intraoral scan (Trios 4; 3shape, Copenhagen, Denmark) was performed on both edentulous jaws. The edentulous scanning strategy (Jamjoom and coworkers 2024) recommended by the scanner manufacturer was used: The maxillary scan started on one side of the tuberosity area and continued along the middle of the residual alveolar ridge to the tuberosity area on the opposite side. Starting from the midline, the entire palate was scanned with smooth side-to-side movements. The third path involved scanning the buccal aspect of the alveolar ridge. The mandible was scanned in the retromolar region lingually across the alveolar ridge to the midline and buccally from the midline to the retromolar region. This procedure was performed in the same way for both halves/parts of the mandible (Lo Russo 2020). The Trios 4 scanner was then used to scan the entire surface of the recently fabricated full denture, including both the denture base and the denture teeth. In addition, the two dentures were scanned buccally in centric occlusion. The two denture bases, now in digital form, were then digitally fused with the intraorally scanned mucosa of the edentulous jaws. This defined the jaw relationship in the virtual patient using the scanned centric occlusion of the full dentures.

A CBCT scan (Orthophos S 2D/3D; Dentsply Sirona, Bensheim, Germany) was performed to evaluate the 3D anatomical bone conditions. During the scan, the patient wore his newly relined complete denture with radiopaque markers (*patient scan* according to the dual-scan protocol). The radiopaque marker balls were placed at seven points on the maxillary complete prosthesis. In addition, the prosthesis with markers was scanned alone in the CBCT (*prosthesis scan* according to the dual-scan protocol). After importing and processing the DICOM data sets and merging them with the IOS data set, virtual implant positioning was performed using the implant planning and design software (coDiagnostiX; Dental Wings) (Figs 6a-c).

Implant placement was determined by the available bone and prosthetic position. Based on the implant position, a mucosa-supported drill guide for fully guided implant placement was designed using CAD and then printed using a 3D printer. The guide was designed with channels for four lateral fixation pins. Maximum intercuspation with the mandibular prosthesis was used for reproducible and unambiguous positioning. For this purpose, corresponding occlusal areas were created in the anterior and posterior regions of the guide (Figs 7a-d). The surgical guide contains sleeves (PEEK self-locking T-sleeve, PEEK, diameter 5 mm, length 5 mm; Institut Straumann AG, Basel, Switzerland) for fully guided implant placement. The selected position of the T-sleeve was H4 with a depth stop at 4 mm.

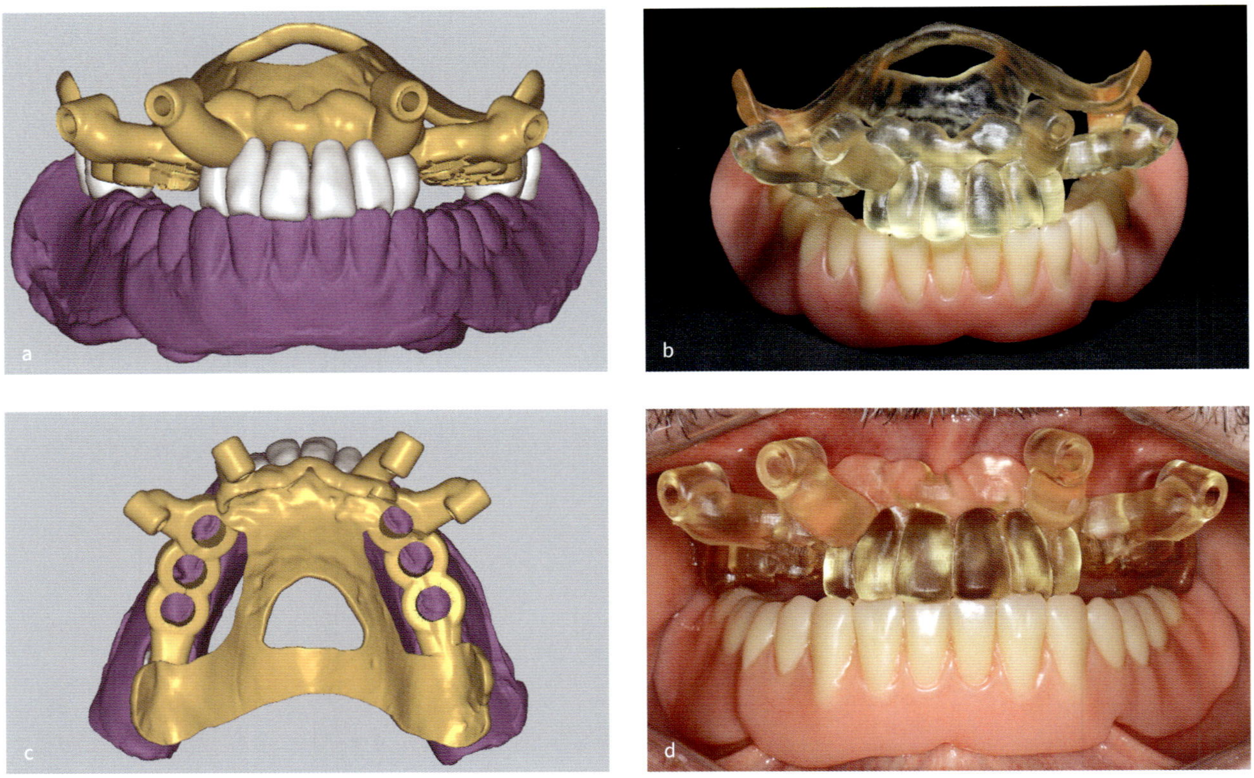

Figs 7a-d Design and fabrication of the surgical guide with occlusal indentations for unambiguous repositioning (fully guided, mucosa-supported, pin-stabilized).

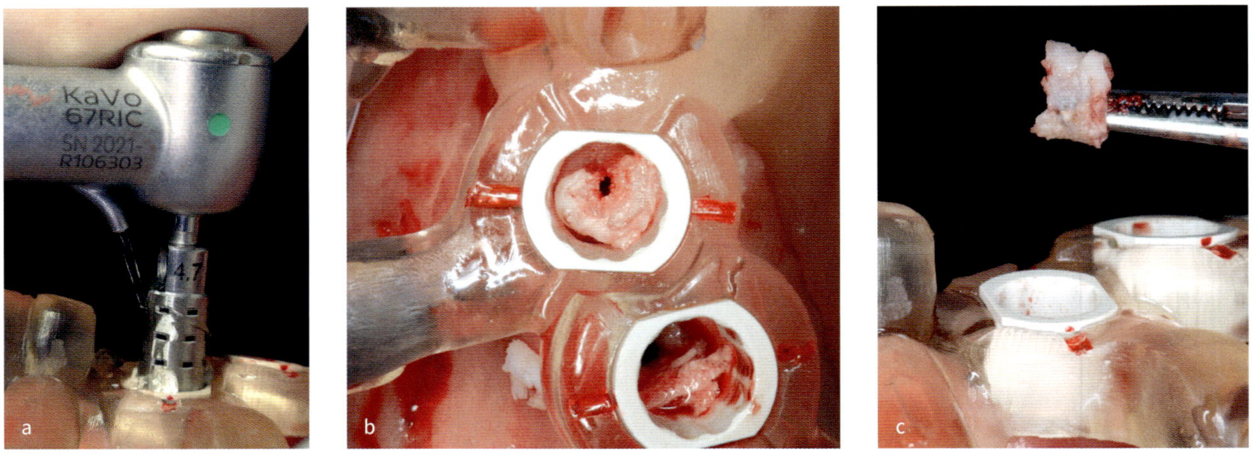

Figs 8a-c Execution and removal of the fully guided mucosal punch.

SURGICAL PROCEDURES

The try-in of the mucosa-supported surgical guide included verification of shape congruence with the mucosa and correct occlusal positioning with the mandibular prosthesis. After verification of the correct fit, the surgical guide was fixed under local anesthesia with four lateral guide fixation pins (Fixation Pin, diameter 1.3 mm, length 28 mm; Institut Straumann AG, Basel, Switzerland) according to the manufacturer's instructions.

Minimally invasive mucosal punches were performed at all implant sites (16, 15, 14, 24, 25, and 26) using the mucosal punch tool guided through the surgical guide (Figs 8a-c).

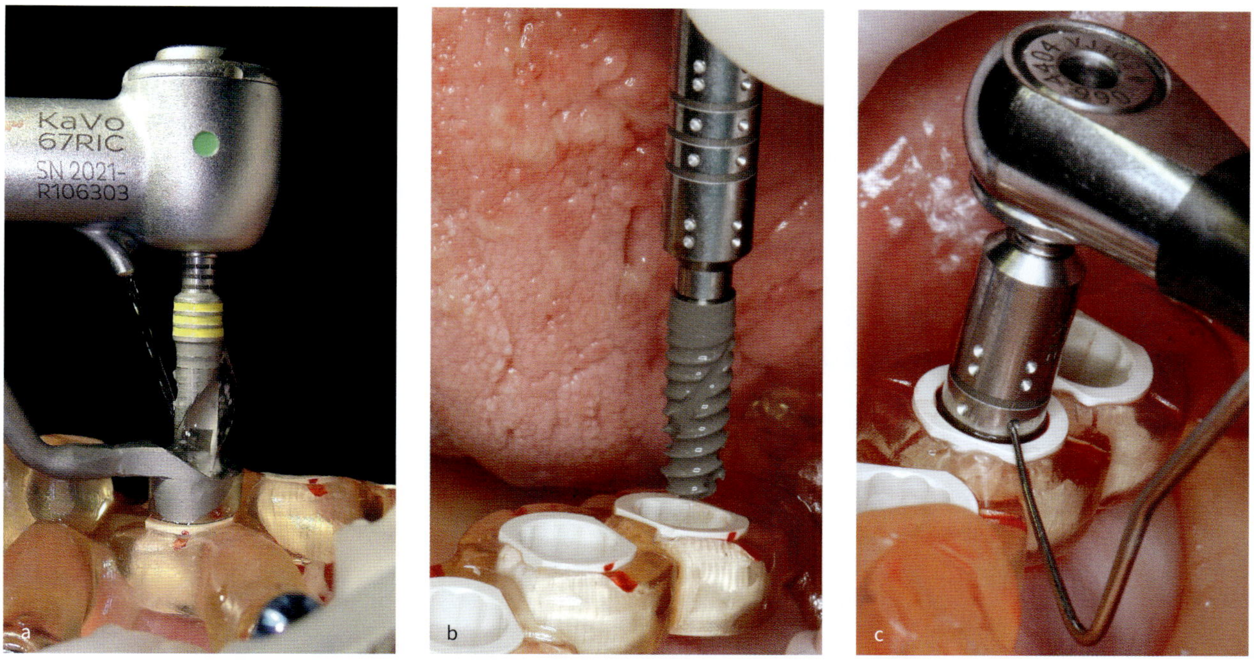

Figs 9a-c Fully guided implant placement according to manufacturer's specifications.

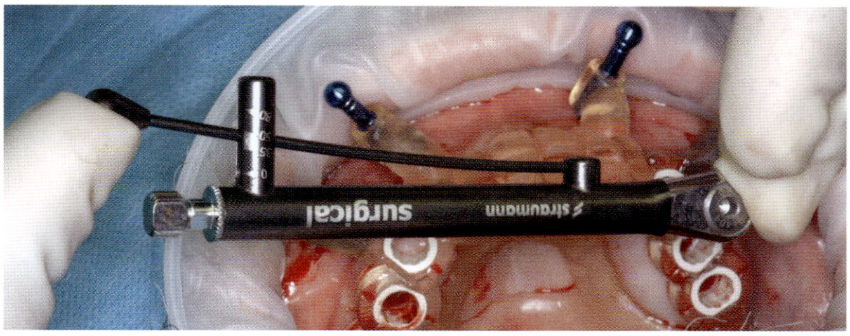

Fig 10 High primary stability of the implants.

The osteotomy protocol using Straumann VeloDrill drills for placement of six Straumann BLX implants was preplanned and defined in the coDiagnostiX implant planning software. Drilling was performed to the vertical stop of the drill. After the osteotomy, six BLX implants (BLX Roxolid, SLA, diameter 3.75 mm, length 12 mm; Institut Straumann AG, Basel, Switzerland) were placed fully guided in D3 bone quality at sites 16, 15, 14, 24, 25, and 26 according to the manufacturer's instructions (Figs 9a-c). The implants demonstrated good primary stability with a torque in excess of 35 Ncm (Fig 10). After removal of the surgical guide, a very small mucosal wound surface was present at the implant sites (Figs 11a-b).

Postoperatively, an intraoral scan (Trios 4; 3shape) of the implant positions of the six BLX implants was taken (Fig 12).

To verify the implant positions and reduce radiation, the STL data set was overlaid with the DICOM data set from the preoperative CBCT (Chmielewski and coworkers 2019; Khaohoen and coworkers 2024) in the software. This eliminated the need for postoperative radiographs in this case.

The healing abutments were hand-tightened onto the implants (Fig 13a).

The existing maxillary prosthesis was adapted and relieved to avoid pressure on the healing abutments and to ensure transmucosal healing. An internal impression was taken with low viscosity silicone to check the fit of the base of the denture (Silasoft; DETAX, Ettlingen, Germany) (Fig 13b).

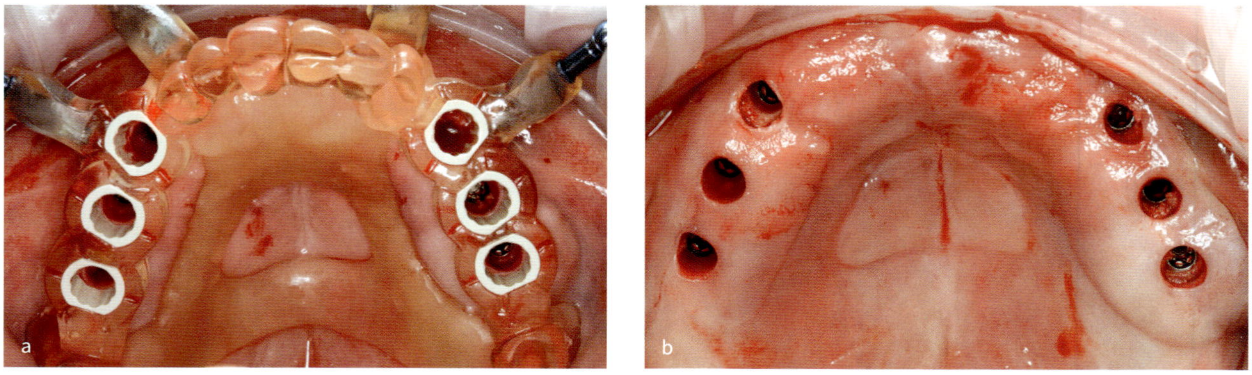

Figs 11a-b Occlusal view of surgical guide and implant sites after implant placement.

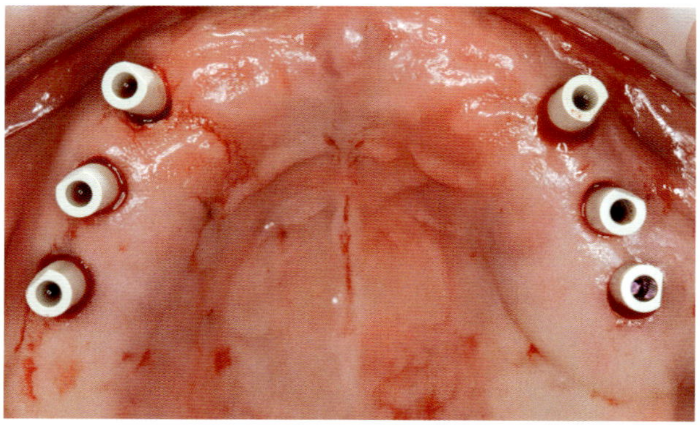

Fig 12 Postoperative digital impression.

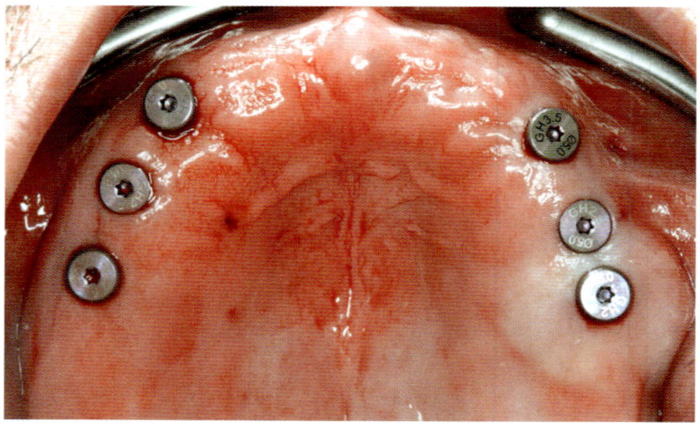

Fig 13a Insertion of healing abutments.

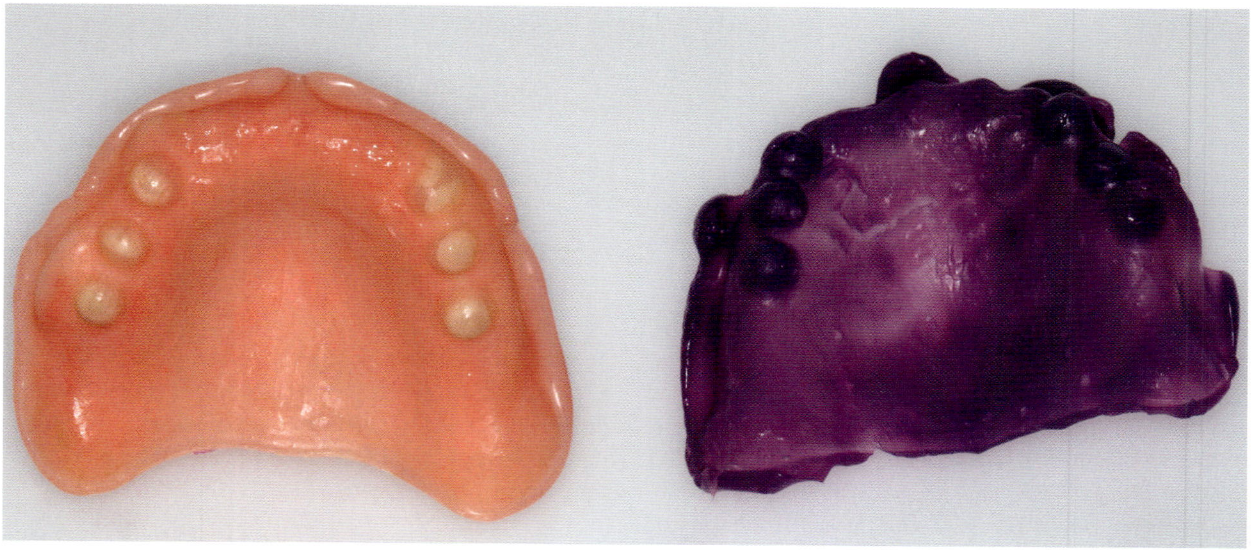

Fig 13b Fitting the base of the complete denture with a low-viscosity silicone control.

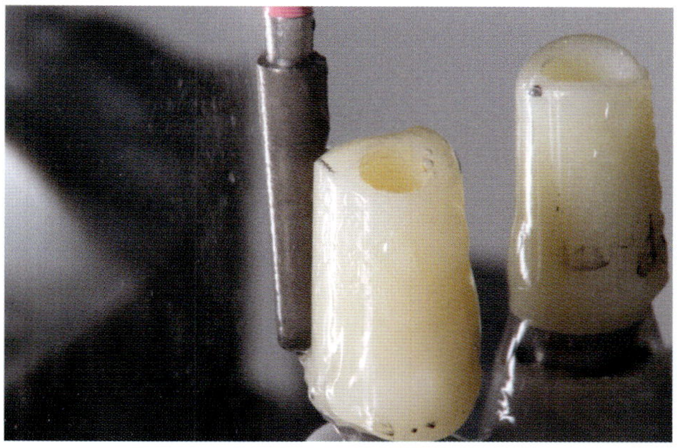

Fig 14 Fabrication of the zirconia hybrid abutments.

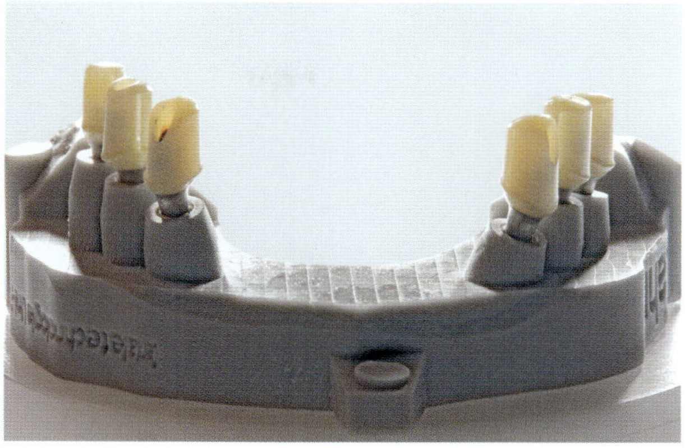

Fig 15 Zirconia hybrid abutments.

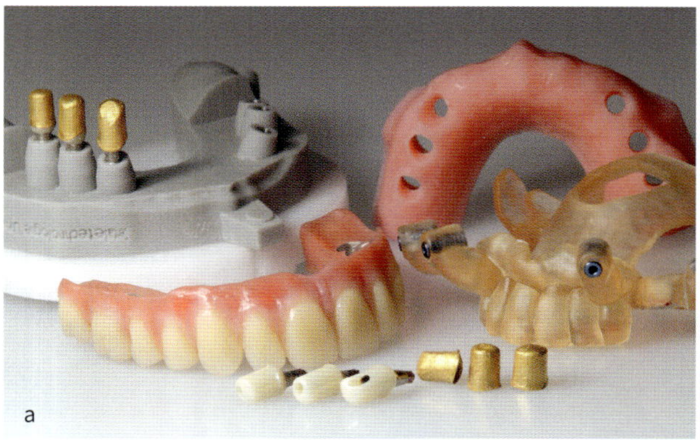

a

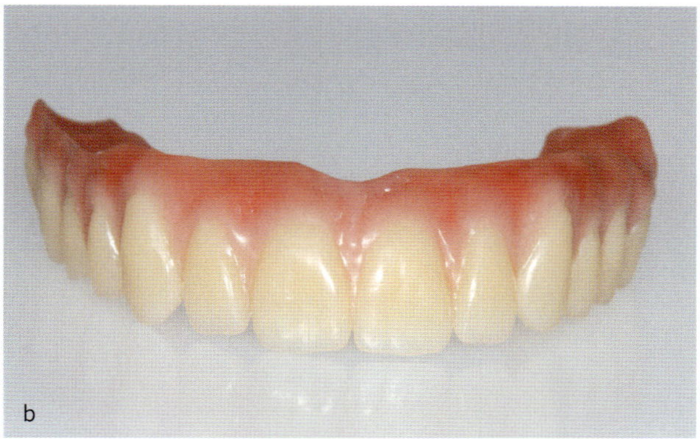

b

Figs 16a-b Design and fabrication of the final telescopic prosthesis (final conical zirconia hybrid abutments and electroplated gold copings, resin-veneered framework, and prosthetic teeth).

LABORATORY PROCEDURES

The final prosthesis was fabricated at the dental laboratory during the healing period.

The STL data set of the postoperative intraoral scan was used to fabricate a high-precision 3D-printed master model with gingival mask and for the subsequent fabrication of the zirconia hybrid abutments (sites 14 and 24: RB/WB Variobase for Crown incl. screw, diameter 3.8 mm, gingival height 2.5 mm, abutment height 5.5 mm; and sites 15, 16, 25, and 26; RB/WB Variobase for Crown incl. screw, diameter 3.8 mm, gingival height 1.5 mm, abutment height 5.5 mm; all Institut Straumann AG, Basel, Switzerland).

The zirconia primary crowns were fabricated from Katana Zirconia High Translucent Multi Layered Plus (Kuraray Noritake, Miyoshi, Aichi, Japan) and cemented in the laboratory. The titanium abutment and the inner surface of the zirconia primary crown were air-abraded according to the manufacturer's instructions (Multilink Automix and Monobond Plus; Ivoclar Vivadent, Schaan, Liechtenstein). The hybrid abutments had a component height of the zirconia primary crowns of approximately 7 mm and a milling with a cone angle of 2 degrees (Figs 14 and 15).

Transfer keys were fabricated for clinical placement of the hybrid abutments. Pure gold copings were then electroplated directly on the original hybrid abutments (Helioform HF 700; C. Hafner, Wimsheim, Germany) to ensure a fit of less than 5 μm between the primary and secondary parts (Weigl and coworkers 2000). A sufficiently sized tertiary framework of the prosthesis was designed using CAD and milled from a CrCoMol alloy. A clearance of 0.7 mm (0.3 mm layer thickness of the electroformed gold coping; 0.4 mm bonding gap) was incorporated between the tapered hybrid abutments and the metal framework. The printed upper master model could be precisely positioned in relation to the printed lower teeth of the mandible using the digitally available jaw relationship. The prosthetic teeth were set and the denture base was fabricated using conventional laboratory techniques (Figs 16a-b).

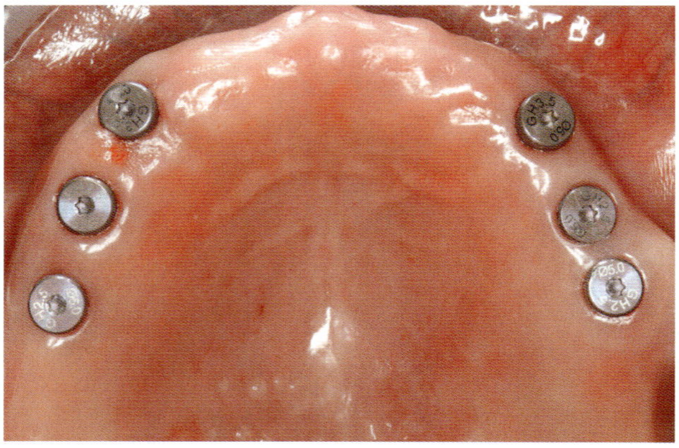

Fig 17 Healing abutments at 3 months.

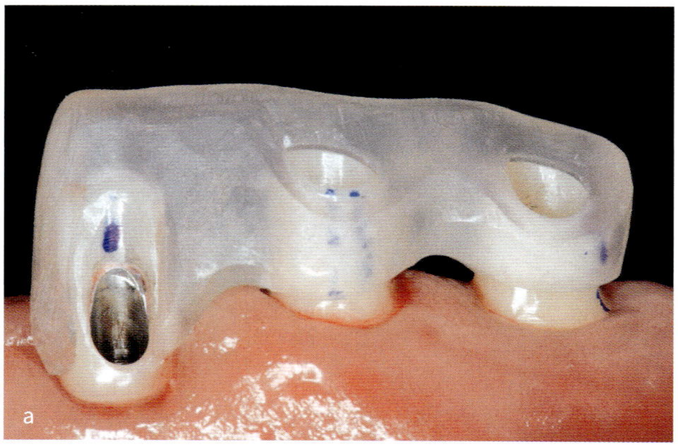

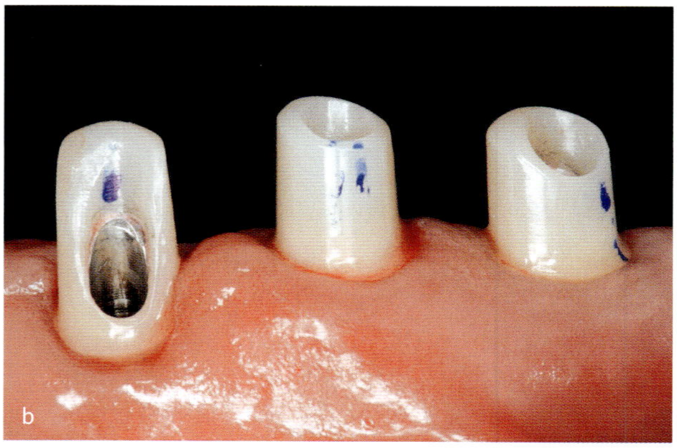

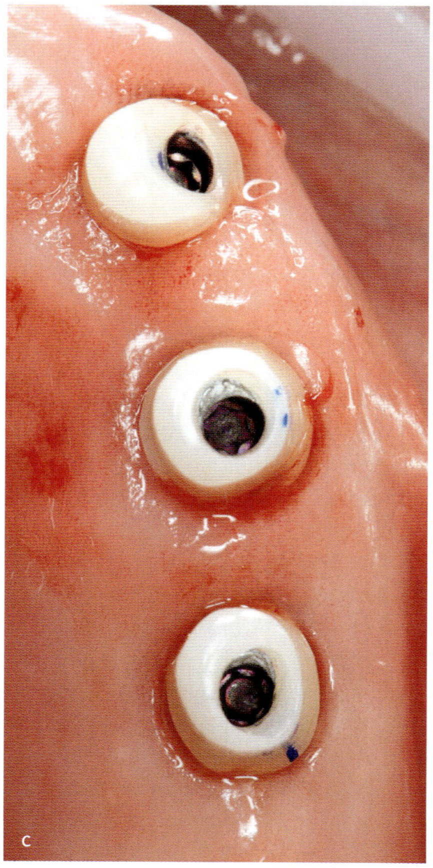

Figs 18a-c Insertion of hybrid abutments (zirconia primary crown) with transfer key to prevent rotational malpositioning.

PROSTHETIC PROCEDURES

The final prosthesis was inserted in a single visit.

After a healing period of 3 months (Fig 17), the osseointegration of the implants was evaluated using an electromechanical testing procedure (Periotest M; Medizintechnik Gulden, Modautal, Germany) and a percussion test, where the implant is struck with a type of hammer (usually the back of a mirror instrument) to produce its characteristic sound. This percussion test assumes that an integrated implant should have a sharper and more defined sound, while a non-integrated implant should have a dull low-frequency sound (Zanetti and coworkers 2018).

The healing abutments were removed and the implants were rinsed with chlorhexidine solution (Chlorhexamed Forte 0.2%; GlaxoSmithKline, Munich, Germany).

The tapered zirconia hybrid abutments 16, 15, 14, 24, 25, and 26 were placed using a customized transfer key for each quadrant to reliably prevent rotational malpositioning of the abutments (Figs 18a-c).

The abutment screws were tightened to the manufacturer's recommended torque of 35 Ncm using a newly calibrated torque ratchet. The screw channel was sealed with sterilized PTFE tape and a temporary filling material (Clip; Voco, Cuxhaven, Germany) (Fig 19).

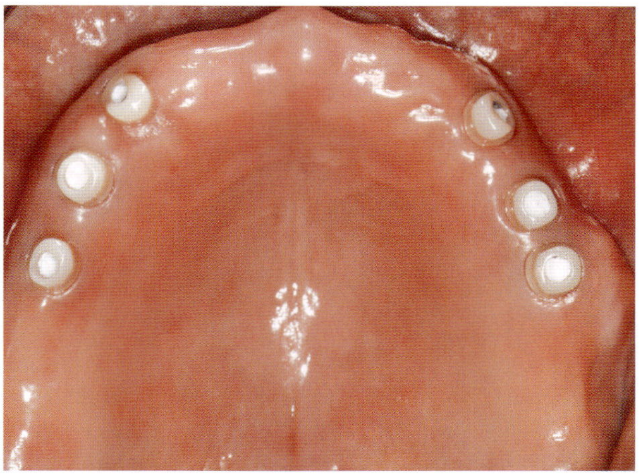

Fig 19 Occlusal view of the hybrid abutments with temporary closure.

The electroplated gold copings were placed on the hybrid abutments without applying any pressure and checked for a tight fit (Figs 20a-b).

Prior to intraoral bonding of the electroplated gold copings, the prosthesis was inserted to verify that the framework was free of tension. This means that the bonding gap between the framework and the fine gold coping must provide a clearance fit.

After a lip and cheek retractor was used to aid in maintaining a dry field (Optragate; Ivoclar Vivadent), the gold copings were degreased with ethanol and the framework was conditioned with a bonding agent (Alloy Primer; Kuraray Noritake). The gold copings, which were positively seated on the abutments, were simultaneously cemented into the denture framework with a self-curing compomer cement (AGC Cem; C. Hafner) (Weigl and Lauer 2000). For this purpose, the recesses of the framework were vertically filled with the adhesive approximately halfway (Fig 21). The prosthesis was then inserted (Fig 22) and fixed in maximum intercuspation while the cement cured. This procedure secures the prosthesis in the correct position relative to the alveolar ridge and the mandibular prosthesis despite the clearance fit with the gold copings.

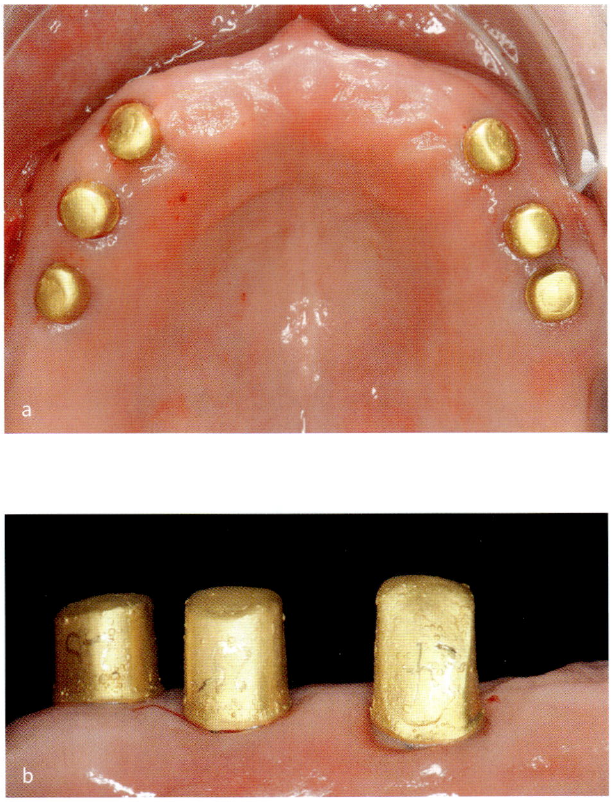

Figs 20a-b Insertion of the electroplated gold copings.

The prosthesis was removed after the cement had set because the pure gold copings can separate from the zirconia hybrid abutments along the common path of insertion.

When cementing the gold copings into the denture framework, it must be ensured that only the occlusal, upper half of the framework is filled with cement (Fig 21). This underfill allows for easy removal of the framework and denture after the cement has set. Occasionally, the adhesive gap between the gold copings and the framework is not completely filled with cement. In this case, freshly mixed cement is placed extraorally into the unfilled gap.

The static and dynamic occlusion was then adjusted (Figs 23 and 24a-b). The patient was instructed on the insertion and removal of the tapered-crown full-arch prosthesis. In particular, oral hygiene measures for the hybrid abutments and cleaning of the denture were demonstrated and briefly practiced with the patient.

FOLLOW-UP AND PATIENT SATISFACTION

The patient regularly attended recall appointments and implant checkups. He felt very comfortable with the prosthesis in place and was very satisfied with the retention of the maxillary denture. Due to the absence of micromovement, the patient experienced the reconstruction as comparable to what he remembered as his natural dentition. The maxillary mucosa showed no signs of bruising or inflammation at the 11-month recall. Clinical signs of mucositis were absent around all six implants (Schwindling and coworkers 2017). The implants showed stable osseointegration radiographically (Nomiyama and coworkers 2023) (Figs 25a-c).

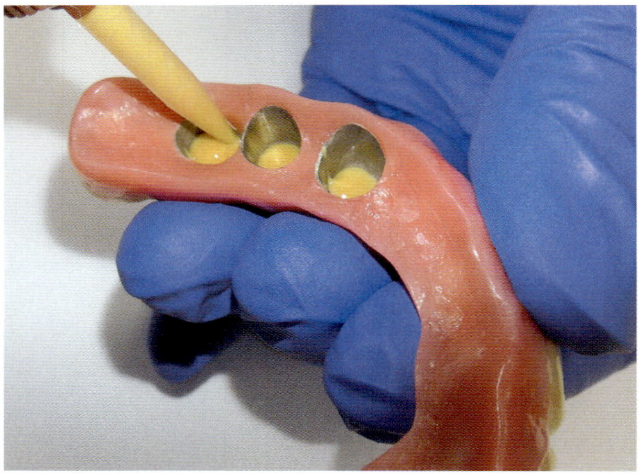

Fig 21 Filling the frame recesses approximately halfway with adhesive.

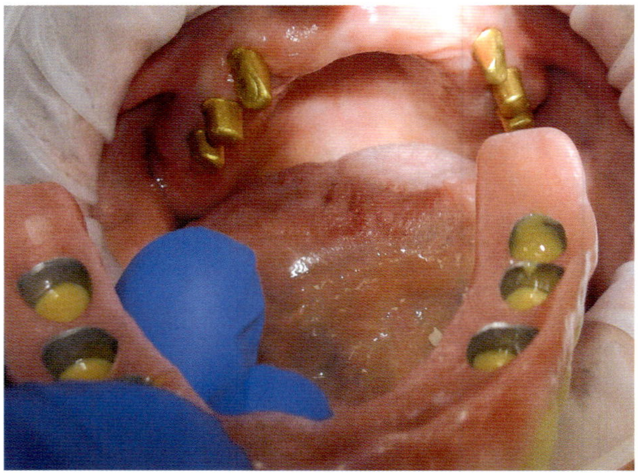

Fig 22 The adhesive-filled prosthesis was placed over the pure gold caps that fit over the abutments and is positioned and fixed with the lower prosthesis in maximum intercuspation.

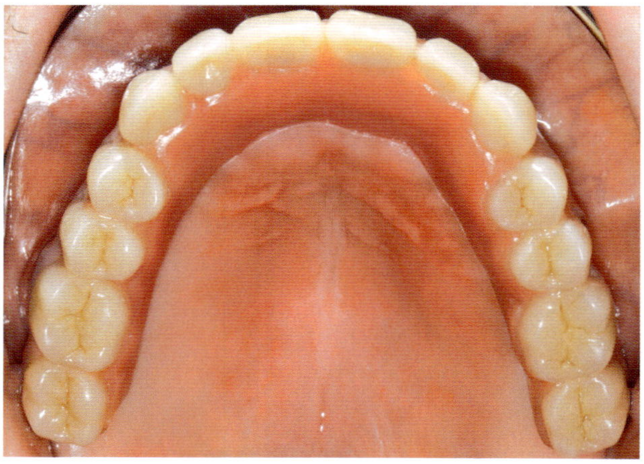

Fig 23 Delivery of the final restoration (occlusal view).

In the future, the patient plans to rehabilitate his mandible with this type of restoration as well, following the treatment workflow presented.

Use this code to watch a highlight video with the patient reporting on his satisfaction with the treatment.

DISCUSSION

The therapy presented in this case report for the full-arch rehabilitation of an edentulous jaw takes advantage of the minimally invasive surgical approach made possible by fully guided implant placement. Flapless access to the bone for implant placement is achieved by circular punching of the mucosa. Punching is performed through the guide and is therefore in exact position relative to the implant. The healing abutments primarily close this minimal mucosal wound. This primary wound closure requires no sutures, does not cause mucosal swelling and reduces or eliminates postoperative pain (Nomiyama and coworkers 2023; Lemos and coworkers 2020). These factors lead to high patient acceptance of this therapy (Lemos and coworkers 2020) and especially meets the patient's risk of a slowed metabolism due to chemotherapy (Nomiyama and coworkers 2023).

The primary stability of more than 35 Ncm achieved in D3 bone quality is due to the macro design of the BLX implant line. The thread design, which initially provides good mechanical anchoring in the cancellous bone, allows these high torques to be achieved predictably based on the osteotomy protocol designed for this purpose. This allows both the transmucosal healing of the implants and the assembly of the abutments immediately after implant placement to assess the clinical position of the implants.

Virtual implant positioning with the coDiagnostiX implant planning software also offers the advantage that the real clinical position of the implants can be compared with the virtual position after a postoperative IOS. This means that

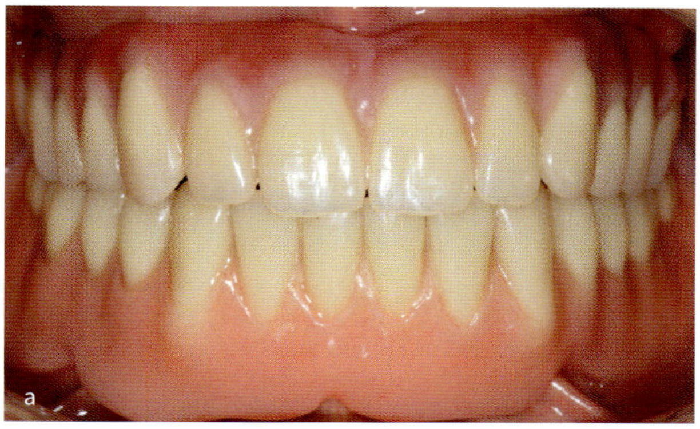

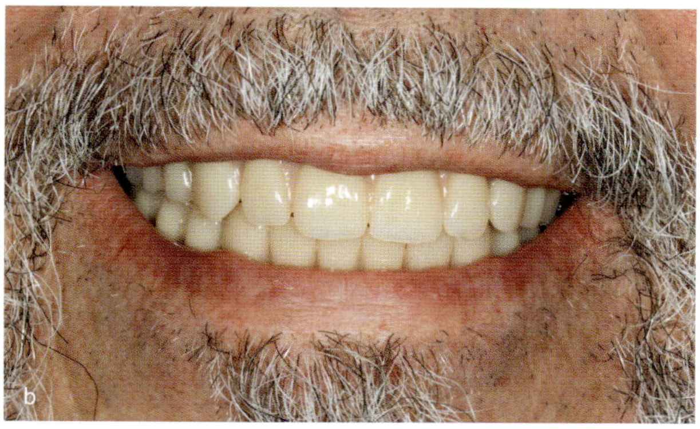

Figs 24a-b Final treatment outcome (frontal view, smile line).

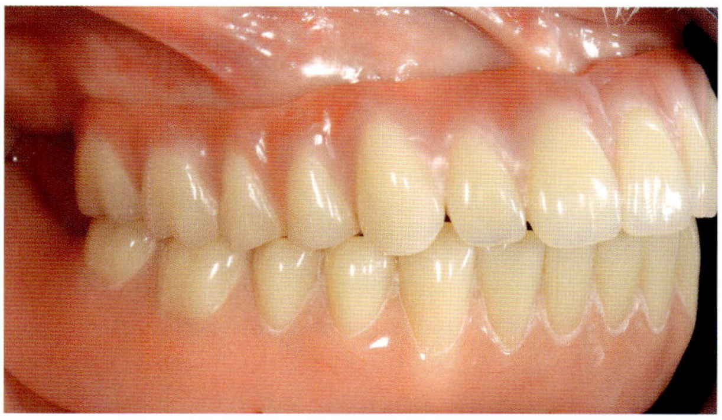

Fig 25a Right lateral view in occlusion at the 11-month follow-up.

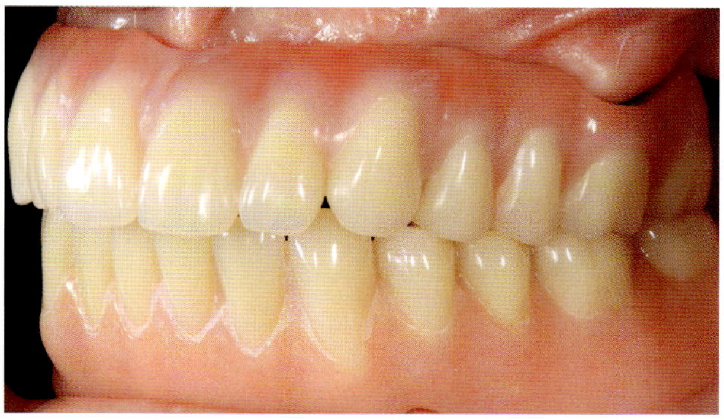

Fig 25b Left lateral view in occlusion at the 11-month follow-up.

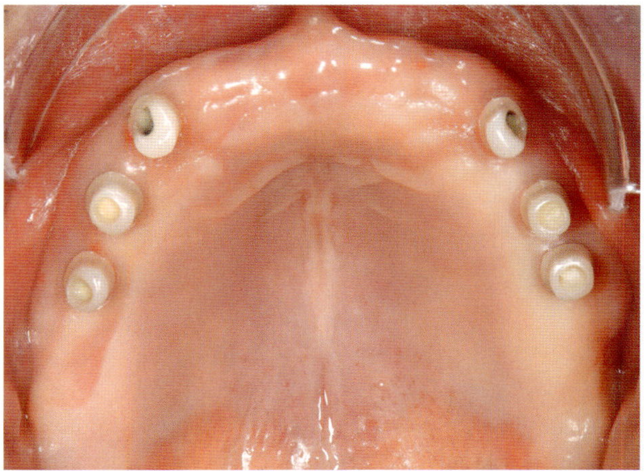

Fig 25c Intraoral occlusal view without final restoration at the 11-month follow-up.

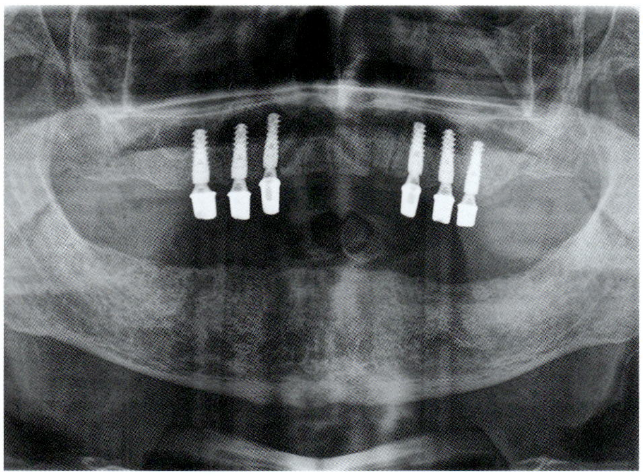

Fig 26 Panoramic radiograph at the 11-month follow-up.

the real implant position can be precisely transferred to the preoperative CBCT and a postoperative radiograph can be avoided in case of a slight deviation between the virtual and the clinical implant position.

The postoperative intraoral scan also allows the final tapered crown-supported overdenture to be fabricated during the healing period of the implants. In particular, the transfer of the correct jaw relationship of very well-fitting full dentures can save a new jaw relationship determination by scanning them and merging the data with the virtual patient. Only the gold copings are bonded in the patient's mouth instead of in the dental laboratory. This significantly reduces the treatment time during the prosthetic phase: only one treatment session is required, which lasts between 1 and 2 hours. In addition, there is no need for the assistance of a dental technician during or after this session, since the prosthesis fits precisely after the gold caps are bonded intraorally, there is no need to adjust the retention force, and the dentist verifies the static and dynamic occlusion. The prosthesis is then complete. There is no need to fabricate a new temporary denture.

Other benefits of an removable maxillary denture are well known:

- It avoids bone reduction (Mijiritsky and coworkers 2021), which is performed for esthetic reasons in cases of fixed bridges, by moving the transition between the fixed bridge and the soft tissue into the invisible area of the alveolar fold. This sometimes significant vertical reduction of the alveolar ridge is used in implant-supported fixed full-arch bridges, especially those with a high smile line (Tonnelini and coworkers 2018).
- Cleaning the peri-implant mucosa is easier for the patient than with screw-retained bridges. This simplified cleaning is also much easier and more time-efficient for third party caregivers, especially if the patient requires care at a later date.
- In the event of implant loss, the removable prosthesis can be adapted quickly and inexpensively; repairs are also straightforward.

A disadvantage of this treatment approach is the high cost for the laboratory to fabricate the tapered-crown full-arch prosthesis. In addition, dental technicians require intensive training to properly fabricate a tapered zirconia hybrid abutment and an electroformed pure gold coping. These two issues have prevented widespread use in oral implantology worldwide. In addition, patients often prefer a fixed full-arch bridge to an overdenture. In particular, fixed full-arch temporaries carry the risk that the patient will also want a fixed prosthesis for the definitive solution and that acceptance of the planned removable denture will decrease. In addition, adequate keratinized mucosa is a prerequisite for flapless implant placement. Keratinized mucosa is less common in the edentulous mandible than in the maxilla.

CONCLUSION

The treatment procedure for a tapered-crown full-arch prosthesis based on fully guided placement of BLX implants, presented in this case report, meets the requirements for safety, minimally invasive surgery, pain reduction, esthetics, and comfort for patients with sufficient bone volume, combined with usually only three short office visits. In particular the target group of elderly and very elderly patients, or patients with slowed metabolisms can benefit from this digital workflow and this type of prosthetic treatment for edentulous jaws.

Patients who wish to have a fixed restoration

5.7 Treatment of a Hopeless Maxillary Residual Dentition with a Fixed Implant-Supported Restoration Using a Staged Approach

T. Ghedini, P. Casentini

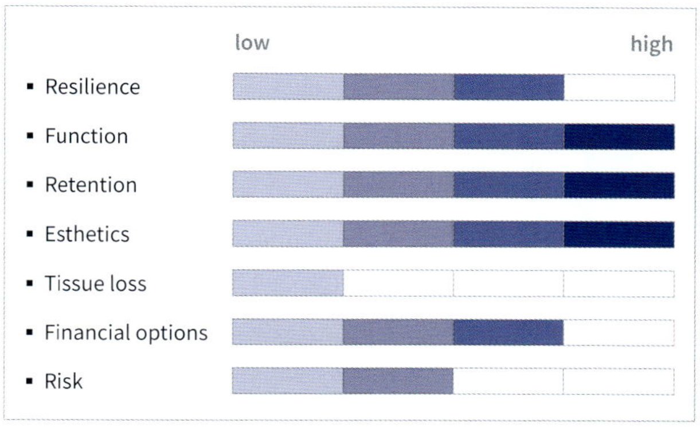

Fig 1 Patient profile.

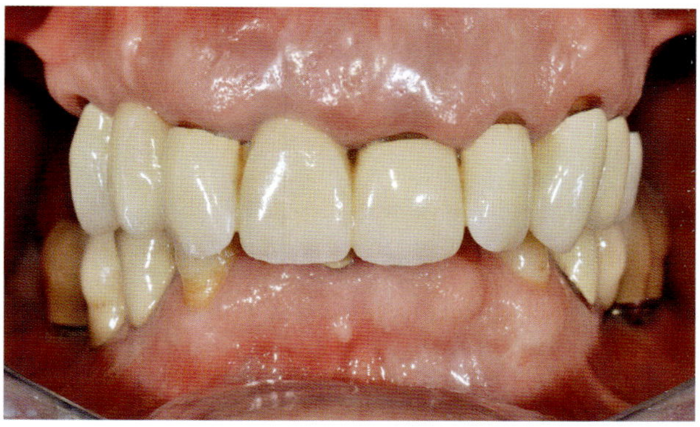

Fig 2 Clinical situation at baseline visit.

PATIENT CHARACTERISTICS AND PATIENT PROFILE

A 62-year-old male patient, a non-smoker, presented after 4 years without recall and with a history of recurrent abscesses on the maxillary central incisors. He was otherwise in good health but had history of periodontitis, so his associated risk was rated as moderate. His main complaint was difficulty with chewing, so he wanted to restore his dentition in the shortest possible time and without any removable provisional prosthesis. The patient wanted a definitive fixed restoration and was looking for an improvement in function, while maintaining the esthetics as much as possible. The patient was a manager in a good financial situation, so the total cost of the procedure was not a primary concern.

Based on this information and the clinical and radiographic evaluation described below, the following patient profile (Fig 1) can be derived for this patient (for more information about patient profiles, see Chapters 2.1.3 and 3.6).

CLINICAL EVALUATION AND TREATMENT PLAN

Clinical examination revealed bilateral absence of maxillary upper molars, a residual root at site 15, mobility of tooth 25, and gingival swelling around teeth 11 and 21 (Figs 2 to 4). Radiographic examination revealed caries in teeth 14 and 23, which were part of a failed fixed dental prosthesis (FDP) extending from site 12 to site 24 (Figs 5a-c). A Straumann Tissue Level implant at site 13 had been placed 10 years previously and showed no evidence of inflammation or bone loss. A periodontal evaluation resulted in a diagnosis of stage IV, grade B periodontitis (Tonetti and coworkers 2018) (Figs 6a-b). Esthetically, the patient exhibited a medium gingival display at full smile and an intact interarch distance (Fig 7). There was a deep bite with complete shadowing of the mandibular incisors due to tooth extrusion.

In the mandible, the patient presented with some implant-supported and tooth-supported metal-ceramic crowns, with tooth 41 requiring extraction.

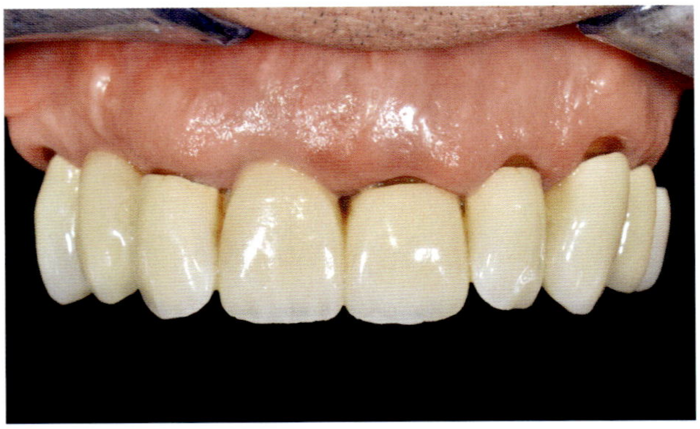

Fig 3 Maxilla at the baseline visit, frontal view.

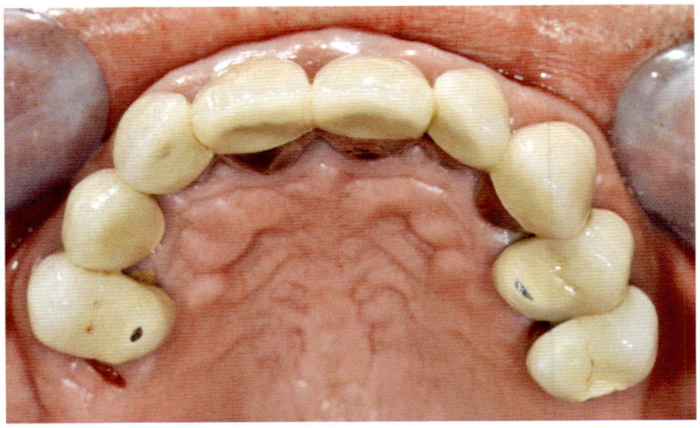

Fig 4 Maxilla at the at baseline visit, occlusal view.

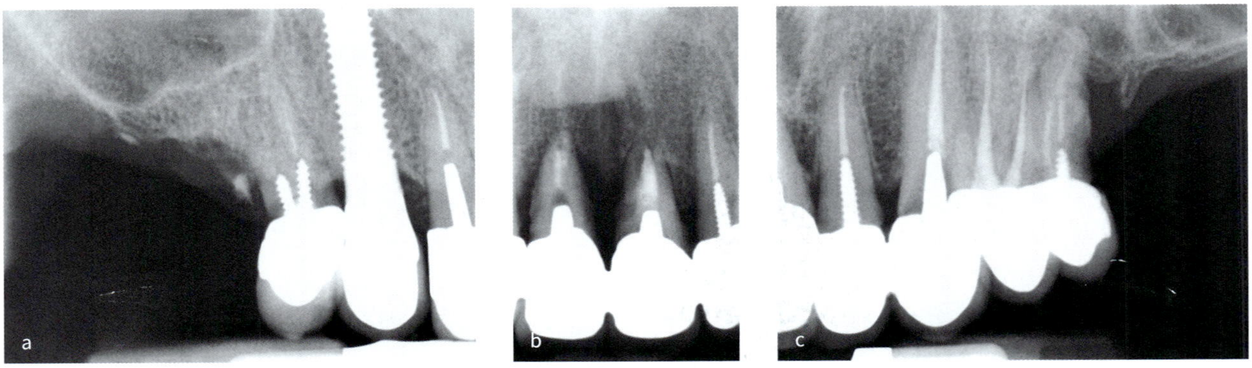

Figs 5a-c Periapical radiographs at the baseline visit.

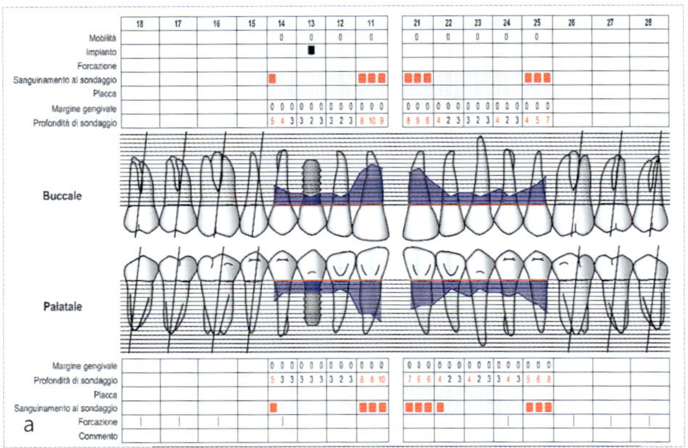

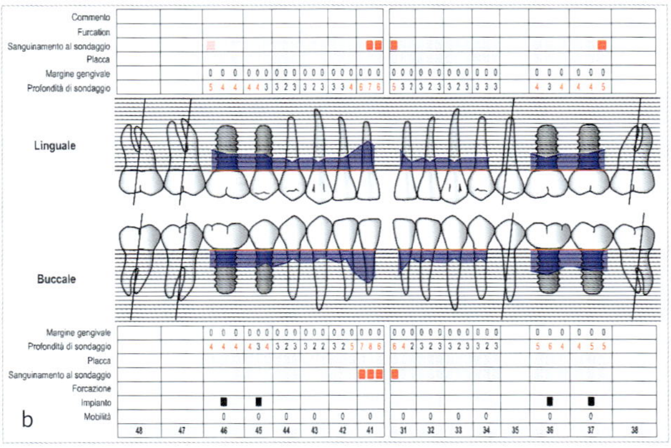

Figs 6a-b Periodontal chart at the baseline visit.

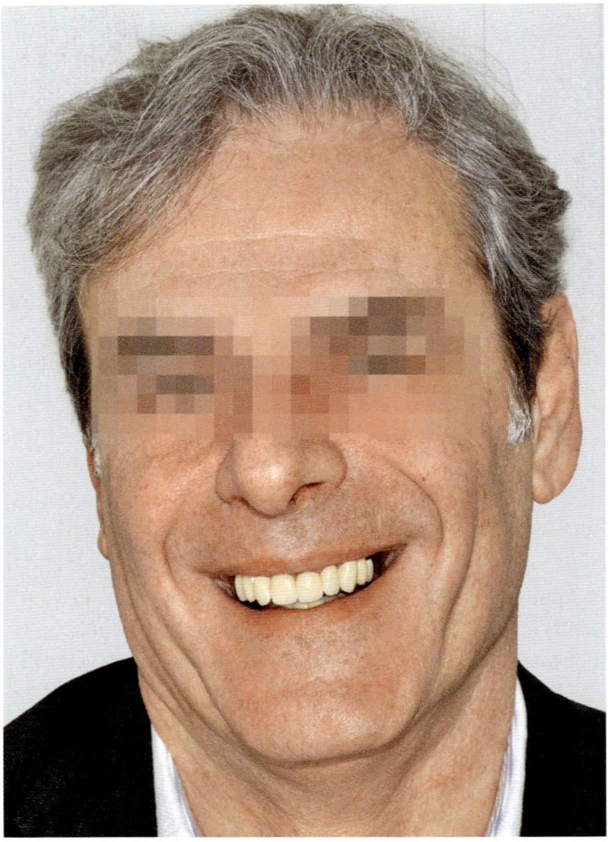

Fig 7 Patient's smile at baseline.

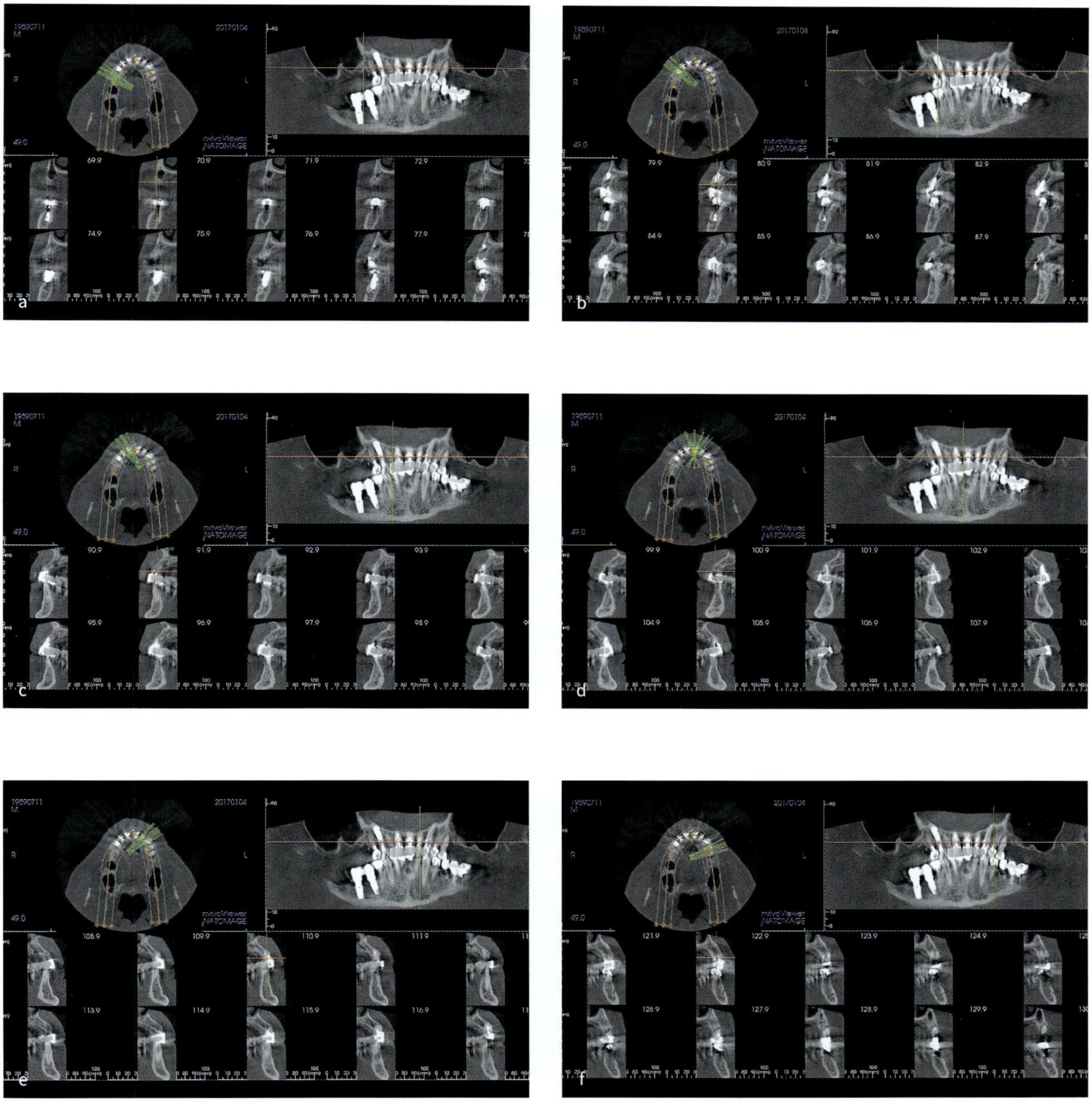

Figs 8a-f Preoperative CBCT.

The patient brought a cone-beam computed tomography (CBCT) and a treatment plan developed *alio loco* (Figs 8a-f). That treatment plan called for a full-arch implant-supported maxillary restoration after extraction with immediate loading. The CBCT scan was of poor quality in that the ostiomeatal complex (OMC) could not be visualized, so we referred the patient to the otorhinolaryngologist for an endoscopic nasosinusal evaluation to avoid repeating a high-dose radiation scan.

The previously proposed treatment plan was rejected for several reasons:

- Clinical evaluation of the residual dentition after removal of the FDP was required before proceeding with tooth extraction.
- Planning for a hypothetical full-arch implant-supported rehabilitation showed limited space for an angled implant at site 14 due to the presence of a hyperpneuma-

tized sinus and of a long implant at site 13. In addition, immediate implant placement at site 25 with active infection was not considered safe, while the reduced anteroposterior spread could cause prosthetic issues with regard to the design and length of the distal cantilever.
- The presence of swelling and infection at sites 11 and 21 could affect the esthetic outcome in the event of uncontrolled tissue shrinkage.

After non-surgical periodontal treatment of the mandibular arch to reduce the overall bleeding on probing and to ensure good plaque control and periodontal stability, teeth 15, 11, 21 and 25, which were considered hopeless for periodontal reasons, were scheduled for extraction. The prognosis of teeth 14 and 23 was considered questionable, so their evaluation was postponed until the FDP was removed. Therefore, an impression was taken for the preparation of a provisional full-arch prosthesis to be relined in the mouth and with teeth 15 and 25 designed as cantilevers (Fig 9).

After extraction of the hopeless teeth, the remaining natural abutments were prepared to support for the provisional acrylic resin-reinforced restoration. The implant abutment at site 13 was also used to support the provisional prosthesis. At this stage, teeth 14 and 23 were not considered restorable due to the depth and extent of the carious lesions, although tooth 14 was still retained at this stage to support the provisional prosthesis (Fig 10). Due to the active infection and the insufficient alveolar morphology, socket preservation was not performed at sites 11 and 21. The pontics of the immediate provisional prosthesis were carefully shaped to minimize the shrinkage of the soft tissue (Bakshi and coworkers 2018) (Fig 11).

During this initial treatment phase, anterior swelling was reduced and partial masticatory function was restored, while scaling and root planing of the remaining teeth was performed.

At this stage, two different treatment options were discussed with the patient:

- **Combined tooth- and implant-supported FDP:** Bilateral sinus floor elevation to compensate for the lack of vertical bone and extraction of tooth 23. After 6 months of healing, implant placement at sites 14, 16, 25, and 26 with fixed implant-supported restorations and preservation of the remaining anterior teeth with a new transitional FDP from site 12 to site 24, with 11, 21, and 23 as pontics.
- **Implant-supported FDP using a stepwise approach:** Bilateral sinus floor elevation and extraction of tooth 23. After complete bone healing (6 months), placement of implants 16, 21, 23 and 26 sites in a single step. Following osseointegration, extraction of the remaining teeth with socket preservation and delivery of an implant-supported resin-reinforced provisional restoration. After tissue maturation, delivery of a definitive metal-ceramic full-arch FDP.

The second treatment plan was selected for the following reasons:

- The remaining natural abutments were considered high-risk because they were all endodontically treated, had poor residual structure, and had previous cemented and screw-retained metal posts (Nevins 1993).
- The anticipated shrinkage in the central incisor region may require soft-tissue augmentation to achieve proper gingival margin alignment. If crown lengthening were required, it would affect the crown-to-root ratio of teeth 12 and 22, which had already experienced some bone resorption.

The case was classified as Complex according to the SAC classification (Fig 12) both surgically and prosthetically (Dawson and coworkers 2009). Challenges were related to the lack of vertical bone volume in the posterior regions, which required grafting of both maxillary sinuses, and to the periodontal susceptibility of the patient. The latter aspect had to be addressed preoperatively, but also—and most importantly—postoperatively, with regular supportive peri-implant care every 3 to 4 months (Heitz-Mayfield and coworkers 2020).

The presence of parafunctions guided the material selection, also for the mandibular prosthesis. A nightguard was planned after the delivery of the final prosthesis to maintain the integrity of the rehabilitation.

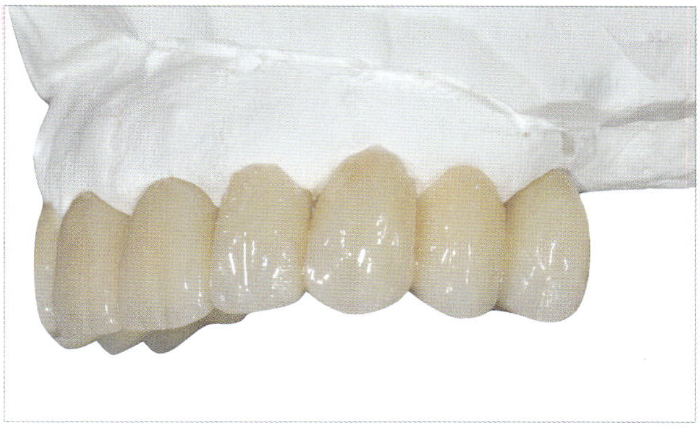

Fig 9 Provisional full-arch prosthesis on the stone cast model.

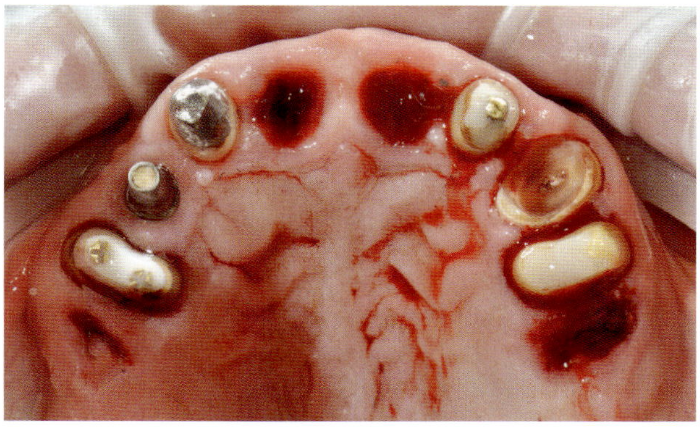

Fig 10 Maxilla after removal of the FDP, occlusal view.

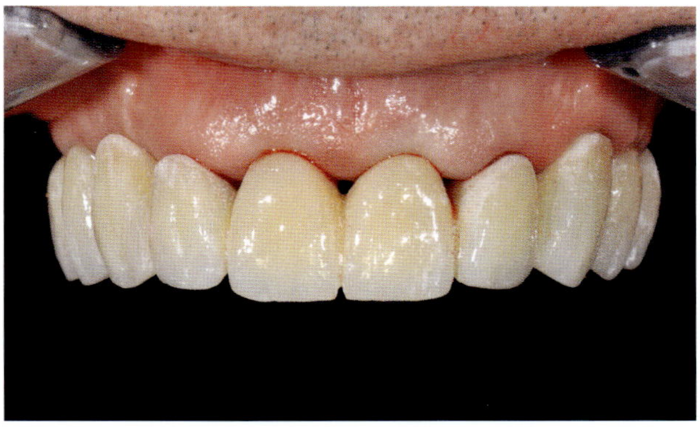

Fig 11 Provisional full-arch prosthesis after relining.

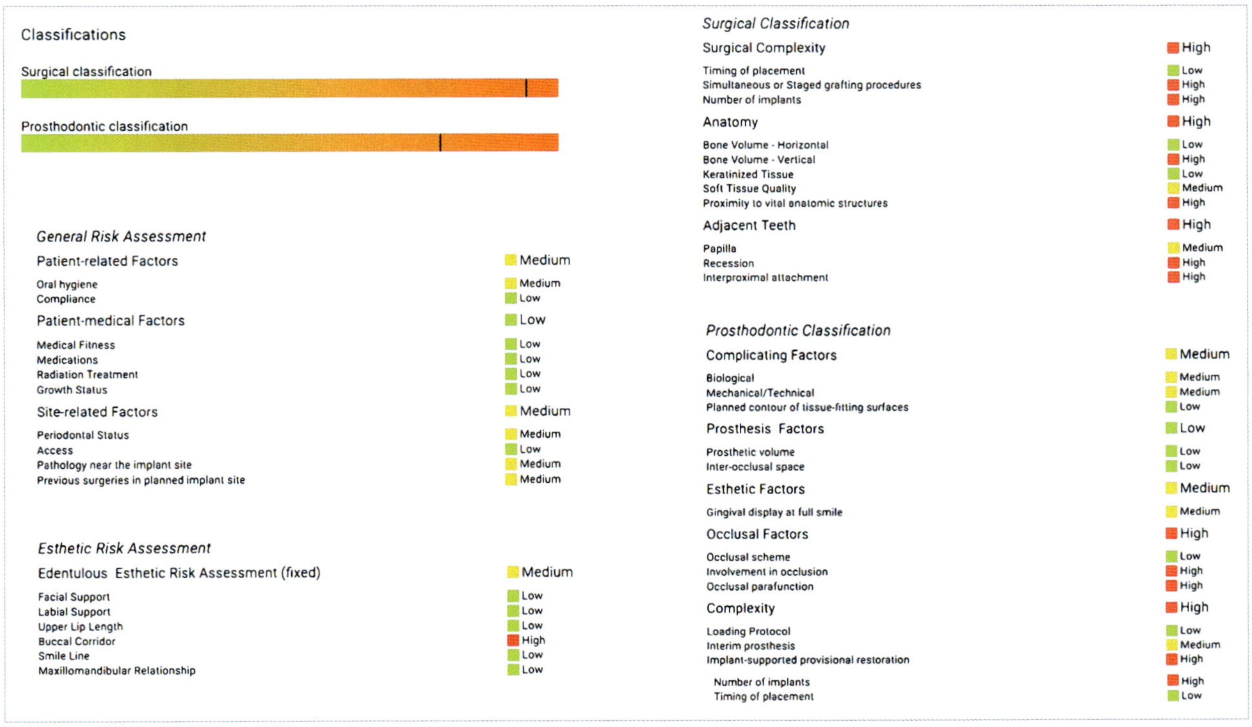

Classifications

Surgical classification

Prosthodontic classification

General Risk Assessment

Patient-related Factors	Medium
Oral hygiene	Medium
Compliance	Low
Patient-medical Factors	Low
Medical Fitness	Low
Medications	Low
Radiation Treatment	Low
Growth Status	Low
Site-related Factors	Medium
Periodontal Status	Medium
Access	Low
Pathology near the implant site	Medium
Previous surgeries in planned implant site	Medium

Esthetic Risk Assessment

Edentulous Esthetic Risk Assessment (fixed)	Medium
Facial Support	Low
Labial Support	Low
Upper Lip Length	Low
Buccal Corridor	High
Smile Line	Low
Maxillomandibular Relationship	Low

Surgical Classification

Surgical Complexity	High
Timing of placement	Low
Simultaneous or Staged grafting procedures	High
Number of implants	High
Anatomy	High
Bone Volume - Horizontal	Low
Bone Volume - Vertical	High
Keratinized Tissue	Low
Soft Tissue Quality	Medium
Proximity to vital anatomic structures	High
Adjacent Teeth	High
Papilla	Medium
Recession	High
Interproximal attachment	High

Prosthodontic Classification

Complicating Factors	Medium
Biological	Medium
Mechanical/Technical	Medium
Planned contour of tissue-fitting surfaces	Low
Prosthesis Factors	Low
Prosthetic volume	Low
Inter-occlusal space	Low
Esthetic Factors	Medium
Gingival display at full smile	Medium
Occlusal Factors	High
Occlusal scheme	Low
Involvement in occlusion	High
Occlusal parafunction	High
Complexity	High
Loading Protocol	Low
Interim prosthesis	Medium
Implant-supported provisional restoration	High
Number of implants	High
Timing of placement	Low

Fig 12 SAC classification.

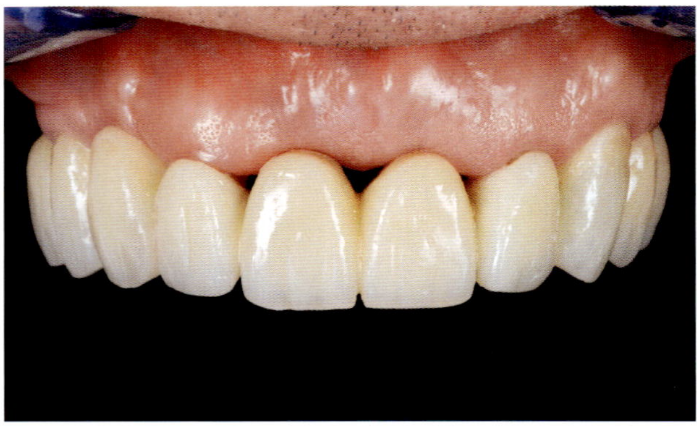

Fig 13 Provisional full-arch prosthesis 2 weeks after delivery.

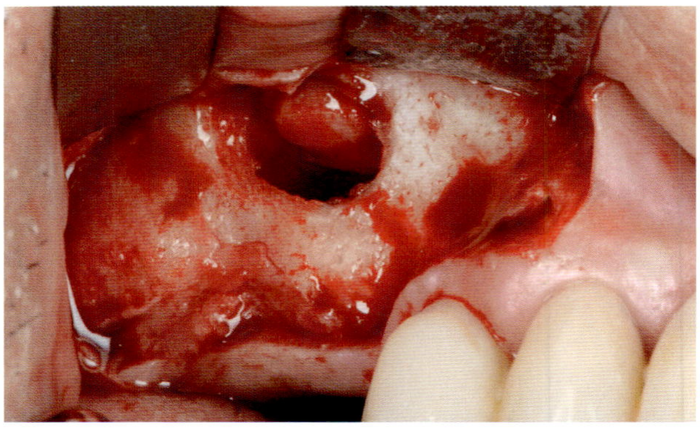

Fig 14 Schneiderian membrane elevation, right upper quadrant.

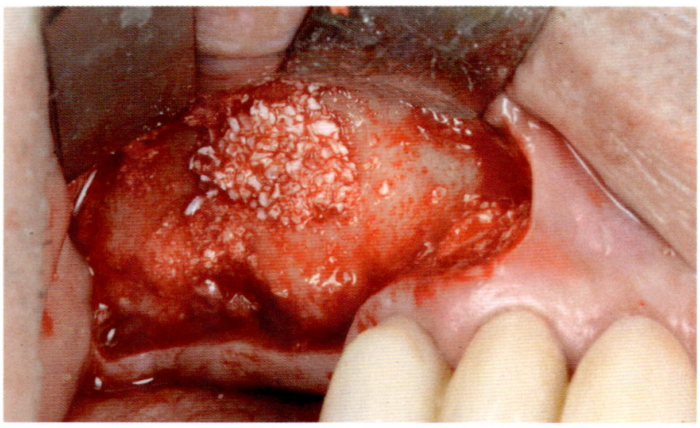

Fig 15 Sinus filling with deproteinized bovine bone material (DBBM).

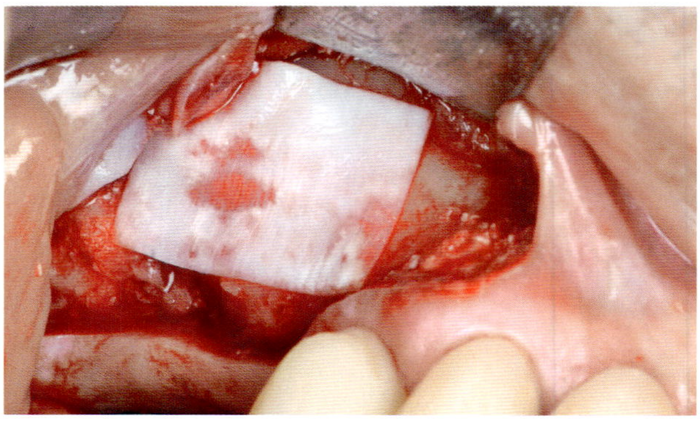

Fig 16 Window coverage with resorbable collagen membrane, right upper quadrant.

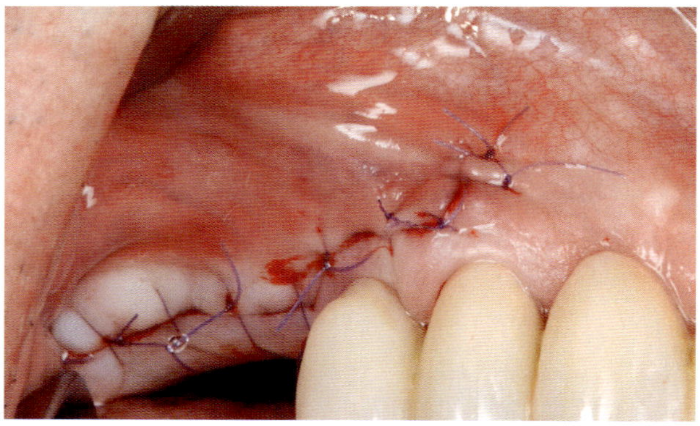

Fig 17 Primary-intention suture.

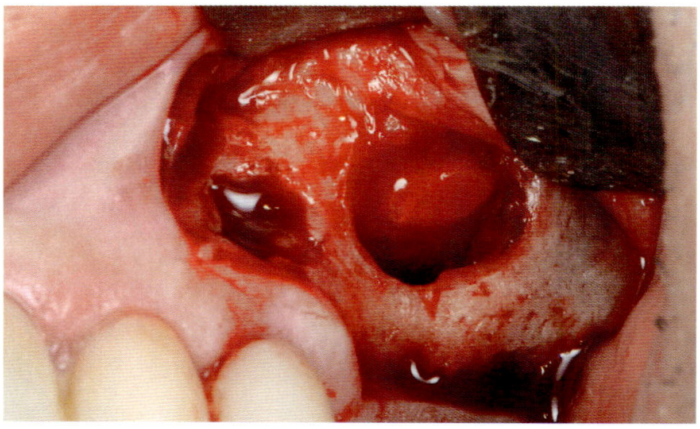

Fig 18 Schneiderian membrane elevation, left upper quadrant.

SURGICAL PROCEDURES AND PROVISIONAL RESTORATION

At 2 weeks after delivery of the provisional prosthesis (Fig 13), bilateral sinus augmentation was performed. A full-thickness flap was elevated under local anesthesia with two releasing incisions. A circumferential fenestration was performed with a round diamond bur in a straight handpiece under continuous irrigation. The Schneiderian membrane was elevated to reach the medial wall and provide sufficient space for bone grafting in the correct mesiodistal position to facilitate future implant placement (Fig 14). The sinus was filled with large (between 1 and 2 mm) granules of deproteinized bovine bone material (DBBM) (Bio-Oss Pen; Geistlich Pharma, Wolhusen, Switzerland) (Fig 15), and the window was covered with a resorbable collagen membrane (Bio-Gide; Geistlich Pharma) (Fig 16). The primary-intention flap was sutured in a tension-free manner with resorbable single sutures (Flysorb 5-0; Butterfly, Cavenago di Brianza, Italy) after releasing the flap (Fig 17).

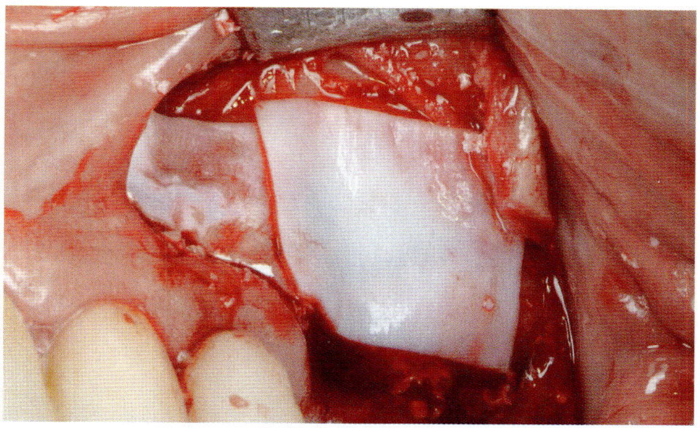

Fig 19 Window coverage with resorbable collagen membrane, left upper quadrant.

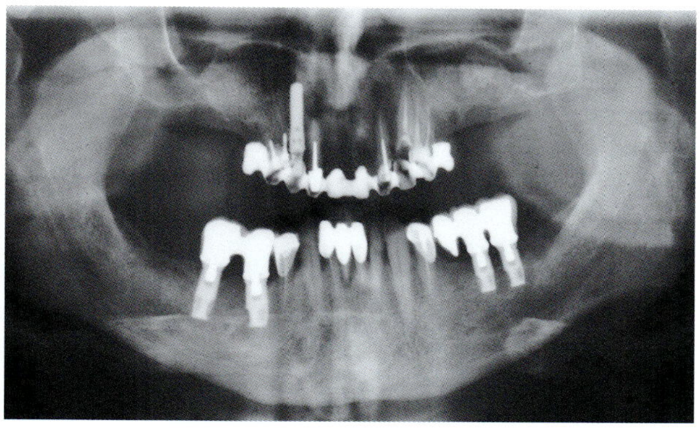

Fig 20 Panoramic radiograph after sinus grafting.

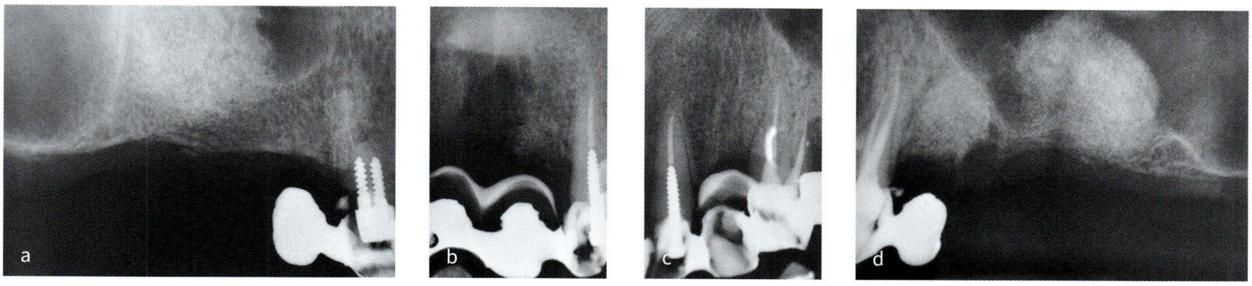

Figs 21a-d Periapical radiographs before implant surgery.

Table 1 Implant types and dimensions

Implant site	Diameter (mm)	Length (mm)	Implant type
16	4.8	10	Wide Neck
13	4.1	12	Regular Neck (previously placed in 2001)
21	4.1	10	Bone Level Tapered
23	4.1	10	Bone Level Tapered
26	4.8	10	Wide Neck

A similar procedure was then performed for the contralateral sinus on the same day (Figs 18 to 20).

At 3 months, a flapless extraction of tooth 23 was performed without grafting to allow complete healing for subsequent implant placement.

At 6 months, after uneventful healing, implants were placed at the grafted sites 16 and 26 and at sites 21 and 23 in a single surgical procedure (Figs 21a-d). Small incisions were made under local anesthesia with a minimally reflected flap. The flap showed good ridge healing at all sites, allowing correct 3D positioning of the implants without grafting. The implant osteotomies were prepared according to the standard protocol for the type of implant selected for each site. The implants were then placed (Table 1) with an average torque of 35 Ncm (Figs 22 to 25). Healing abutments were screwed on top to promote non-submerged healing

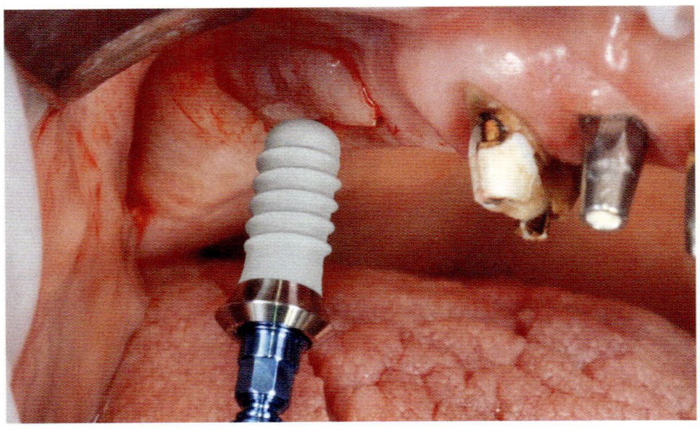

Fig 22 WN implant at site 16.

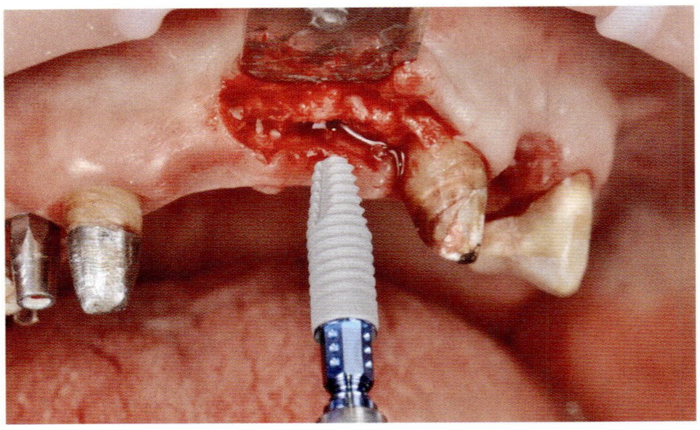

Fig 23 BLT implant at site 21.

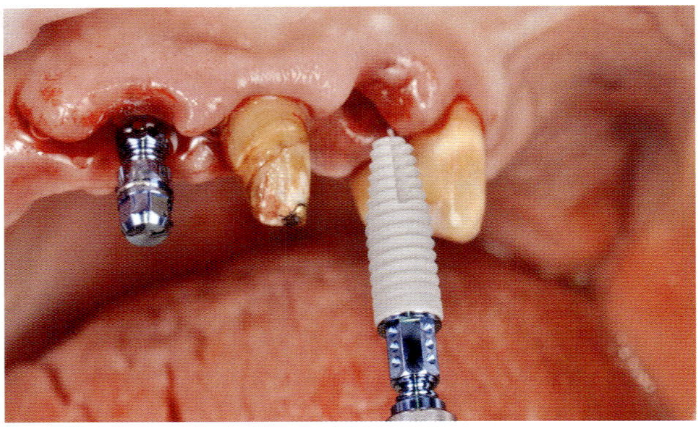

Fig 24 BLT implant at site 23.

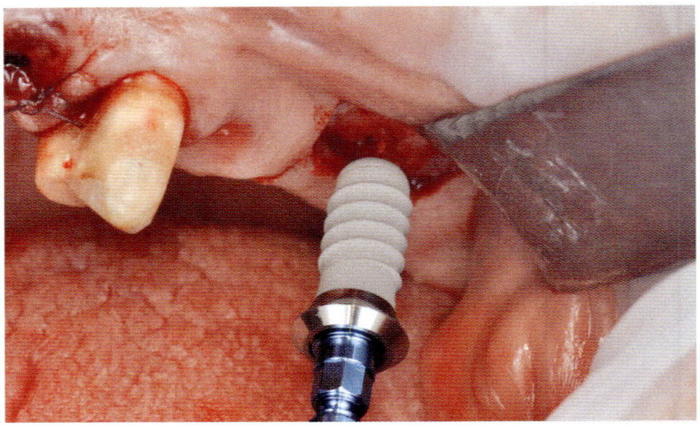

Fig 25 WN implant at site 26.

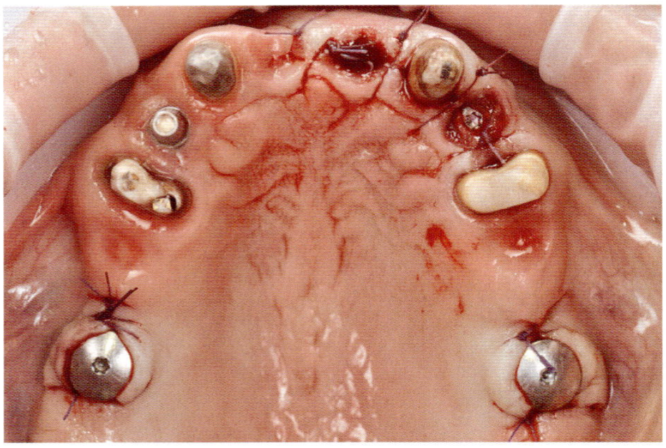

Fig 26 Occlusal view after implant insertion.

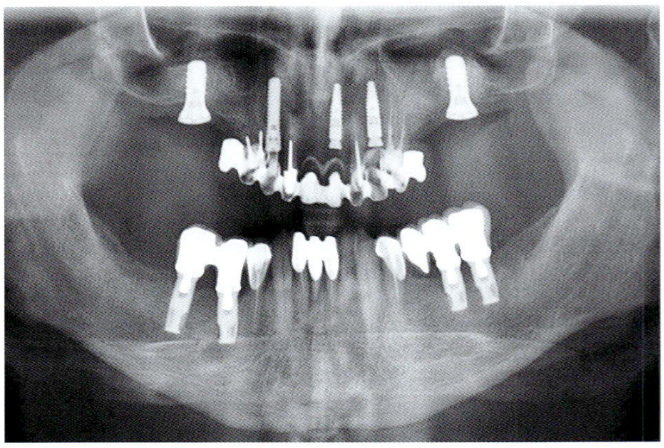

Fig 27 Panoramic radiograph following implant placement.

and avoid an additional surgical procedure. The flaps were sutured with resorbable sutures (Flysorb 5-0; Butterfly) (Fig 26). The provisional FDP was provisionally cemented and adapted to avoid pressure on the tissues and implant abutments during the healing period (Fig 27).

PROSTHETIC PROCEDURES

After implant osseointegration (3 months later), the provisional prosthesis was removed and an analog impression of the implants was taken (Fig 28). After approximately 2 weeks, the remaining natural abutments 14, 12, 22 and 24 were extracted flaplessly under local anesthesia with socket preservation at each site (Fig 29). The extraction

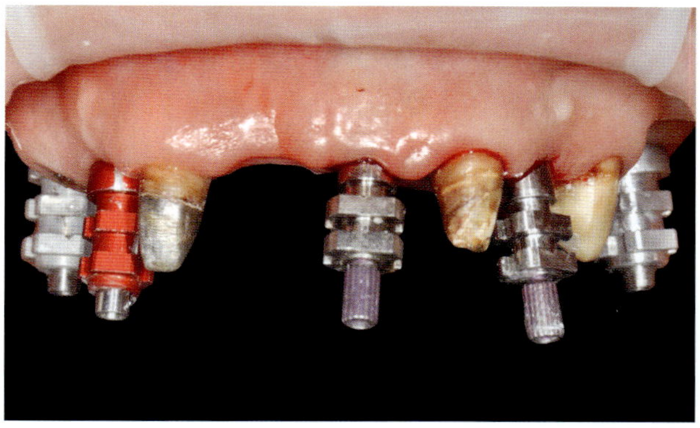

Fig 28 Analog impression for fixed implant-supported provisional restoration.

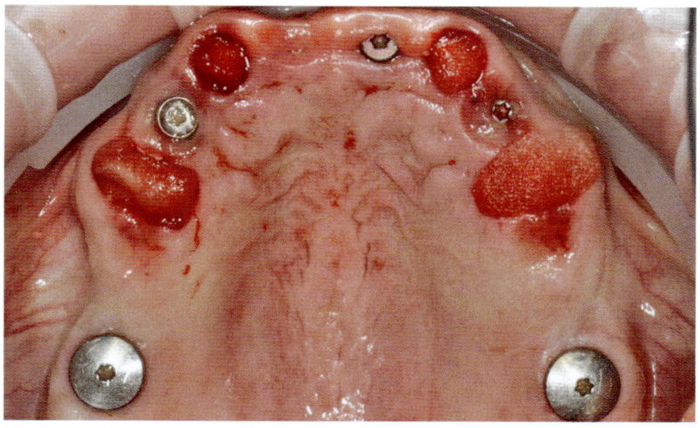

Fig 29 Socket preservation after tooth extractions.

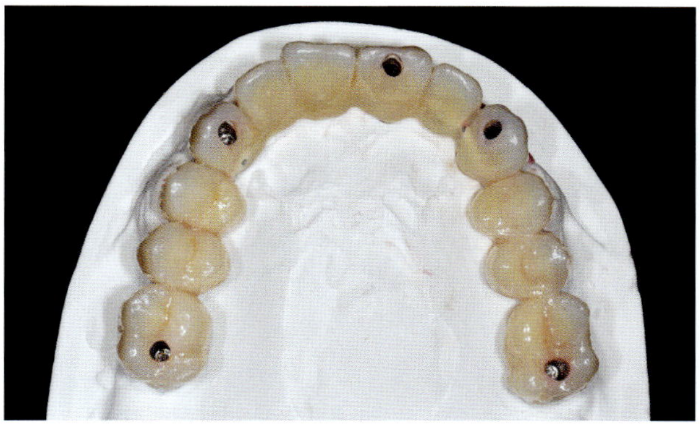

Fig 30 Implant-supported provisional restoration on the stone cast occlusal view.

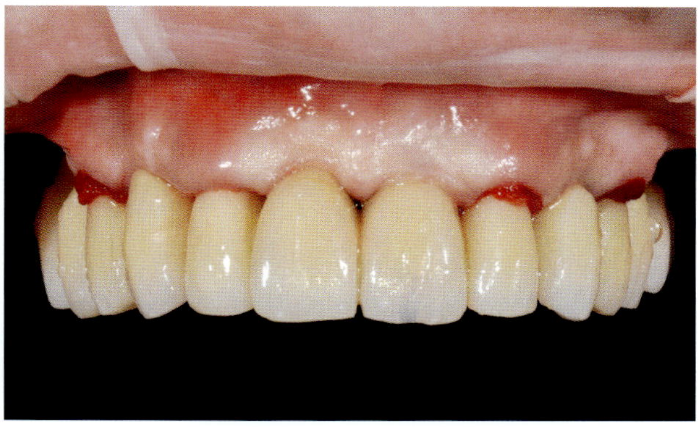

Fig 31 Delivery of the implant-supported provisional restoration.

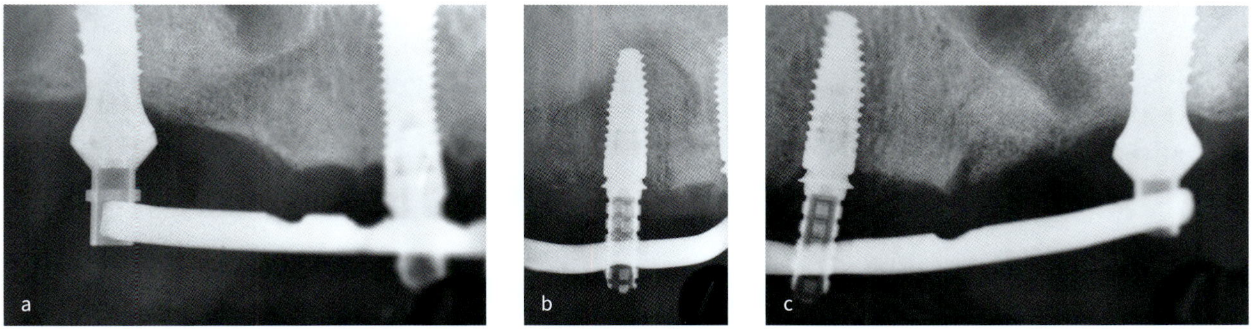

Figs 32a-c Periapical radiographs after delivery of the implant-supported provisional restoration.

sockets were filled with DBBM containing 10% collagen (Bio-Oss Collagen; Geistlich Pharma) and sealed with collagen sponges and the fixed implant-supported provisional restoration (Figs 30 to 32a-c). This approach is considered useful for preserving the soft- and hard-tissue architecture beneath the pontic areas (Schlee and Esposito 2009).

After final soft-tissue conditioning (3 months later), a definitive one-step/two-viscosity polyether impression (Permadyne; 3M ESPE, St. Paul, MN, USA) of the five implants was taken for the fabrication of a screw-retained metal-ceramic FDP (Figs 33 to 37). The cobalt-chromium metal framework was tried in and checked for passive seating on intraoral radiographs (Figs 38a-c). To improve the support for the cera-

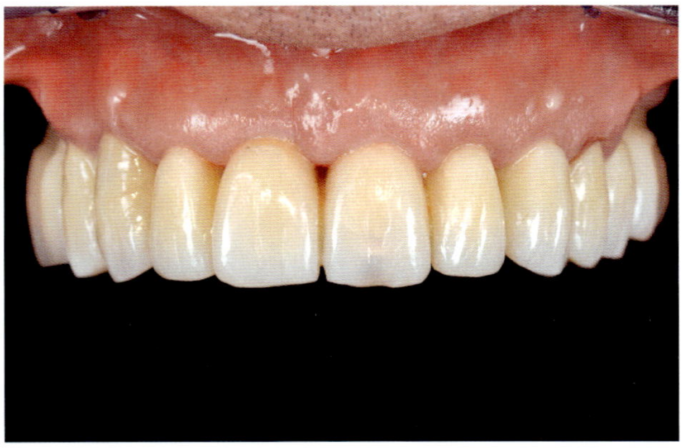

Fig 33 Implant-supported provisional restoration after 3 months in function.

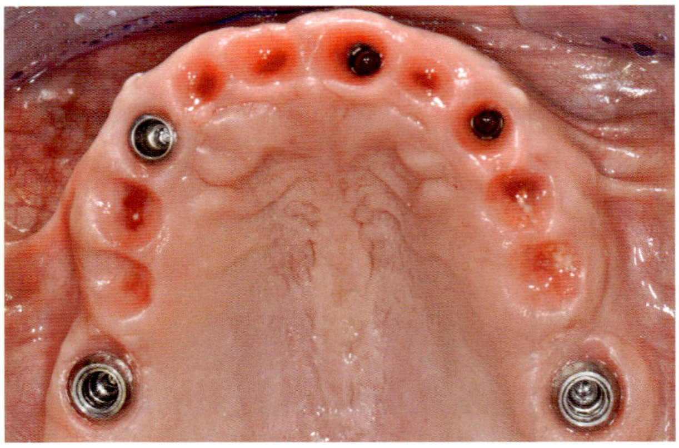

Fig 34 Soft tissue conditioning before definitive impression.

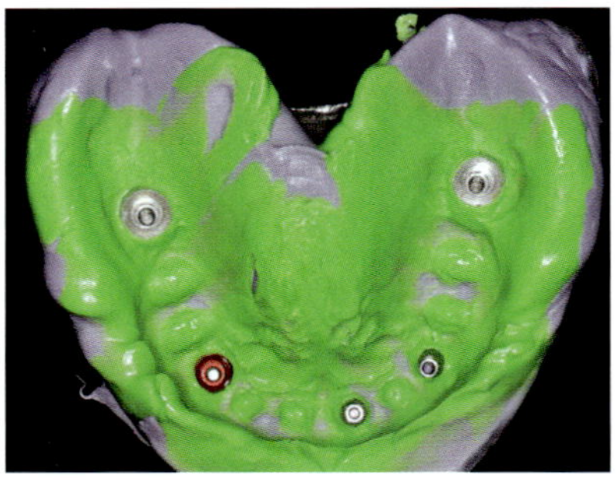

Fig 35 Definitive one-step/two-viscosity polyether impression.

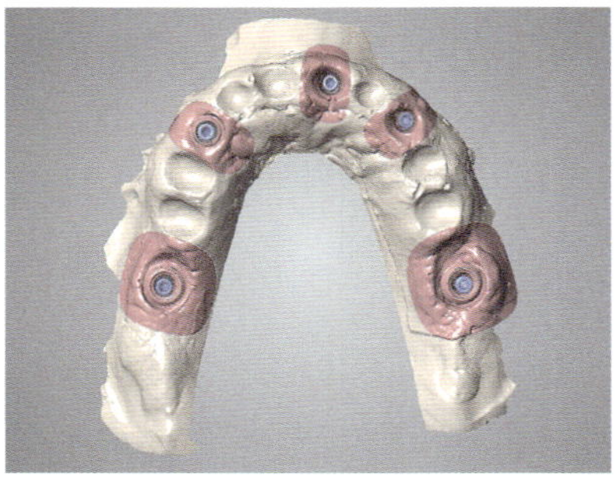

Fig 36 Digital model, occlusal view.

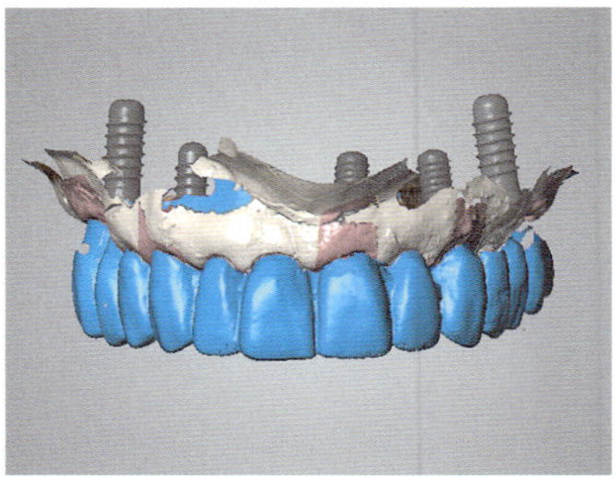

Fig 37 Digital model, frontal view.

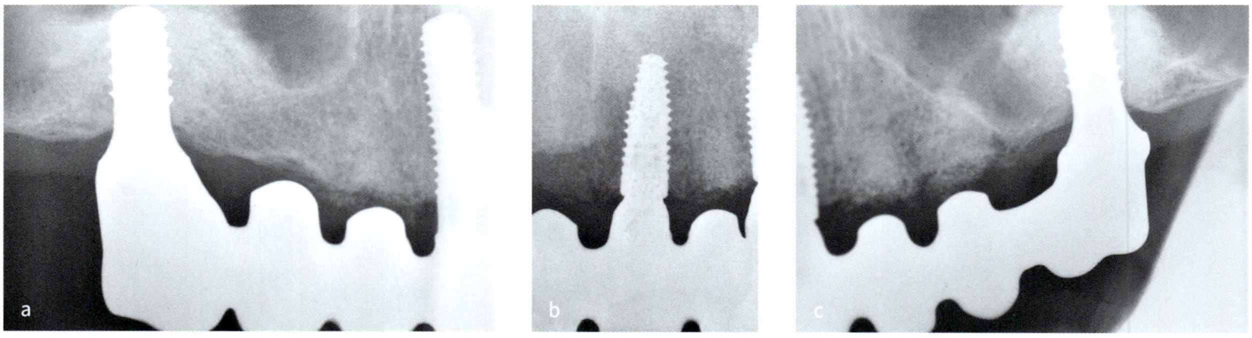

Figs 38a-c Periapical radiographs to check the fit of the cobalt-chromium metal framework.

mic layer and to prevent chipping or other technical complications, the screw access holes in the anterior implants were angulated using dynamic screws (Fig 39).

The final screw-retained full-arch FDP was then delivered, and the occlusion and mandibular excursion movements were checked (Figs 40 to 48).

FOLLOW-UP AND PATIENT SATISFACTION

Clinical (Figs 49 to 51) and radiographic (Figs 52a-d) evaluations at the 5-year follow-up revealed stable peri-implant hard and soft tissues. These interim results bode well for the anticipated long-term success of the rehabilitation.

Use this code to watch a highlight video with the patient reporting on his satisfaction with the treatment.

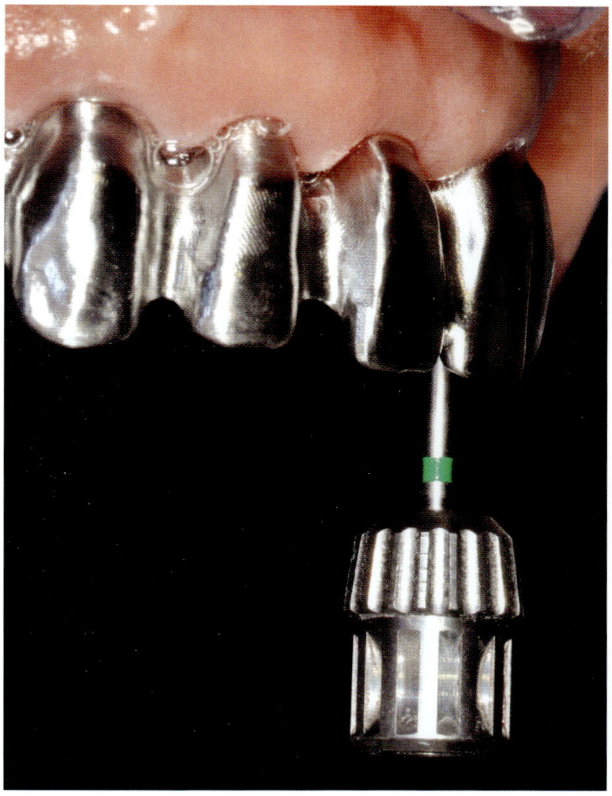

Fig 39 Angled screw access holes using dynamic screws.

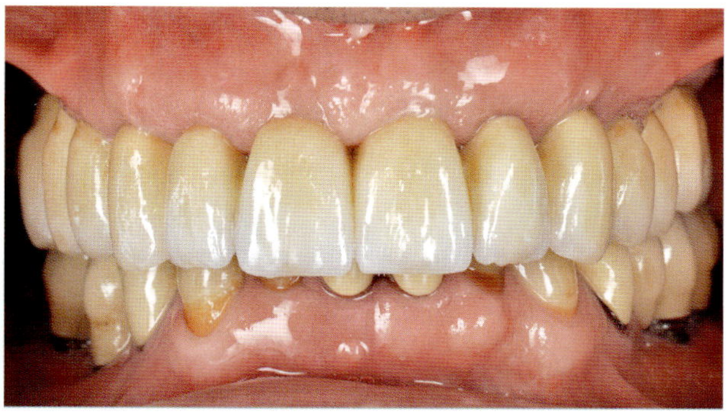

Fig 40 Clinical situation at the delivery of the final restoration.

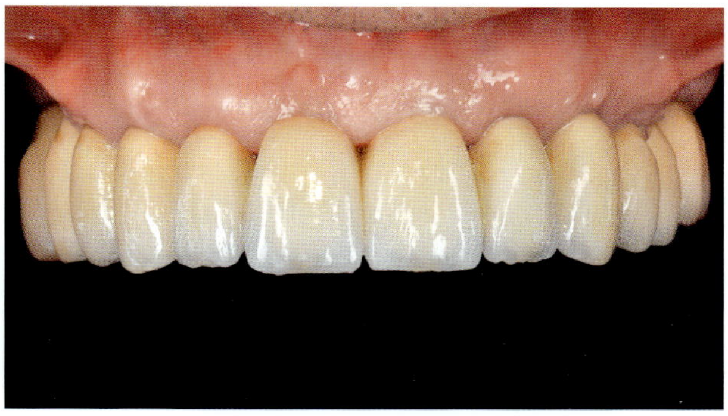

Fig 41 Maxilla at the delivery of the final restoration, frontal view.

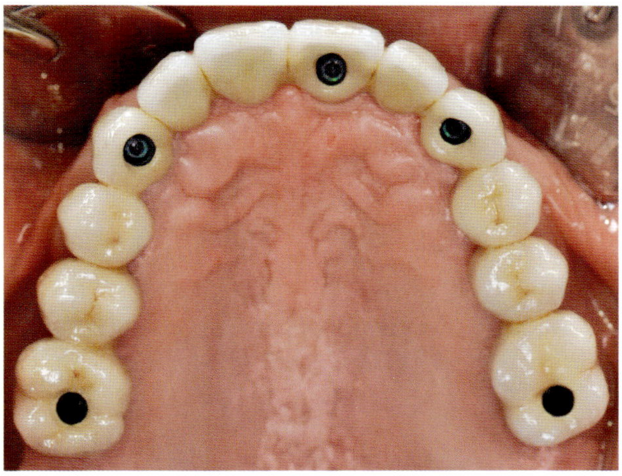

Fig 42 Maxilla at the delivery of the final restoration, occlusal view.

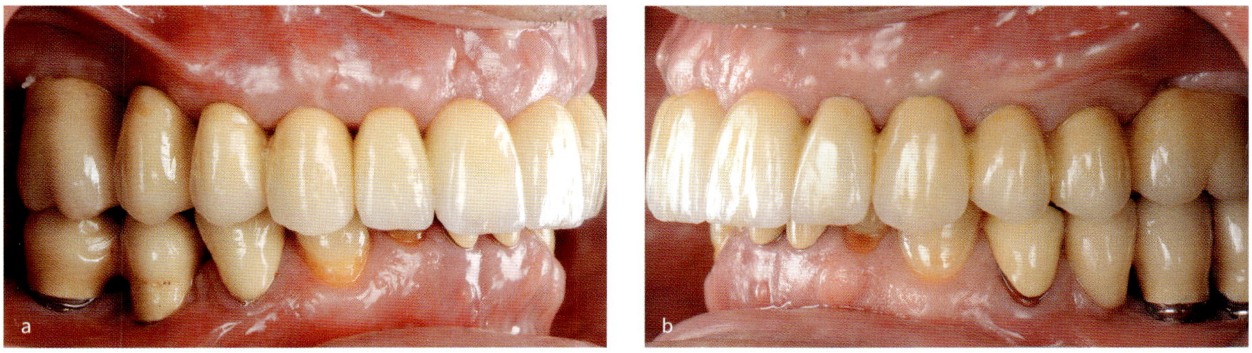

Figs 43a-b Maxilla at the delivery of the final restoration, lateral views.

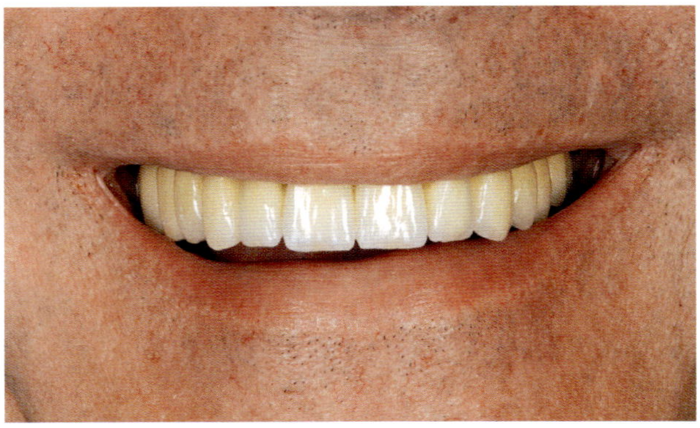

Fig 44 Extraoral frontal view after delivery.

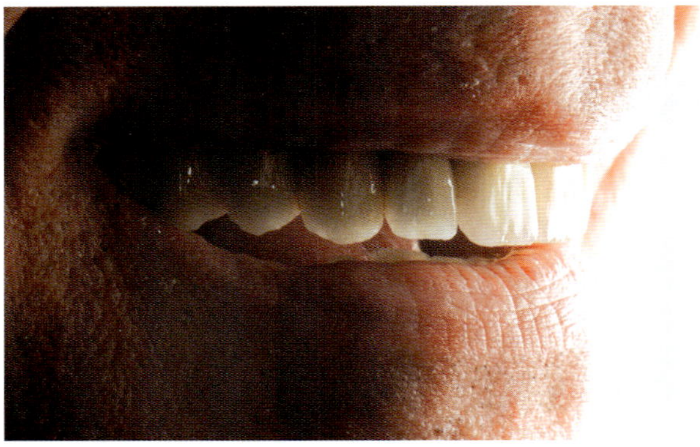

Fig 45 Close-up of the patient's smile.

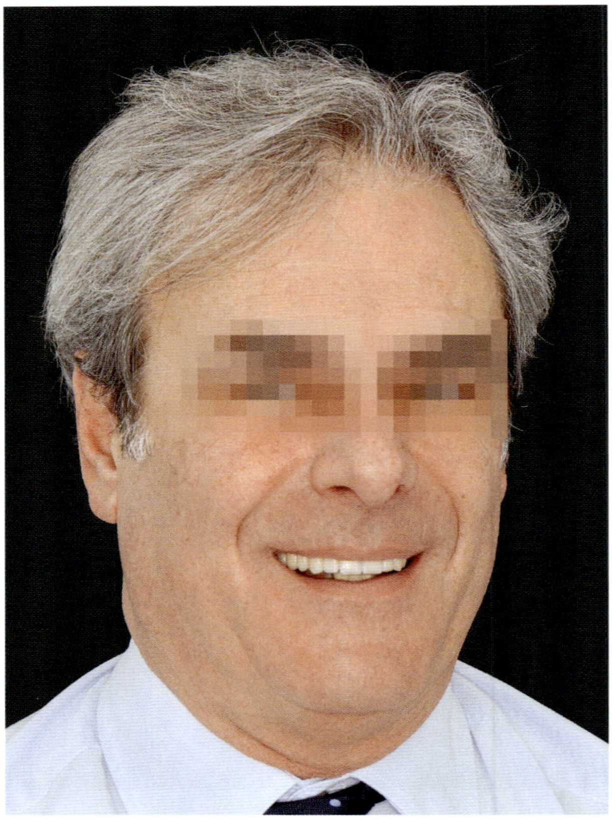

Fig 46 Patient's smile after delivery.

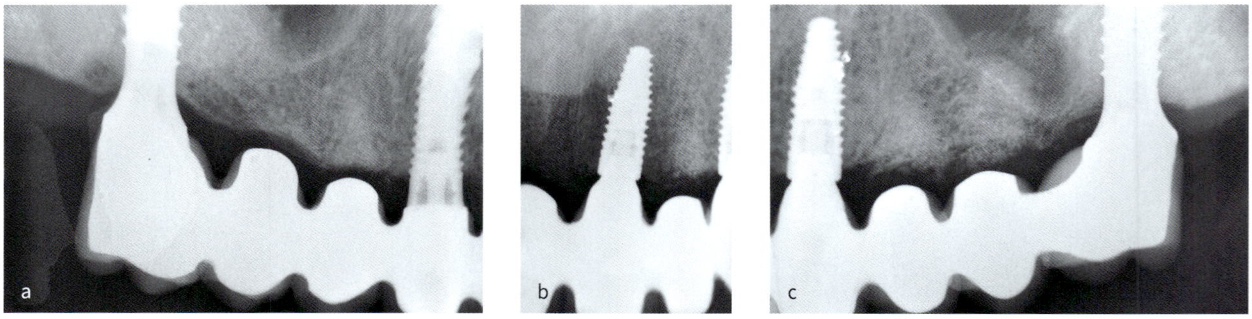

Figs 47a-c Periapical radiographs after delivery.

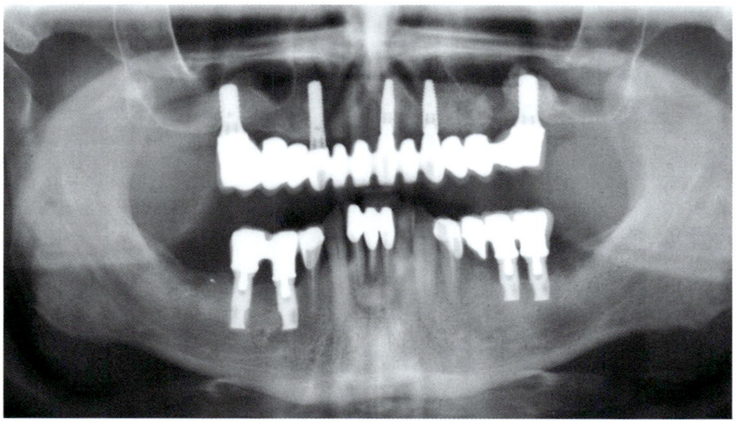

Fig 48 Panoramic radiograph 3 months after delivery.

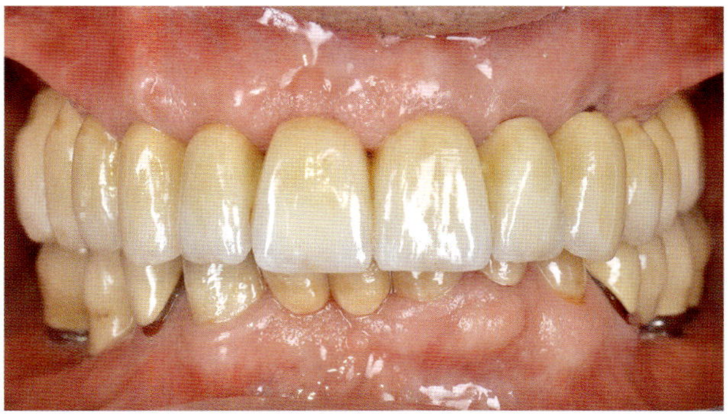

Fig 49 Clinical situation at the 5-year follow-up.

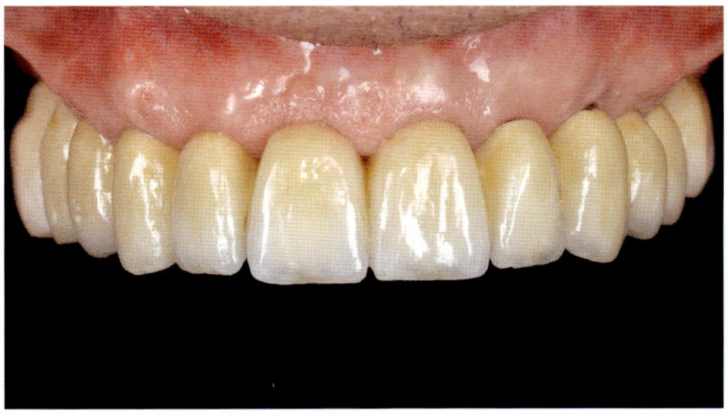

Fig 50 Maxilla at the 5-year follow-up, frontal view.

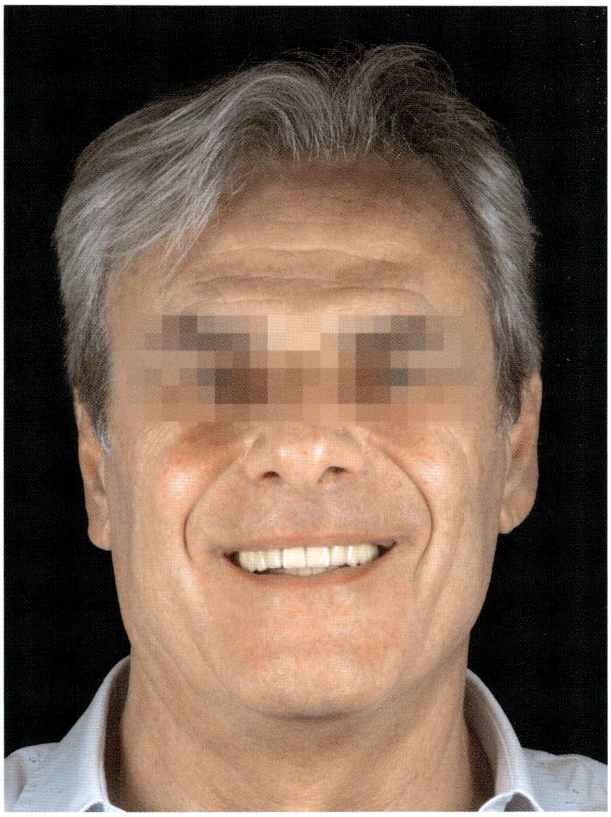

Fig 51 Patient's smile at the 5-year follow-up.

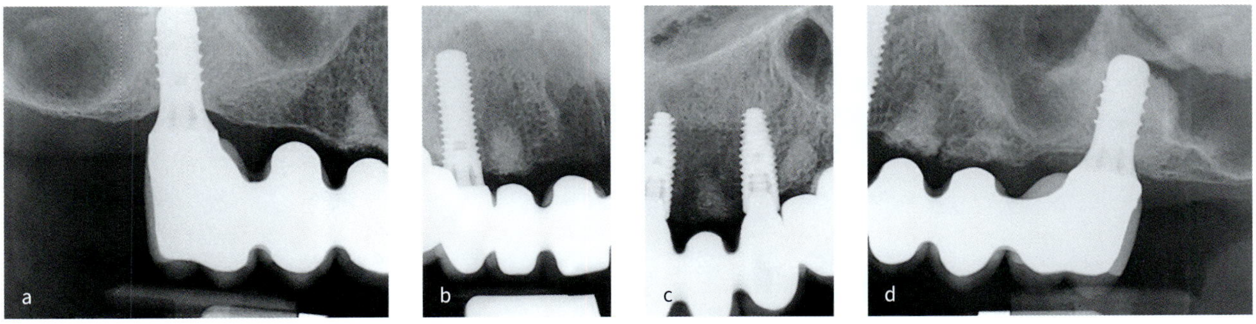

Figs 52a-d Periapical radiographs at the 5-year follow-up.

Table 2 Treatment sequence with timing

T0	Strategic tooth extraction and relining of immediate fixed provisional
After 2 weeks	
T1	Bilateral sinus lift with grafting
After 6 months	
T2	Implant placement
After 3 months	
T3	Extraction of the residual dentition, socket preservation, and insertion of a temporary implant-supported FDP
After 4 months	
T4	Impression for the definitive full-arch FDP
After 1 month	
T5	Delivery
Overall treatment time: 14 months	

DISCUSSION

The staged approach (Cordaro and coworkers 2007) has advantages and disadvantages. Advantages include the possibility of avoiding a removable provisional prosthesis, which enhances patient comfort but may also improve clinician efficiency. Implants can heal without the direct or indirect pressure of a removable prosthesis. Most importantly, however, esthetics and function can be maintained, minimizing the risks associated with immediate implant placement and loading.

A recent meta-analysis (Chen and coworkers 2019) showed a higher risk of failure for immediately loaded implants compared with conventionally loaded implants, with no difference in marginal bone level changes and probing depths.

The suggested timing for implant placement in this clinical scenario is usually of type 2/type 3 (Morton and coworkers 2014) to minimize the horizontal resorption of the alveolar bone, but also the soft-tissue contraction. In this case, a type 4 protocol was followed because of the time needed for the sinus graft to mature; no soft- or hard-tissue augmentation was performed.

Disadvantages of this staged approach include the need for multiple surgical procedures, extended treatment time (Table 2), and a slight increase in cost. In this case, the treatment took longer, but the patient achieved the same occlusion that would have been achieved with immediate loading, from day one. In addition, immediate loading of the immediate implants was ruled out because of excessive anteroposterior expansion spread due to the hyperpneumatization of the paranasal sinuses, which could have compromised the longevity of the prosthesis.

In addition, the staged approach can reduce the complexity of the treatment but is only applicable when implants can be placed in strategic positions bilaterally.

ACKNOWLEDGMENTS

Laboratory procedures

Laboratorio C&P SNC – Roberto Colli e Carlo Pedrinazzi

5.8 Treatment of a Fractured Edentulous Mandible Following Extraction of All Residual Teeth Using Computer-Guided Surgery and Immediate Loading

P. Casentini

PATIENT CHARACTERISTICS AND PATIENT PROFILE

A 65-year-old female patient was referred to our clinic by another patient for evaluation and treatment of her compromised dental clinical situation.

The patient presented with a pessimistic attitude and declared she had no confidence in the possibility of improving her oral situation. Her main complaint was discomfort, inability to chew, and collapse of the facial tissues related to her medical history. The patient had a serious domestic accident 18 months before the consultation and suffered from a head injury, followed by 4 months in a coma. She then gradually progressed toward almost complete neurological recovery, although, at the time of the consultation, she still had difficulty walking. The patient suffered a mandibular fracture in that accident, but because her life had been in danger, the fracture had been ignored. Since the patient was immobilized at the hospital for 4 months, the mandibular fracture had healed spontaneously, but the fragments reossified in an incorrect position, which resulted in a complete discrepancy between the positions of the remaining mandibular teeth and the maxillary teeth.

In consideration of the patient's disheartened attitude, her resilience was evaluated as low (level 1). Because of the absence of an occlusion, the severe discomfort, and the inability to chew, her expectations regarding function and retention were also rated as low (level 1). Since the patient did not express any esthetic request, esthetic expectations were evaluated as low (level 1). After the preliminary radiographic examination, the degree of tissue loss was considered moderate (level 2). The patient's son proved willing to cover the financial costs of treatment and no significant limitations were detected (Level 3). The risk of implant loss was initially difficult to evaluate.

The patient did not smoke. She was taking antidepressants.

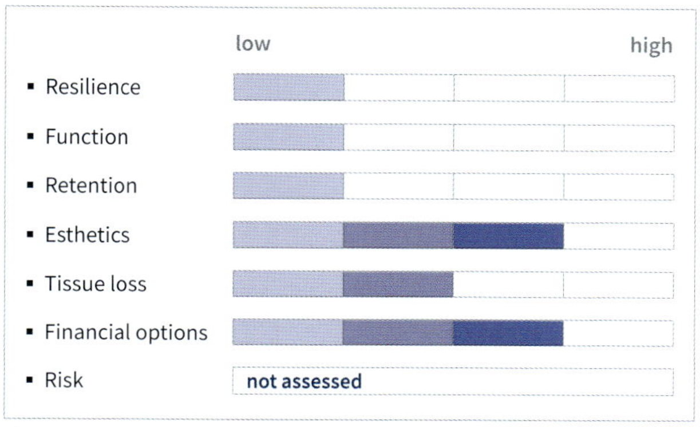

Fig 1 Patient profile.

Based on this information and the clinical evaluation described below, the following patient profile (Fig 1) can be derived for this patient (for more information about patient profiles, see Chapters 2.1.3 and 3.6).

CLINICAL EVALUATION

Extraoral examination revealed a collapse of the perioral facial tissues, with a partial introflexion of the lower lip (Figs 2 and 3).

Intraoral examination revealed the following clinical situation:

- In the maxilla, the loss of the molars was noted, with a residual dentition from tooth 15 to tooth 25. The remaining teeth appeared to be partially migrated and showed gingival recession, but no pathological probing depth was recorded despite the presence of bacterial plaque deposits. Teeth 15 and 25 showed class II mobility.

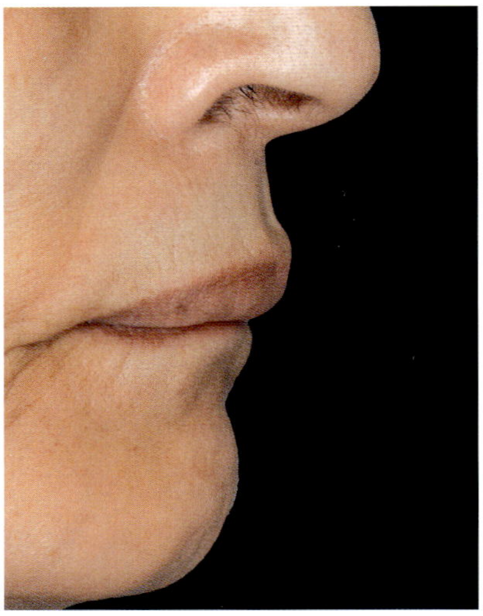

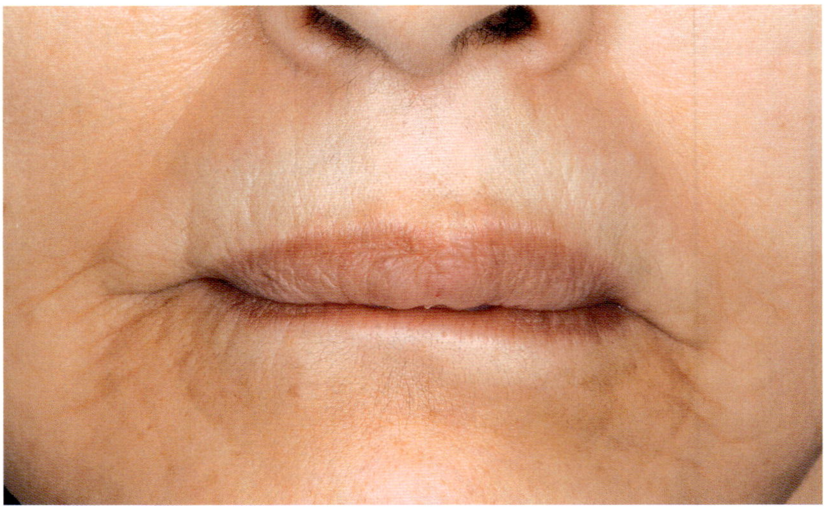

Figs 2 and 3 Extraoral baseline situation.

- In the mandible, most of the teeth were still present except for teeth 48, 44 to 41, 34 and 38. Teeth 47, 46, and 35 to 37 had been restored with metal-ceramic crowns; all crown margins were exposed and poor fit was evident. Two implants had been placed at sites 33 and 34 and connected to unidentified temporary abutments, which were covered by calculus. There was no residual keratinized tissue in this area. The patient reported that implants had been placed and partially restored prior to the trauma. All remaining natural teeth and prosthetic crowns appeared to be poorly located and tilted lingually, with limited and incorrect contacts with the opposing arch. Teeth 31 to 33 exhibited a combination of significant extrusion and lingual inclination and were in contact with the maxillary palatal mucosa. Due to their position and axis, and the unidentified prosthetic connections, the two implants were considered non-restorable (Figs 4 and 5).
- The degree of mouth opening was considered normal and the patient reported no pain in the temporomandibular joint area.

Digital impressions were taken with an intraoral scanner (Trios 3; 3Shape, Copenhagen, Denmark) to verify an altered interarch relationship and to define the contacts between the two arches. In particular, the internal view of the two arches in occlusion confirmed the complete absence of normal contacts between the maxillary and mandibular teeth and the presence of contact between the anterior mandibular teeth and the palatal mucosa (Figs 6 to 8).

PRELIMINARY RADIOGRAPHIC EXAMINATION

A panoramic radiograph was taken at the initial consultation to obtain a general radiographic overview of the oral cavity (Fig 9). The radiograph confirmed poor fit of the mandibular crowns, peri-implant bone loss around the mandibular implants, and generalized horizontal bone loss around the remaining maxillary teeth.

PRELIMINARY TREATMENT PLAN

Non-surgical periodontal treatment was planned, and the patient was instructed and motivated to improve her oral hygiene.

The patient's primary care physician and neurologist were consulted in order to determine her general medical status, the type of medications she was taking, and possible contraindications to dental care and oral surgical techniques.

DIAGNOSIS AND PROPOSED INITIAL TREATMENT PLAN

The mandibular teeth and implants were considered hopeless and unusable for any type of prosthetic rehabilitation due to their malposition and condition. Given the total loss of a stable occlusion, extraction of all the mandibular teeth and implants and temporary restoration with a complete mandibular removable dental prosthesis was considered the safer and more predictable way to restore the correct occlusal plane. Planning for a possible implant-supported restoration was deferred.

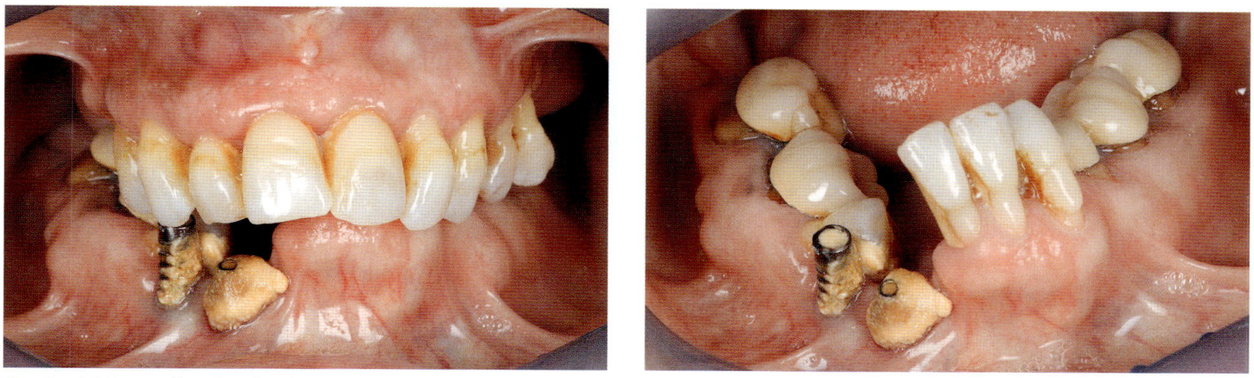

Figs 4 and 5 Intraoral baseline situation.

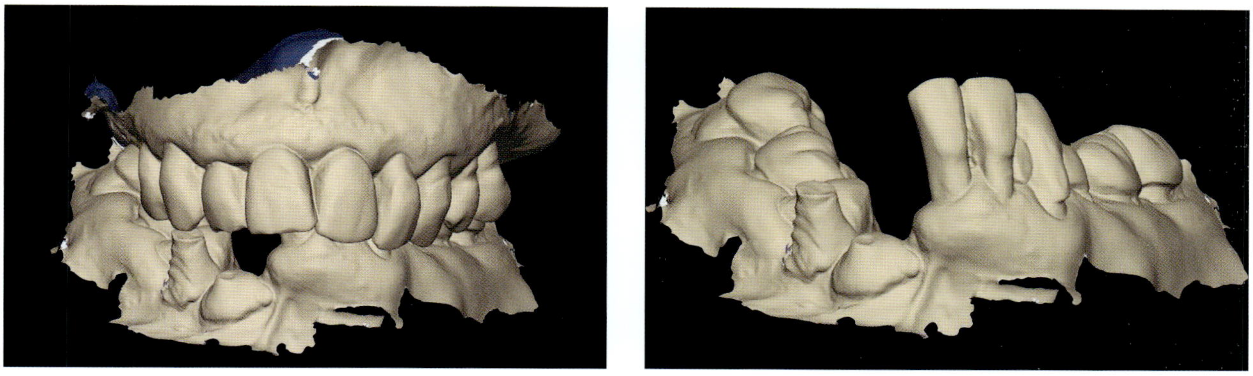

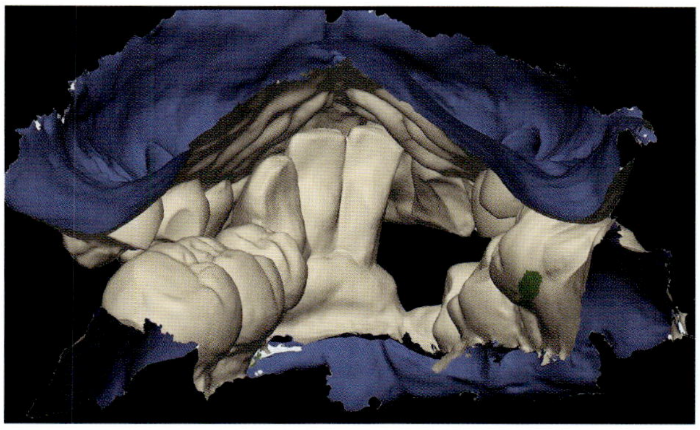

Figs 6 to 8 Intraoral scans at baseline.

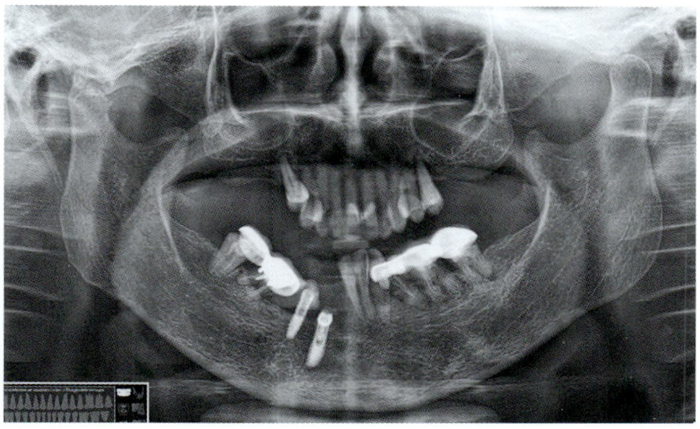

Fig 9 Radiological situation at baseline.

The remaining maxillary teeth had an improved prognosis after non-surgical periodontal treatment and were considered salvageable, except for teeth 15 and 25, which still showed class I mobility and were considered questionable. In any case, the mobility could be partially related to the malocclusion, so it was decided to retain the second premolars and re-evaluate them later. In addition, their presence could contribute to the stability of the mandibular prosthesis and increase the patient's chewing ability. Meanwhile, teeth 21 and 24 required endodontic treatment due to pulpal necrosis.

The decision to limit the extended treatment to the mandible was also in accordance with the patient's wishes.

EXTRACTION OF MANDIBULAR TEETH, REMOVAL OF IMPLANTS AND DELIVERY OF THE MANDIBULAR DENTURE

The attending physician and the neurologist who were following the patient approved the proposed treatment plan, and did not identify any specific medical contraindications.

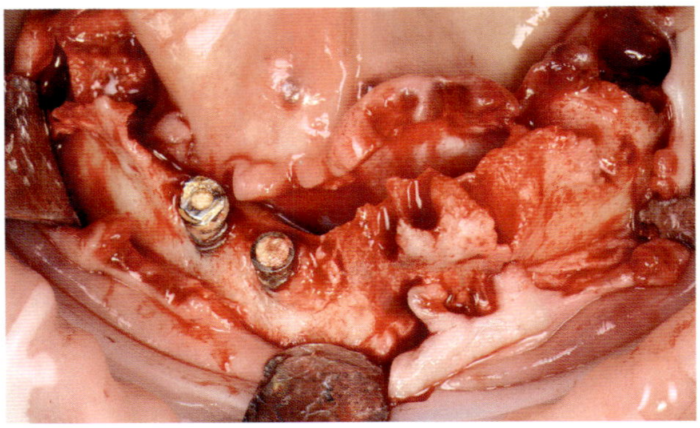

Fig 10 Irregular bone profile after extraction of hopeless teeth and flap elevation.

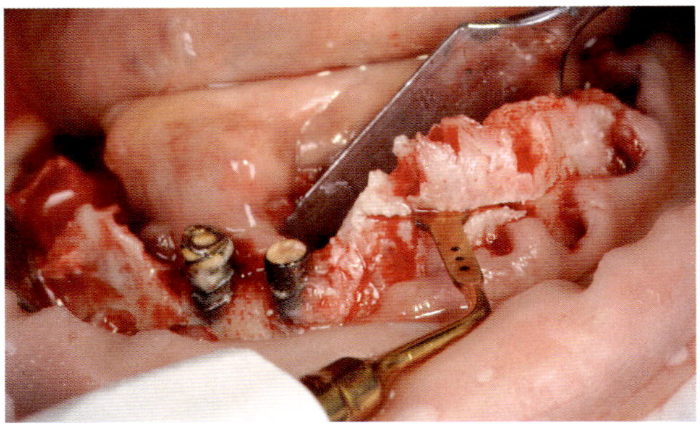

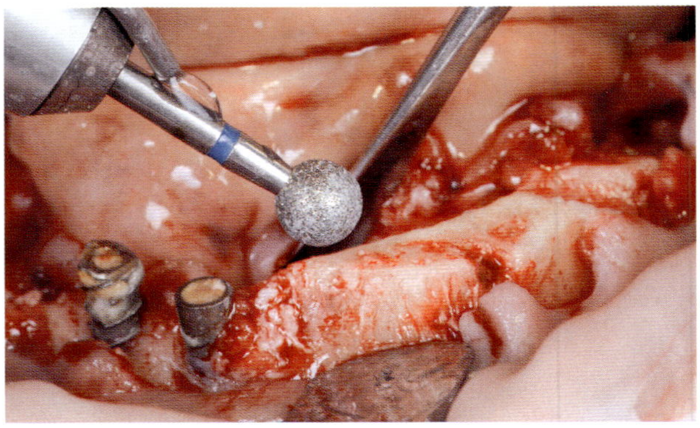

Figs 11 and 12 Surgical bone remodeling with a piezoelectric instrument and a diamond round bur.

The mandibular extractions were performed under sedation with the assistance of an anesthesiologist, who evaluated the patient's medical status.

After removal of the fixed mandibular restorations and extraction of the mandibular teeth, a full-thickness muco-periosteal flap was elevated to facilitate removal of the two implants and surgical remodeling of the bone crest. Bone reduction and implant removal were facilitated by piezosurgical instruments (Piezo-Surgery; Mectron, Carasco, Italy) combined with the use of a round diamond bur mounted on a surgical handpiece. The surgical procedure was completed by closing of the mucoperiosteal flaps with single PTFE sutures (5-0; Omnia, Fidenza, Italy) (Figs 10 to 15).

Chlorhexidine mouth rinses were prescribed for 2 weeks along with a non-steroidal anti-inflammatory drug for pain relief.

The sutures were removed after 2 weeks. Favorable soft-tissue healing allowed an early start of traditional prosthetic procedures to obtain the mandibular prosthesis (Fig 16), which was delivered 4 weeks after the extractions (Figs 17 and 18).

REEVALUATION AT 6 MONTHS

The patient was re-evaluated at 6 months and complete soft-tissue healing was confirmed (Fig 19). The patient's feedback after the first part of the treatment was positive, as her chewing ability and comfort had increased significantly. In addition, the patient reported a significant improvement in her facial appearance because the new prosthesis provided more support to the perioral tissues.

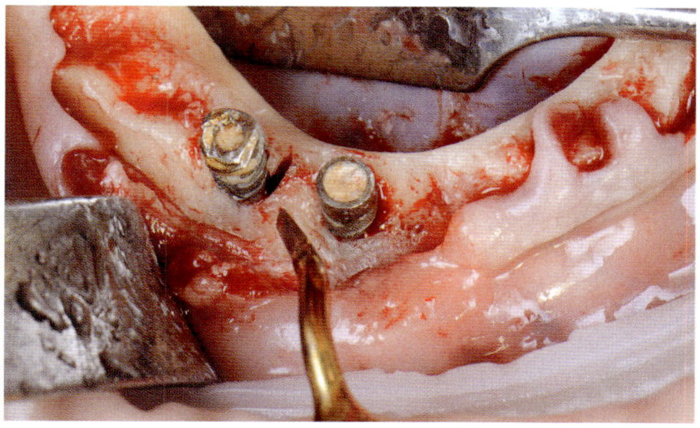

Fig 13 Implant removal assisted by a piezoelectric instrument.

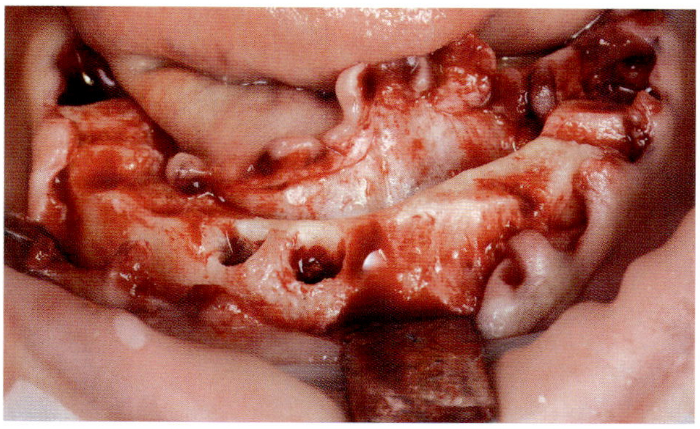

Fig 14 Final aspect of the remodeled bone crest.

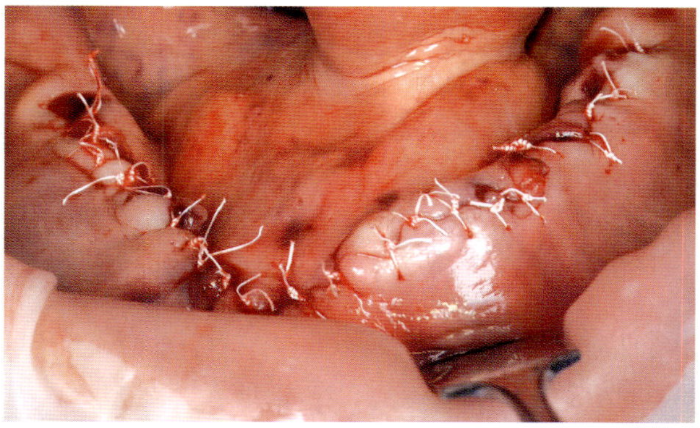

Fig 15 Final aspect of the surgical field after suture.

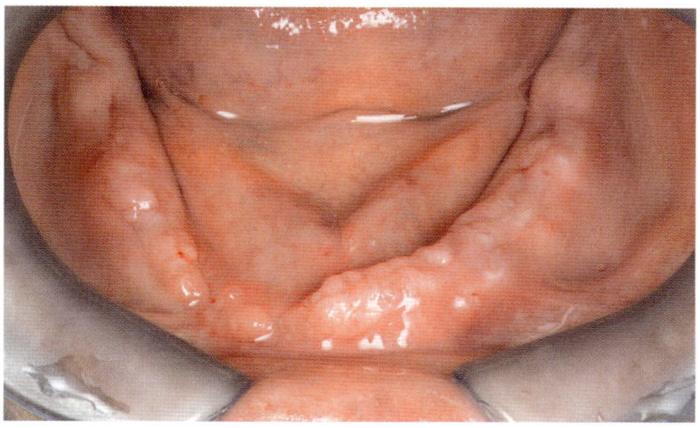

Fig 16 Healing of the soft tissues after 2 weeks.

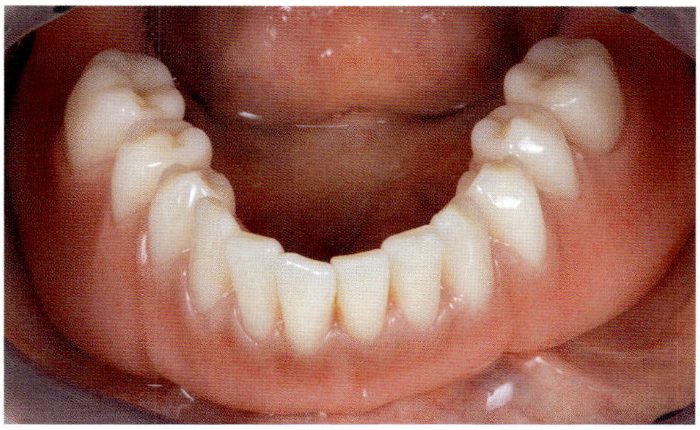

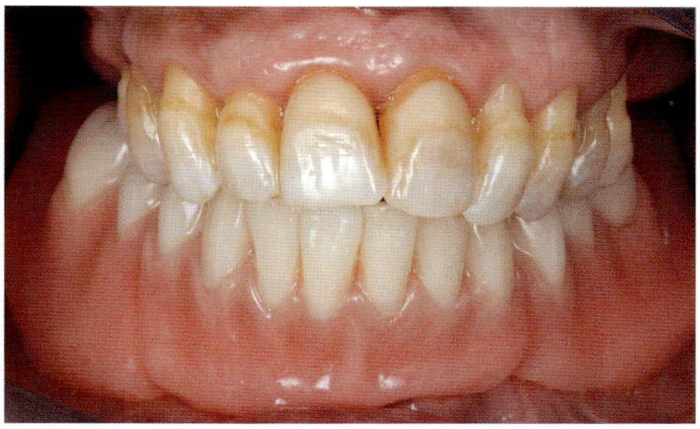

Figs 17 and 18 Delivery of the mandibular prosthesis after 4 weeks.

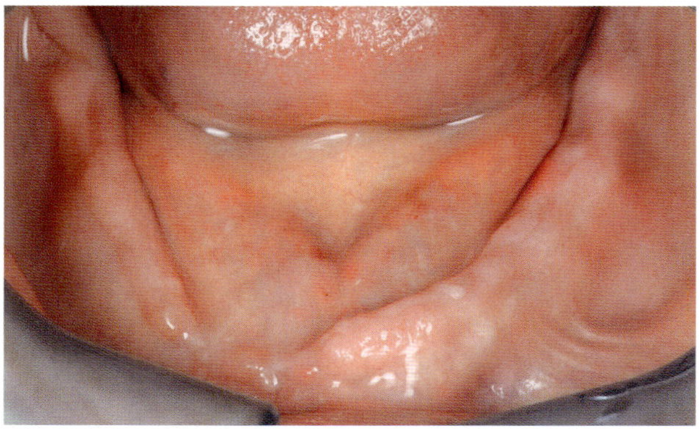

Fig 19 Healing of the mandibular ridge after 5 months.

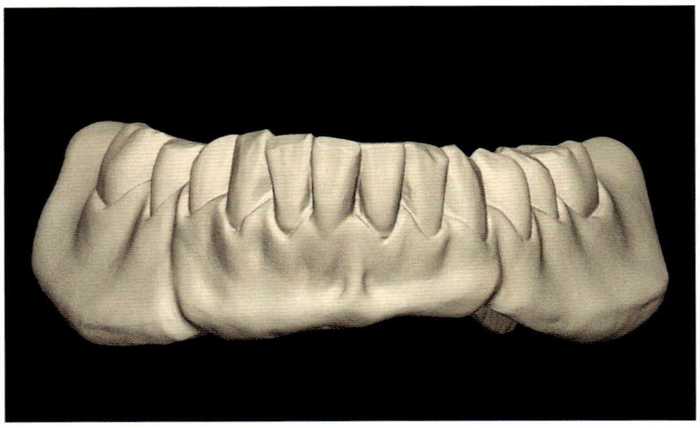

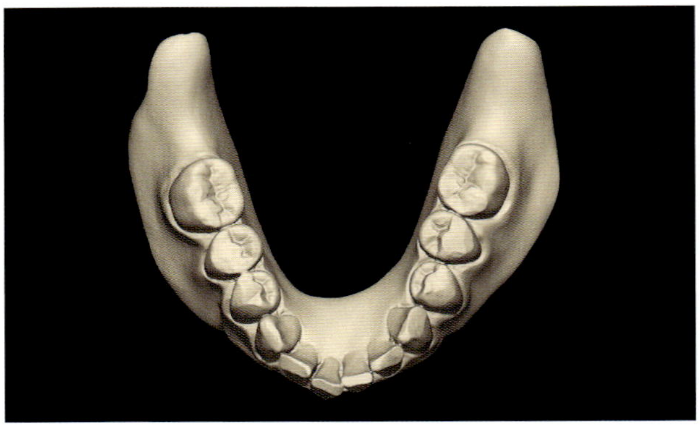

Figs 20 and 21 Extraoral scans of the mandibular denture.

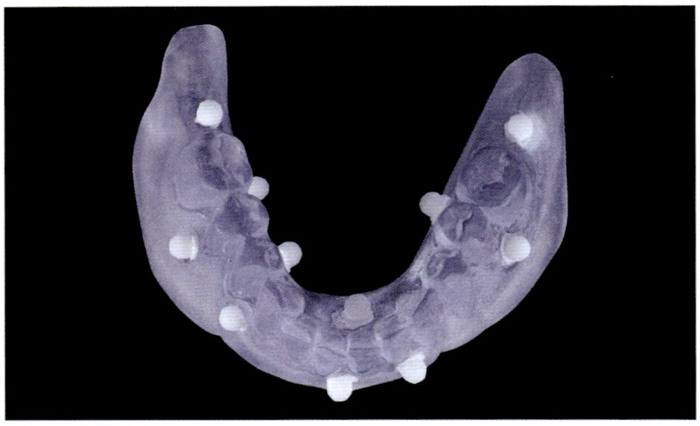

Fig 22 Radiographic guide with radiopaque markers.

The periodontal situation of the maxillary teeth was considered stable: (full-mouth plaque score, 15%; full-mouth bleeding score, 5%). Whilst teeth 15 and 25 still showed class I mobility, the probing depth was less than 4 mm at all residual maxillary teeth. It was therefore decided to retain these teeth. However, the patient complained about instability of the mandibular prosthesis and asked if it was possible to achieve greater stability or even facilitate a fixed restoration with implants.

DIGITAL DIAGNOSTIC WORKFLOW

An extraoral digital impression of the mandibular prosthesis was taken with an IOS (Trios 3; 3Shape) (Figs 20 and 21) and the STL file was sent to the dental laboratory.

The laboratory created a 3D-printed resin duplicate of the mandibular denture, added some radiopaque markers (a mixture of resin and barium sulfate) to the duplicate and created a diagnostic guide for 3D radiography (Fig 22). The diagnostic guide was scanned by the dental laboratory before delivery to the clinic and an STL file was obtained. A CBCT was then performed with the patient wearing the diagnostic guide. The DICOM files from the CBCT were then imported into planning software (coDiagnostiX; Dental Wings, Montréal, Canada) and combined with the STL file of the diagnostic guide.

Matching the DICOM and STL files in the software allowed verification of the relationship between the prosthetic volumes and the residual bone volume.

A preliminary evaluation of the bone volume confirmed the feasibility of the two main treatment options proposed to the patient:

- **Implant-retained overdenture supported by two interforaminal implants:** The main advantages of this solution are the reduction of cost for the patient and the ease of cleaning. In this particular case, since the patient already had a mandibular prosthesis, it only had to be adapted to the implants by incorporating the overdenture retainers. Scientific evidence supports an overdenture stabilized by two implants as a valid long-term treatment option (Rentsch-Kollar and coworkers 2010; Mosnegutu and coworkers 2015) that can improve the denture stability and the patient's quality of life (Kuoppala and coworkers 2013; Mishra and coworkers 2015).
- **Fixed screw-retained prosthesis supported by four implants:** Although this solution is more expensive and requires greater patient compliance, complete prosthetic stability and greater comfort can be achieved with this type of restoration (Brennan and coworkers 2010; Borges and coworkers 2022). Scientific evidence supports the use of four implants to provide adequate support for a fixed restoration in the long term (Daudt Polido and coworkers 2018; Morton and coworkers 2018). With favorable local conditions and adequate primary stability, implants can be loaded immediately after placement, and this option is usually appreciated by patients (Papaspyridakos and coworkers 2014b; Gallucci and coworkers 2014).

Computer-guided implant placement is a reliable evidence-based technique that can increase precision and reduce invasiveness, especially when flapless surgery is performed (Tahmaseb and coworkers 2018; Wismeijer and coworkers 2018).

FINAL TREATMENT PLAN

As the patient had indicated her preference for a fixed prosthesis, the following treatment plan was proposed and accepted by the patient who gave her written consent.

- Computer-guided placement of four implants in the edentulous mandible to support an immediately loaded fixed temporary screw-retained prosthesis. Computer-guided implant placement was considered important to minimize invasiveness, increase precision, and expedite the prosthetic steps, since the temporary restoration can usually be delivered immediately after the surgery.
- Reconstruction of a band of keratinized tissue at sites 44 and 43, as the absence of keratinized tissue around implants has been suggested to be a risk factor for peri-implantitis (Schrott and coworkers 2009; Lin and coworkers 2013; Roccuzzo and coworkers 2016; Thoma and coworkers 2018). Soft-tissue reconstruction was planned in the absence of keratinized tissue, after implant osseointegration and before final restoration.
- Final fixed composite resin restoration supported by a CAD/CAM titanium framework.

COMPUTER-GUIDED PLANNING

The combination of DICOM and STL files allowed four implants to be planned at sites 46, 43, 33, and 36 to support a screw-retained restoration. Because the bone volume allowed the placement of parallel implants, tissue-level implants were chosen in order to simplify the prosthetic treatment. The implant axis was planned to achieve the best position for screw access holes.

Another planning goal was to achieve a direct connection between the implants and the restoration without the need for intermediate abutments. Straumann TLX implants, with their more retentive thread design, were selected in order to improve primary stability, as immediate loading was planned. Three anchor pins were also planned and the surgical guide was designed using the same software. A two-piece modular guide was planned to verify the correct positioning of the guide in relation to the opposing arch (Figs 23 to 28).

FABRICATION OF THE TEMPORARY FIXED PROSTHESIS

The same planning software (coDiagnostiX; Dental Wings) allowed the dental technician to export the master model and the surgical guide in STL format.

An initial STL file was used to create a 3D-printed master model of the mandible with replicas of the planned implants in place. The dental technician then selected and fitted temporary abutments and fabricated the temporary prosthesis in acrylic resin. A tolerance space was left between the temporary abutments and the resin framework in order to accommodate discrepancies between the planned and actual implant positions. Retromolar flanges were also placed to increase the stability of the prostheses during the relining procedures (Figs 29 to 31).

A second STL file was used to print the surgical guide, which was completed with the addition of PEEK and metal sleeves for the implant sites and anchor pins (Figs 32 and 33).

COMPUTER-GUIDED SURGERY

The surgical procedure was again performed under sedation with the assistance of an anesthesiologist. A local anesthetic with a vasoconstrictor was administered buccally and lingually. The surgical guide was first fixed with the anchor pins and the soft tissues were marked with a circular mucotome according to the Straumann Guided Surgery protocol. The surgical guide was then removed and soft-tissue morphology was evaluated in relation to the surgical approach. At the distal sites 46 and 36, removal of the marked soft tissue allowed for preservation an adequate band of keratinized tissue, and the soft tissue operculum was removed with a 15C blade and surgical forceps. There was no residual keratinized tissue at site 43, so the alveolar mucosa was simply removed. At site, 33 a mini-flap was elevated in order to preserve an adequate band of keratinized tissue around the future implant (Fig 34).

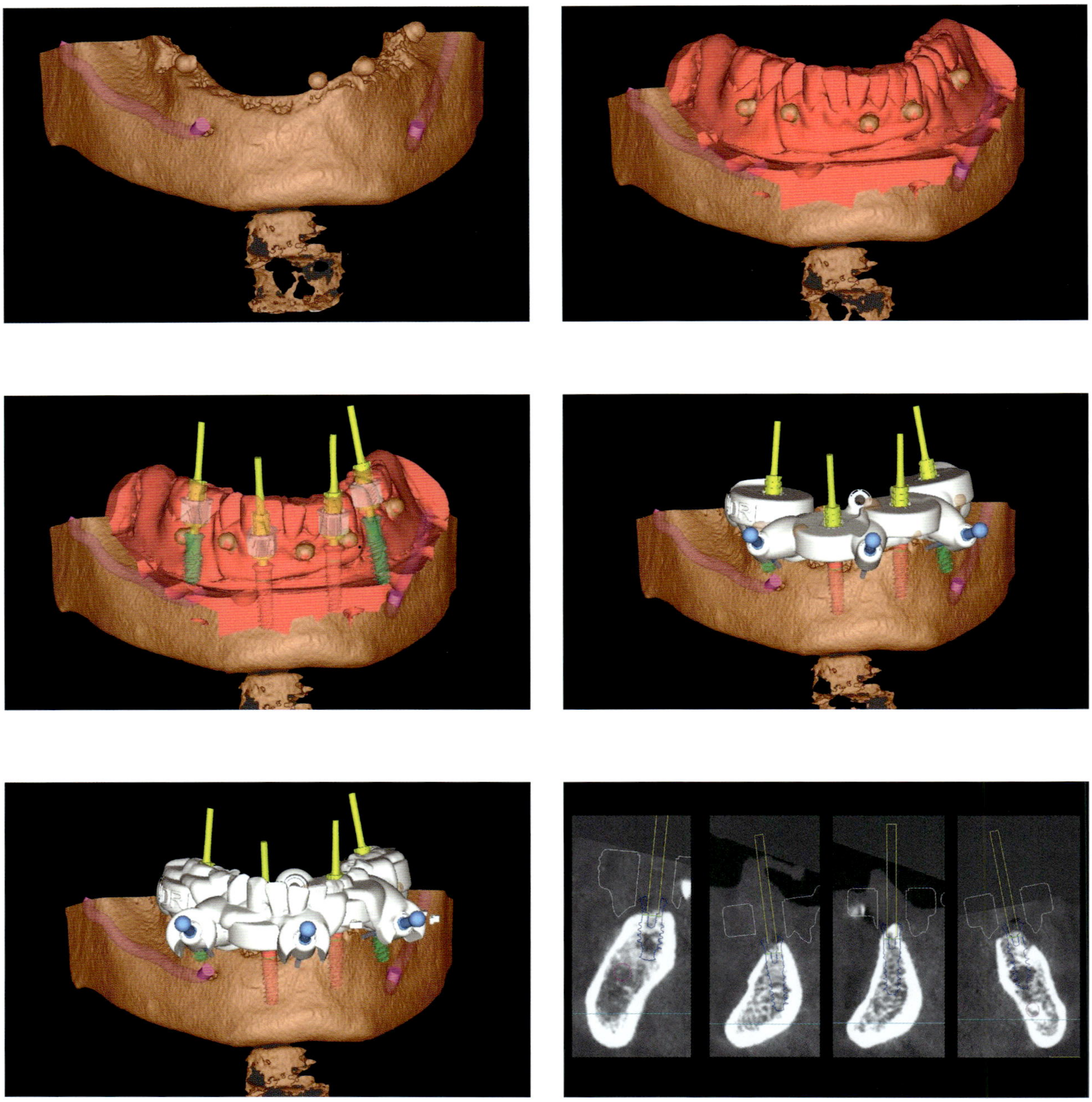

Figs 23 to 28 Prosthetically-driven implant planning using the coDiagnostiX software after matching the DICOM and STL files.

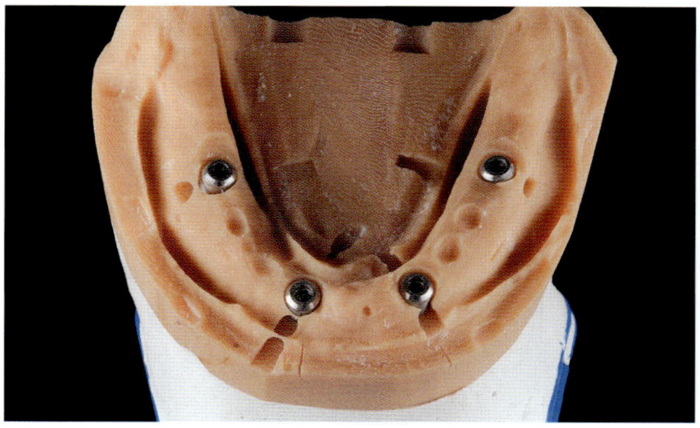
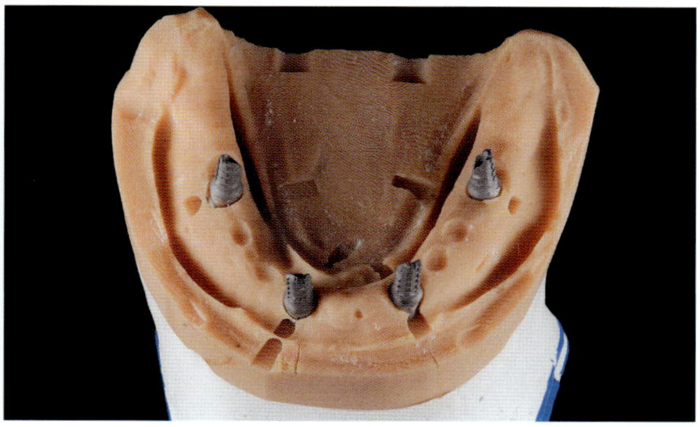
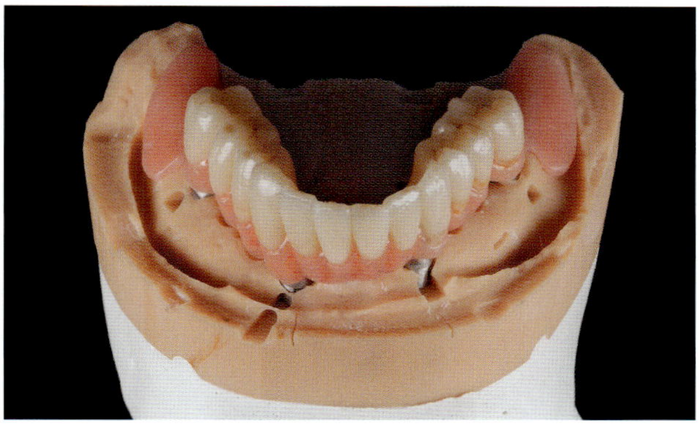

Figs 29 to 31 3D-printed model obtained in a digital workflow; temporary prostheses for immediate loading based on the same model.

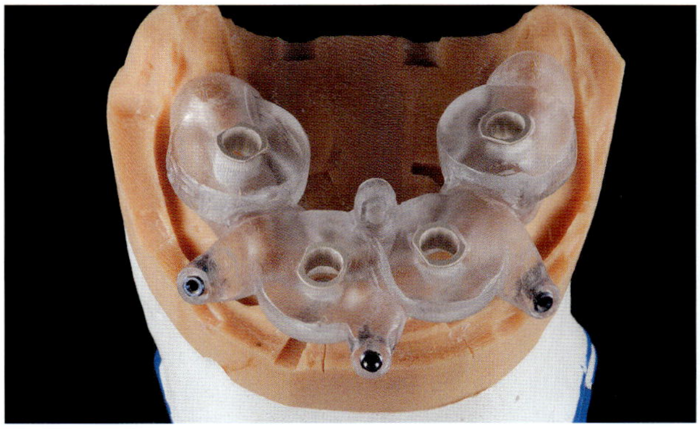
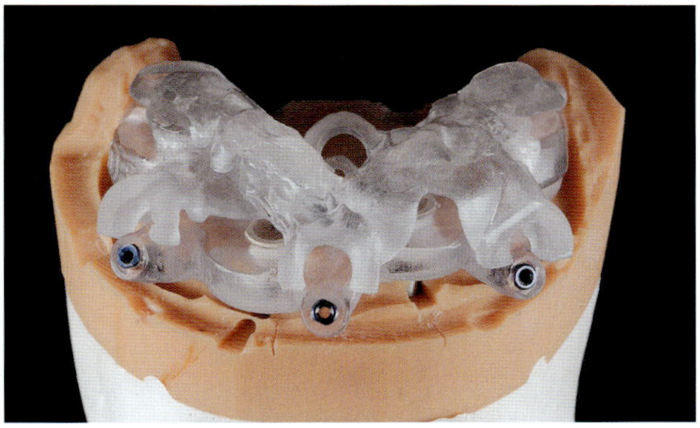

Figs 32 and 33 Surgical guide for computer-guided implant placement. To improve the stability of the surgical guide during fixation with pins, a second, superimposed guide was used, which had a precise relationship to the opposite arch.

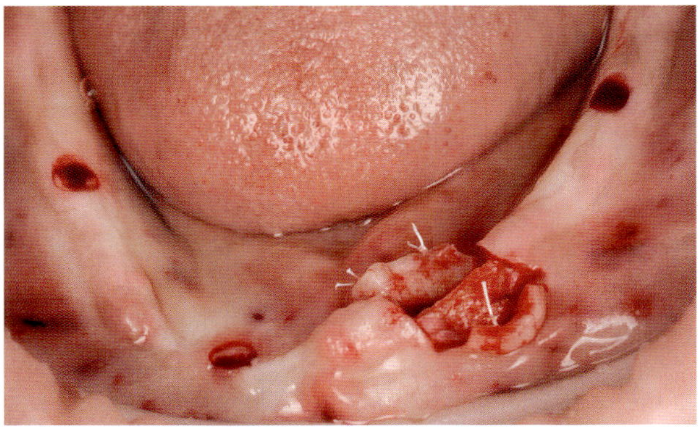

Fig 34 Flapless and flap surgery based on local conditions.

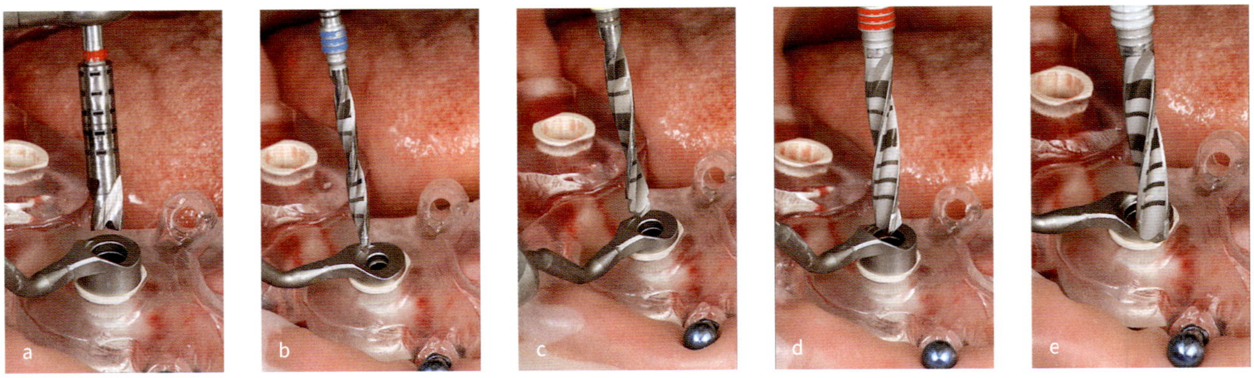

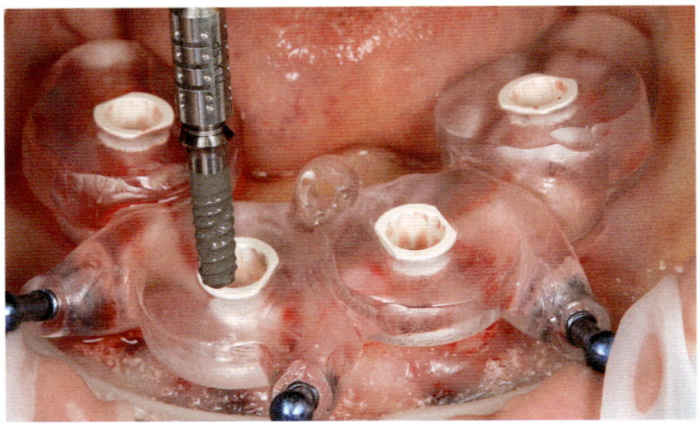

Figs 35a-e and 36 Guided implant site preparation and implant placement.

After soft-tissue removal and access to the bone surface, the surgical guide was repositioned and fixed with the anchor pins.

Osteotomies and implant placement were then performed according to the surgical sequence indicated by the planning software for each implant site (Figs 35a-e and 36). All implants were inserted with a torque greater than 35 Ncm.

The surgical guide was then removed and a correct relationship between the implants and the surrounding soft tissues was verified (Fig 37). The flap at site 33 was sutured with single PTFE sutures (5-0; Omnia).

IMMEDIATE LOADING

Sandblasted titanium temporary abutments were immediately screwed onto the implants (Fig 38) and the complete seating of the temporary prostheses in the correct relation to the opposing arch was verified. Autopolymerizing resin was used to bond the titanium abutments to the temporaries. When the resin had reached a sufficient degree of polymerization, the restoration was unscrewed and removed from the oral cavity (Figs 39 and 40).

The metal wire-reinforced provisional restoration was refined chairside by the dental technician (Figs 41 and 42) and screwed to the implants with a torque of 15 Ncm. The screw access holes were sealed with PTFE tape and a temporary filling material (Cavit; 3M ESPE, St. Paul, MN, USA) (Fig 43). The occlusion was checked and minor adjustments were made. A panoramic radiograph confirmed correct placement of the restoration (Fig 44). Postoperative medication included antibiotics for 6 days, chlorhexidine rinses for two weeks, and non-steroidal anti-inflammatory drugs for pain.

The patient was discharged and recalled at 1, 2, 4, and 8 weeks. Sutures were removed at 2 weeks. No biological or mechanical complications were noted.

The patient reported a more comfortable occlusion and a further significant improvement in her quality of life after receiving the implant-supported prosthesis.

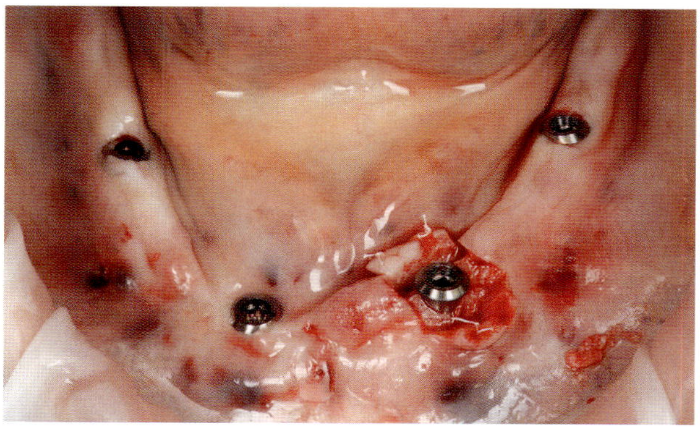

Fig 37 After implant placement.

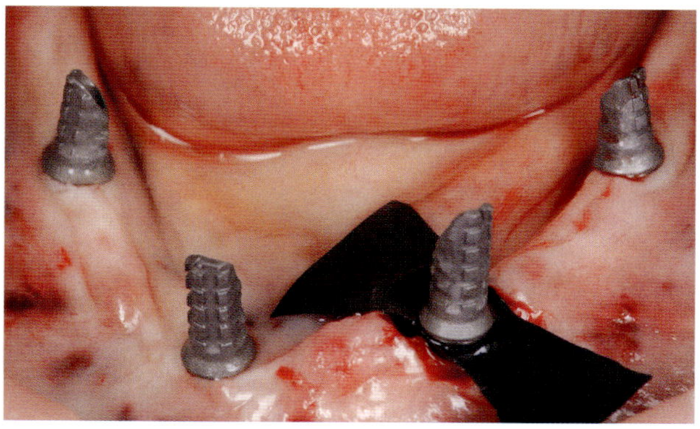

Fig 38 Connection of temporary abutments.

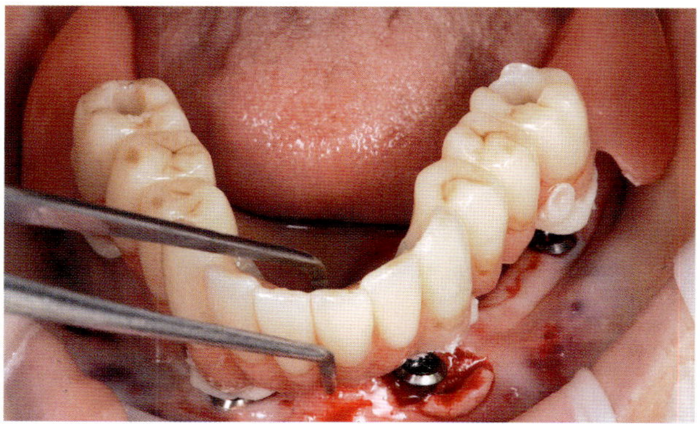

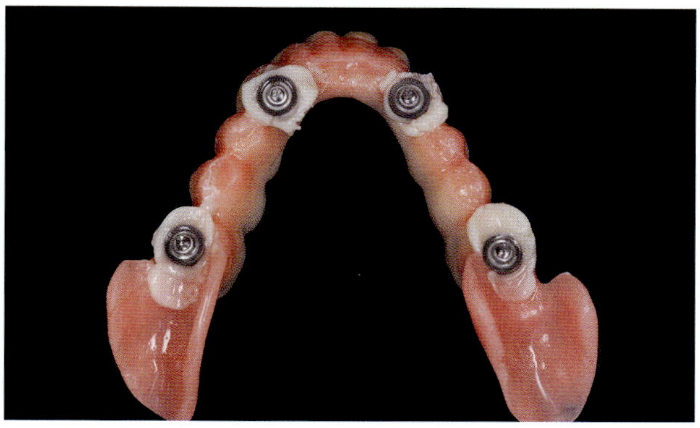

Figs 39 and 40 Removal of the temporary restoration after resin relining.

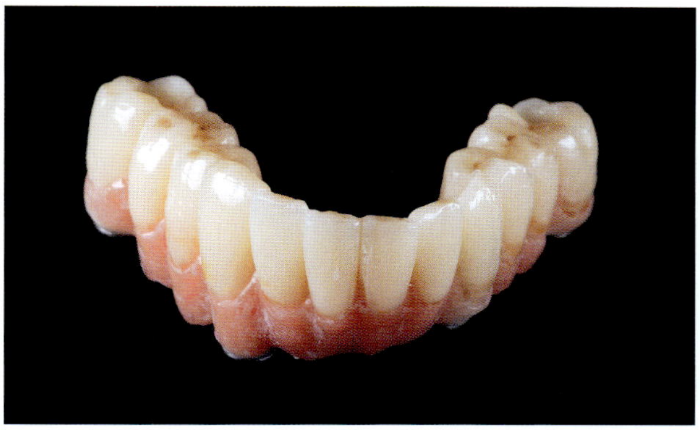

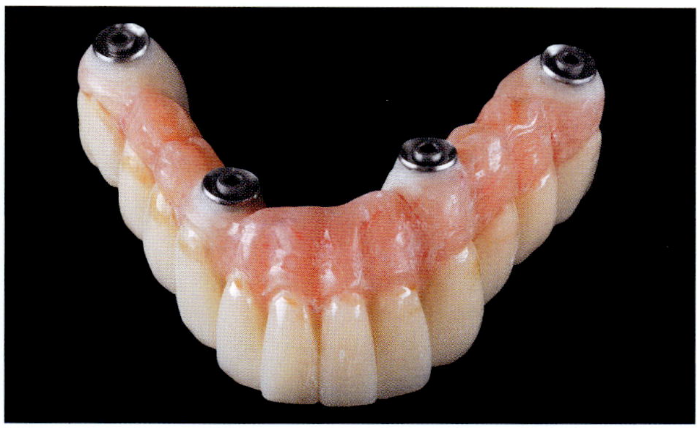

Figs 41 and 42 Extraoral view of the screw-retained restoration before delivery.

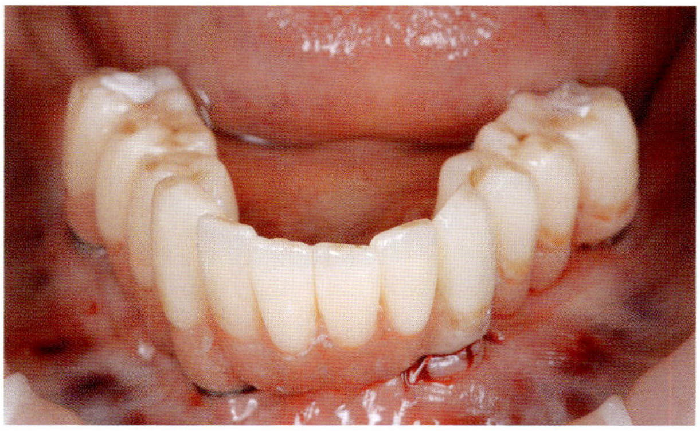

Fig 43 Intraoral view of the screw-retained restoration after delivery.

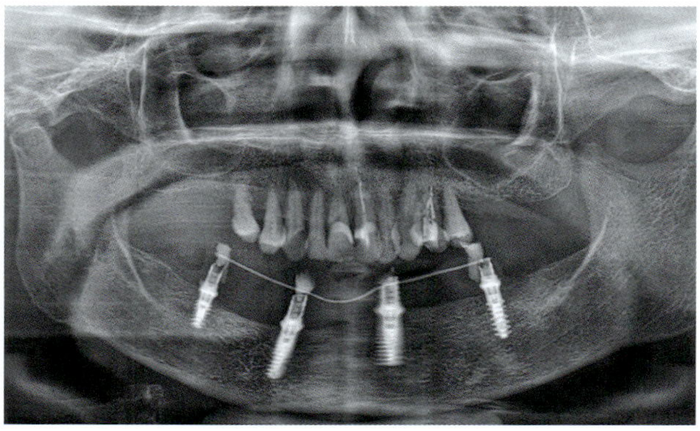

Fig 44 Panoramic radiograph after immediate loading.

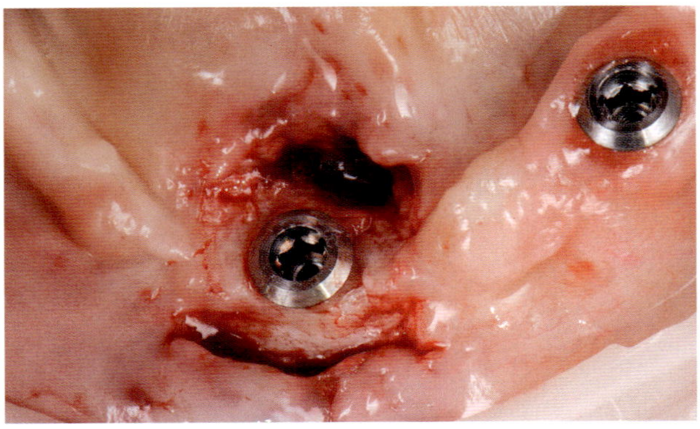

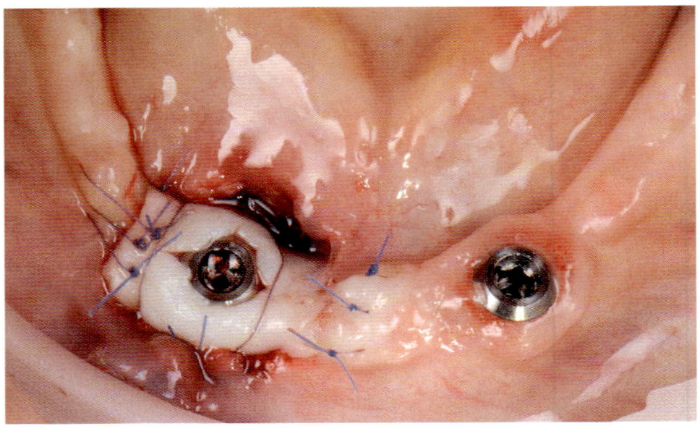

Figs 45 and 46 Peri-implant free gingival graft at site 43.

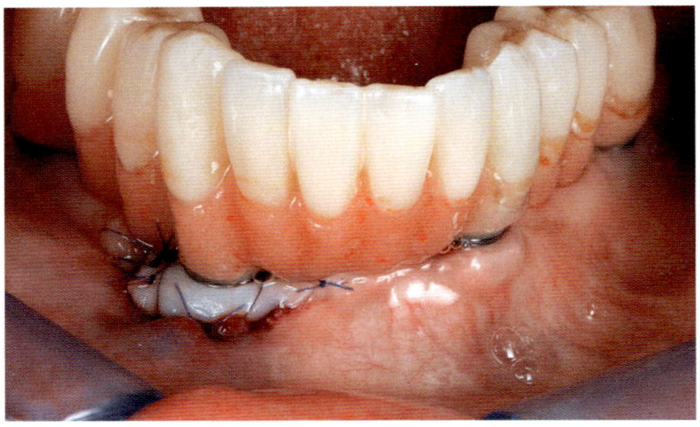

Fig 47 Reinsertion of the temporary restoration after free gingival graft.

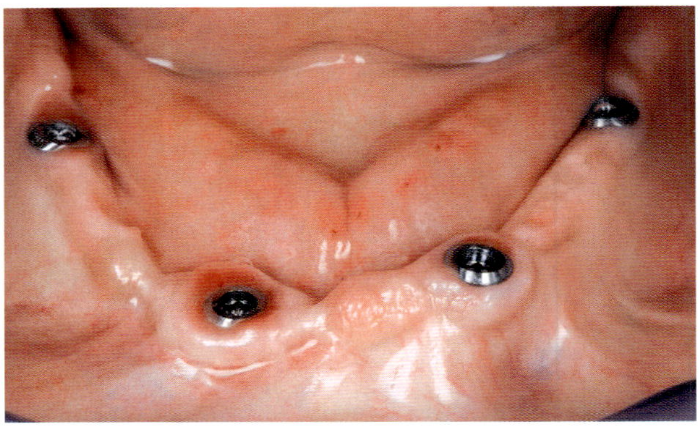

Fig 48 Healing of the grafted site after 8 weeks.

RECONSTRUCTION OF THE KERATINIZED TISSUE

After 8 weeks, a free gingival graft was performed to obtain an adequate band of keratinized tissue at site 43. A peri-implant partial-thickness flap was elevated buccally and lingually, and a free gingival graft was harvested from the palate, adapted to the machined collar of the implant with a "poncho design," and stabilized with resorbable sutures (Vicryl Ethicon 5-0; Johnson & Johnson Medical, New Brunswick, NJ, USA) (Figs 45 and 46) The temporary restoration was reinserted immediately after the surgery (Fig 47). The patient was advised to avoid brushing the surgical site for 3 weeks.

Postoperative medication included chlorhexidine rinses for 2 weeks and non-steroidal anti-inflammatory drugs for pain.

The sutures were removed after 2 weeks. No complications were noted, and the patient reported no significant symptoms.

FINAL RESTORATION

Healing was verified 8 weeks after soft-tissue surgery (Fig 48) and prosthetic procedures for the final restoration could begin. After removal of the temporary fixed restoration, the internal cavities of the implants were disinfected with 1% chlorhexidine gel, and an open-tray polyether impression (Impregum; 3M Espe, Seefeld, Germany) was taken after metal transfer copings were connected to the implants (Figs 49 and 50).

A master cast was fabricated by the dental laboratory and its accuracy was validated using a plaster verification index (Figs 51 and 52). To define the interarch relationship, the temporary restoration was used for a chairside cross-mount procedure.

The dental laboratory then designed and fabricated a CAD/CAM screw-retained titanium bar using an external milling center (Createch, Mendaro, Spain) (Fig 53). A hybrid resin-composite framework (Ambarino Multilayer; Smart Gate, Milan, Italy) was also fabricated by CAD/CAM (Fig 54) and layered with different colored resin composites.

Finally, the composite framework was luted to the titanium bar with a dual-polymerizing adhesive (Bifix Hybrid Abutment; Voco, Cuxhaven, Germany) (Figs 55 and 56).

The design of the final restoration included adequate spaces for oral hygiene and cleanable convex surfaces.

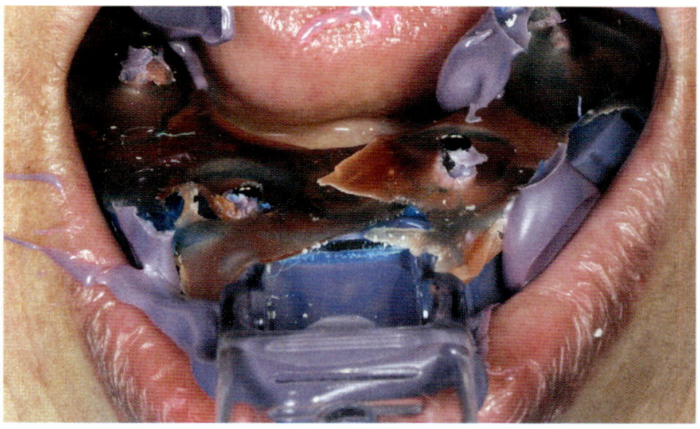
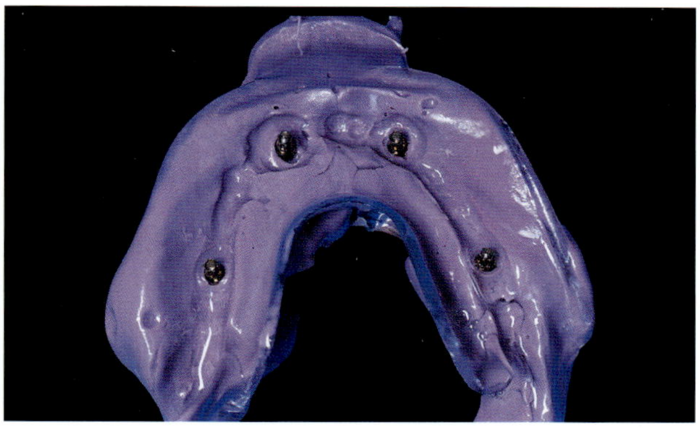

Figs 49 and 50 Open-tray polyether impression for the final restoration.

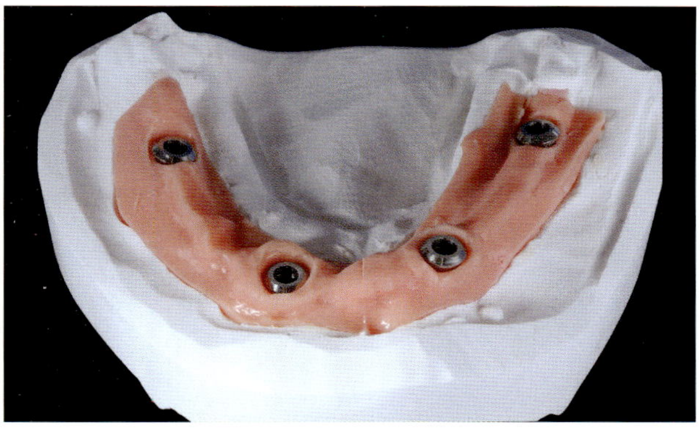

Fig 51 Master cast for the final restoration.

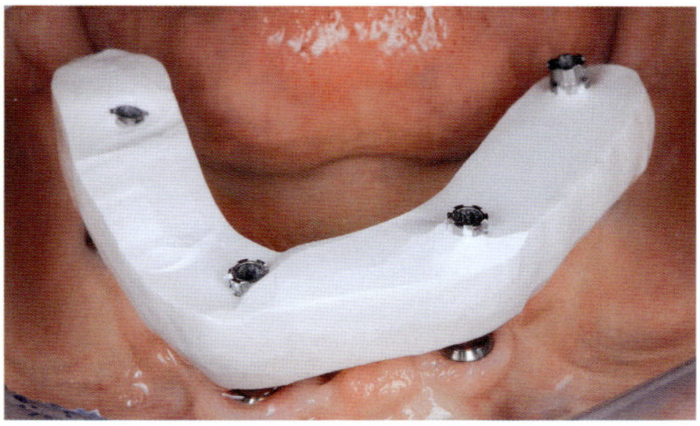

Fig 52 Dental stone verification index screwed onto the implants.

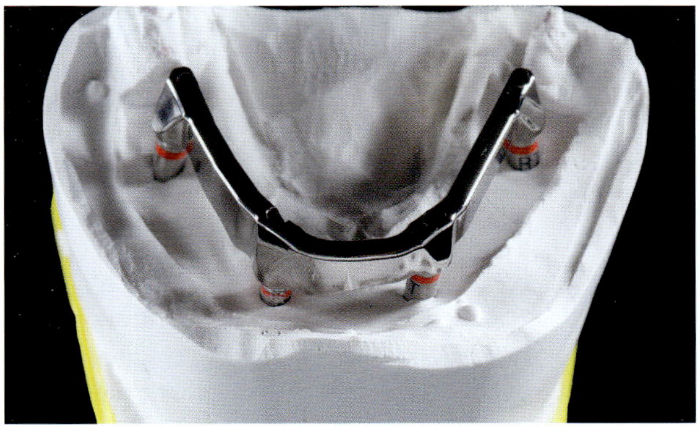

Fig 53 CAD/CAM titanium bar screwed onto the model.

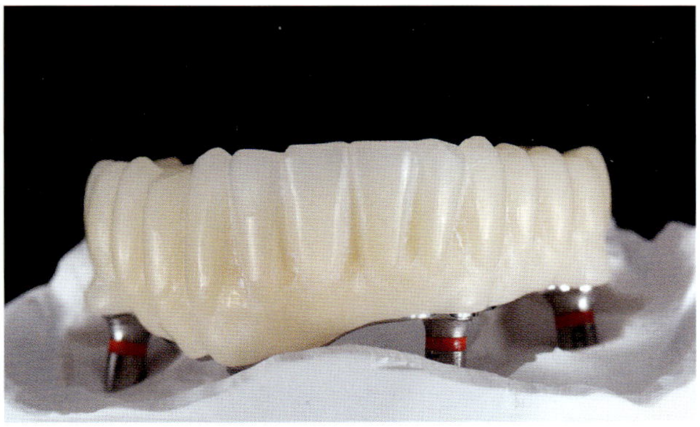

Fig 54 Hybrid resin-composite framework placed on the titanium bar.

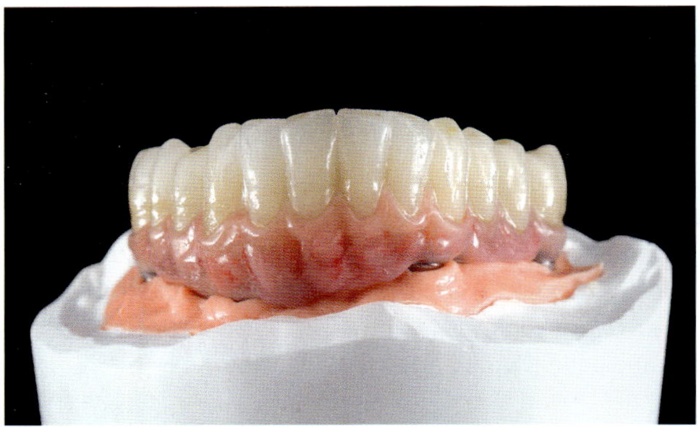
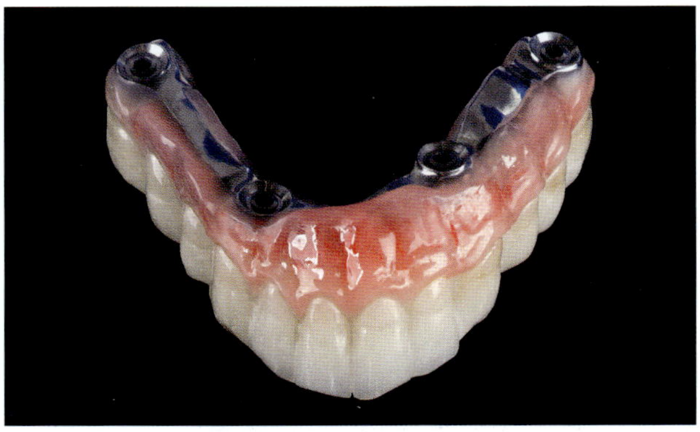

Figs 55 and 56 Final appearance of the glued titanium bar and hybrid resin-composite framework.

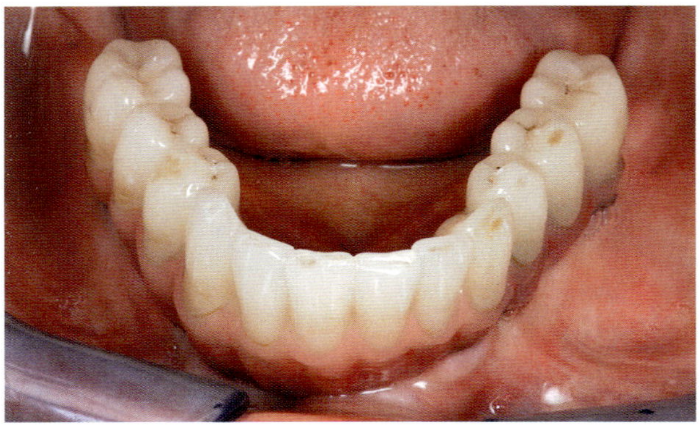

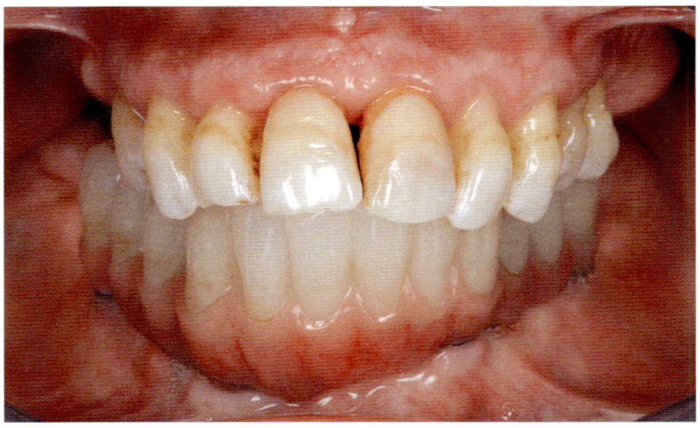

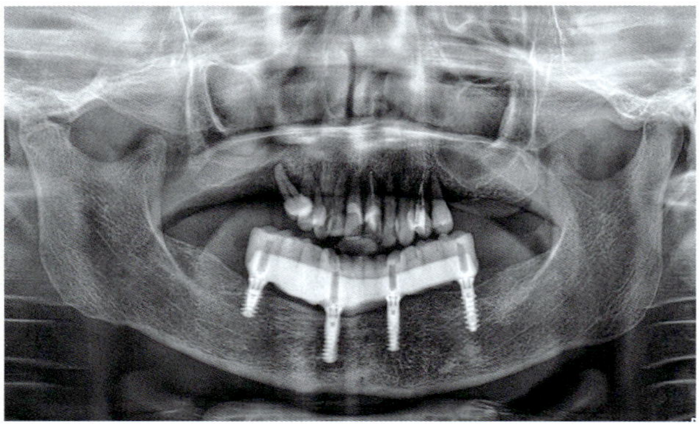

Figs 57 to 59 Clinical and radiographic control 1 year after loading.

DELIVERY

After removal of the temporary restoration, the internal cavities of the implants were disinfected with a 1% chlorhexidine gel. Peri-implant probing depths were recorded, in order to facilitate monitoring. After the patient approved the esthetic appearance of the prosthetic restoration, the restoration was tightened to 35 Ncm. The occlusion was checked and slightly adjusted. The access holes were sealed with PTFE tape and flowable composite.

The periodontal status of the maxilla was considered stable. The patient was given specific oral hygiene instructions, including brushing instructions and guidance for the use of interproximal brushes.

FOLLOW-UP AND PATIENT SATISFACTION

After delivery of the final restoration, the patient was enrolled in a periodic recall system, returning every 4 months for professional tooth cleaning.

At 1 year after loading, the prosthesis showed a favorable esthetic appearance and a stable clinical and radiographic situation, together with a precise fit of the prosthetic framework (Figs 57 to 59).

The patient reported complete satisfaction with the final treatment outcome (Figs 60 and 61).

DISCUSSION

This case report describes the treatment of a patient with a severely compromised clinical situation using a combined analog and digital workflow. Digital technology was used in the initial diagnostic phase, in the creation of a diagnostic guide, in implant planning and in the subsequent computer-guided surgery, and in the CAD/CAM fabrication of temporary and definitive implant-supported restorations.

Although the digital workflow is now an established reality that can help assist clinicians manage complex cases, some

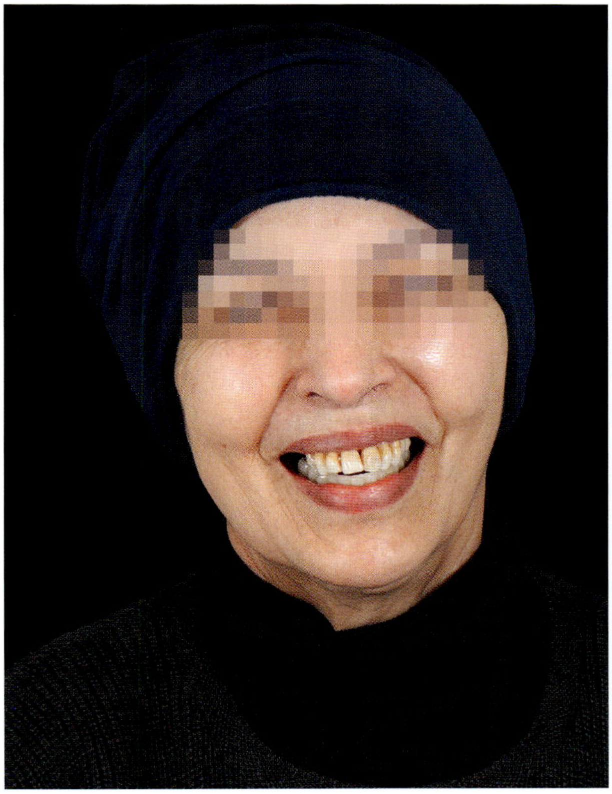

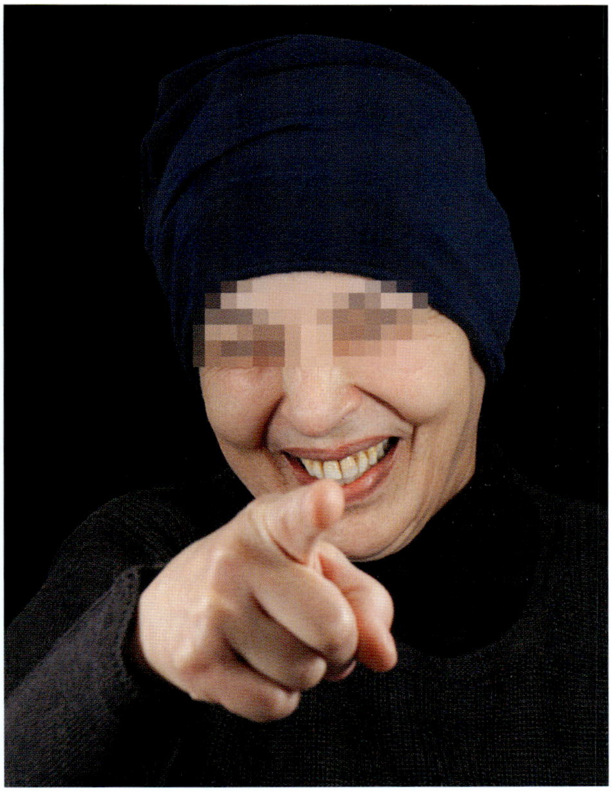

Figs 60 and 61 Facial view after treatment.

conventional prosthetic and surgical steps are still required during the treatment. In fact, the use of a complete digital workflow for the treatment of a fully edentulous patient has not been validated (Joda and coworkers 2017; Bernauer and coworkers 2023).

The use of flapless computer-guided surgery represents a significant improvement and helps shorten the surgery and reduce its invasiveness, which represents a great benefit for the patient (Tahmaseb and coworkers 2018; Wismeijer and coworkers 2018). The residual amount of keratinized tissue, however, should always be evaluated. For this reason, a small flap at site 46 would have helped to maintain a greater amount of keratinized tissue. In any case, the site is constantly monitored, the patient is able to clean it, and no significant issues have been detected.

Digital impressions in fully edentulous patients, with or without implants still have a higher degree of inaccuracy and are not yet supported by the scientific evidence (Joda and coworkers 2017; Bernauer and coworkers 2023). This applies especially to the mandible, and particularly to this case where a limited amount of keratinized tissue exists on the edentulous crest between implants. For this reason, the realization of a complete denture during the initial phases of treatment and the final impression that was made using conventional procedures—as in the case presented here—still represents the gold standard.

The choice of an immediate loading protocol is supported by the scientific literature (Papaspyridakos and coworkers 2014b; Gallucci and coworkers 2014). This allows reduction in discomfort and avoids uncontrolled loading of implants under a removable prosthesis.

As an insertion torque of more than 30 Ncm is usually recommended for immediate loading (Gallucci and coworkers 2014), the use of Straumann TLX implants helped achieve adequate primary stability of the implants.

A free gingival graft was used at implant site 43 to create an adequate band of keratinized tissue prior to fabrication of the final restoration. Indeed, the presence of a band of keratinized tissue is considered important for comfortable brushing, long-term implant maintenance, and the prevention of peri-implantitis (Schrott and coworkers 2009; Lin and coworkers 2013; Roccuzzo and coworkers 2016; Thoma and coworkers 2018).

Furthermore, once the soft tissue has been augmented, it is possible to maintain the soft-tissue volume in the long term (Stefanini and coworkers 2023).

In conclusion, the presented case demonstrates the advantages of a digital workflow, even if a strategic alternation of digital and conventional surgical and prosthetic steps may represent the gold standard in the treatment of complex cases today.

ACKNOWLEDGMENTS

Laboratory procedures

Alessandro Giacometti – Genova, Italy

5.9 Simultaneous Maxillary and Mandibular Full-Arch Fixed Rehabilitation: Extractions, Immediate Implant Placement and Loading, and Definitive Zirconia Prostheses

D. Morton, A. A. A. Alehaideb. W. D. Polido

PATIENT CHARACTERISTICS AND PATIENT PROFILE

An alert and ambulatory 60-year-old male patient presented with a desire to "repair or replace his teeth." A detailed clinical evaluation revealed multiple missing teeth. Generalized severe calculus and biofilm accumulation was noted, associated with poor oral hygiene. All remaining teeth were mobile and showed more than 50% attachment loss. All molars showed furcation involvement. Caries was prevalent throughout the remaining dentition. The patient reported intolerance of his existing removable partial prosthesis, which had been fabricated more than 20 years previously.

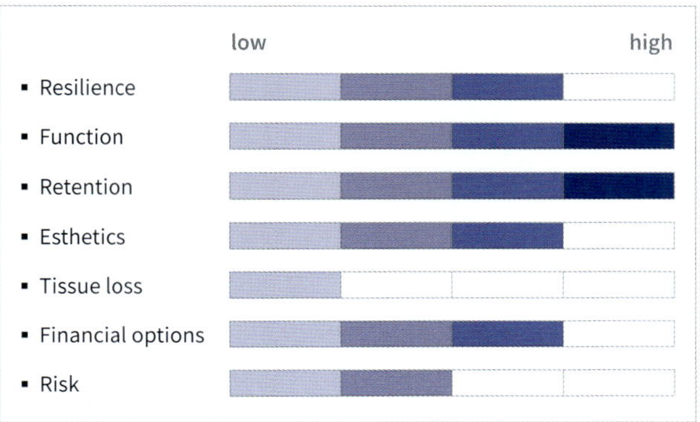

Fig 1 Patient profile.

Diagnoses:

- Partial edentulism
- Generalized dental caries
- Generalized stage IV, grade 3 periodontitis
- Poor oral hygiene
- Failed existing removable partial dentures
- Dental phobia

The patient was anxious and apprehensive about dental care, citing this as a reason for avoiding treatment in the past. He requested that procedures be performed under sedation or general anesthesia if possible. An assessment of his health status specific to sedation and anesthesia revealed no contraindications, and no additional aspect of the patient's general health was considered significant to dental treatment. He was a former smoker (20 cigarettes per day for more than 30 years), although he had not smoked for more than 12 months. The patient was motivated to seek treatment and improve his oral health. He expressed a strong preference for fixed restorations in the maxilla and mandible.

Based on this information, the clinical evaluation, and the risk assessment analysis described below, the following patient profile (Fig 1) can be derived for this patient (for more information about patient profiles, see Chapters 2.1.3 and 3.6).

CLINICAL EVALUATION AND TREATMENT PLAN

Pretreatment data collection included intraoral and extraoral photographs (Figs 2 to 5), a full-face CBCT, a full-mouth series of periapical radiographs (Fig 6), a panoramic radiograph (Fig 7) and intraoral scans of his remaining dentition (Figs 8 to 10). The treatment team determined that his remaining dentition could not be managed with any degree of periodontal or restorative predictability.

Although the patient had expressed a desire for fixed restorations in both arches, removable full-arch removable dental prostheses with or without implant support were discussed as treatment options. However, the patient reiterated his strong reluctance to accept removable treatment options. Considerations specific to fixed restorative alternatives mostly related to the timing of extractions and of implant placement and loading, in addition to commitment and maintenance requirements. Fixed restorative options that were discussed included:

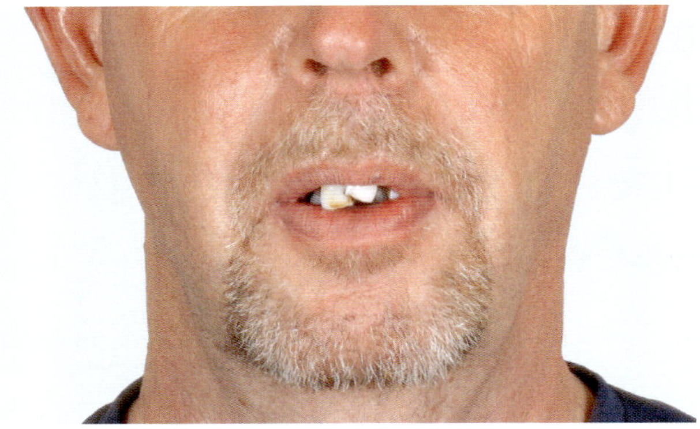

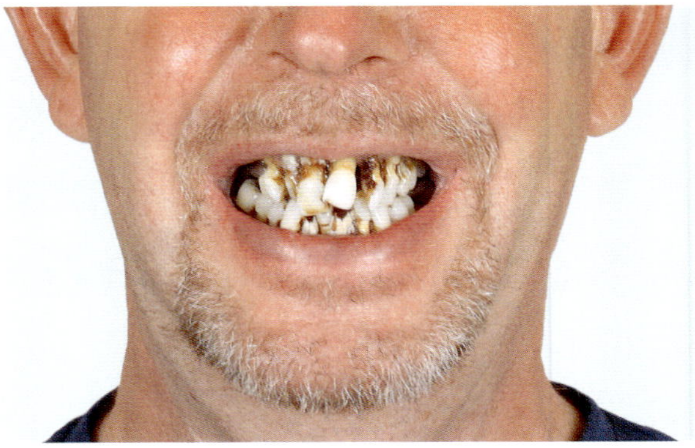

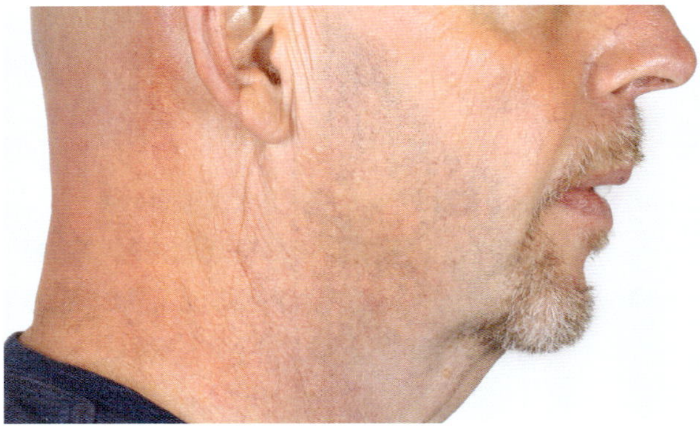

Figs 2 to 4 Pretreatment frontal and profile views.

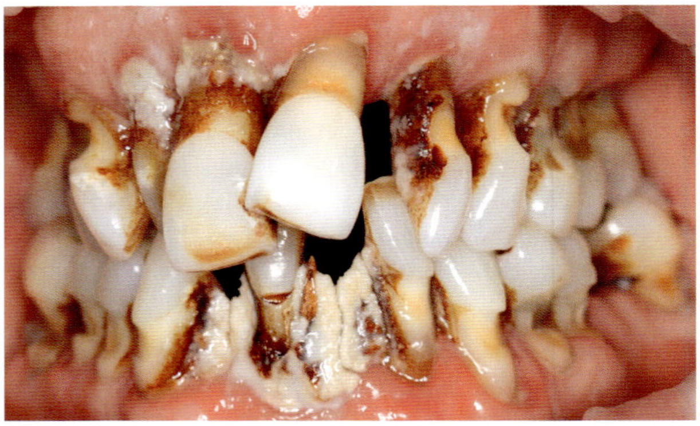

Fig 5 Intraoral frontal view.

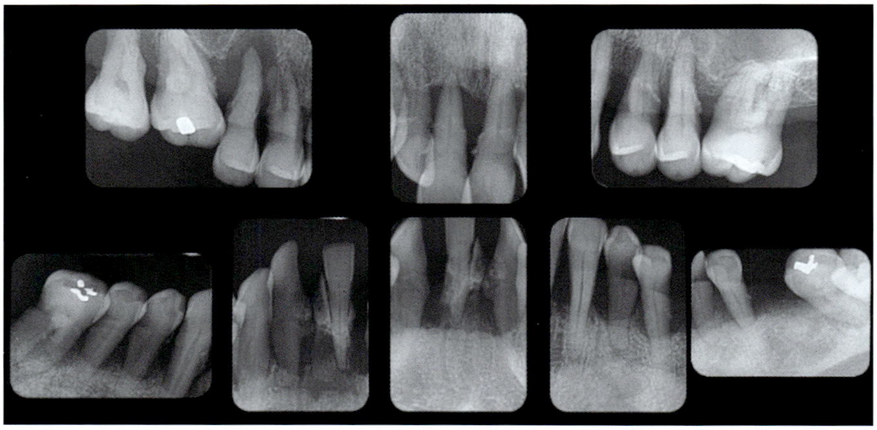

Fig 6 Periapical radiographs.

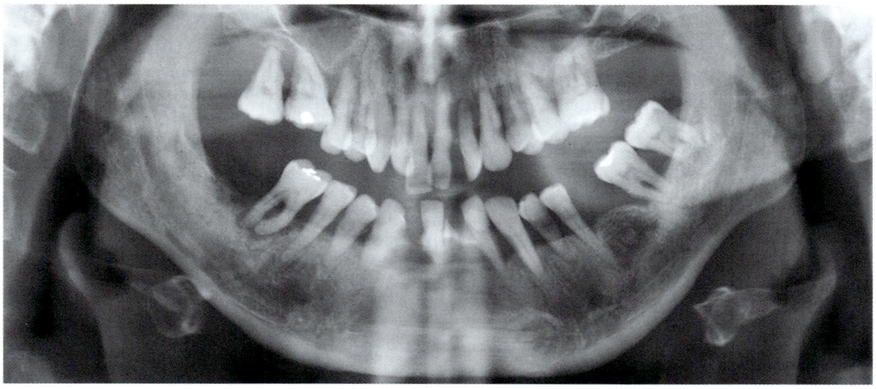

Fig 7 Panoramic radiograph.

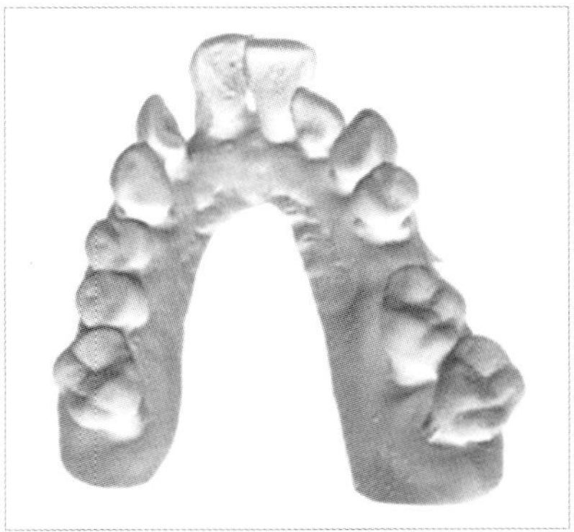
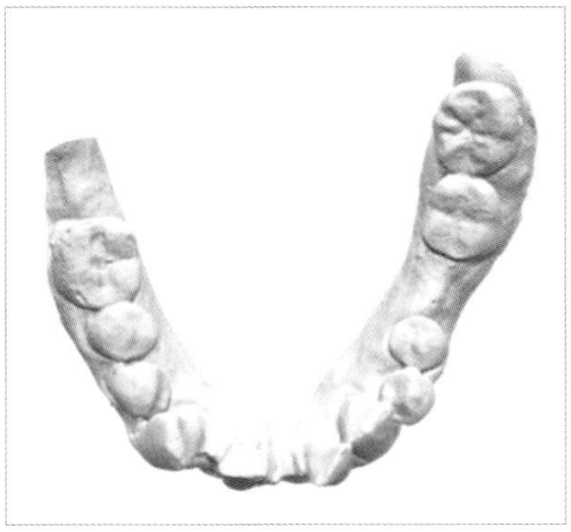
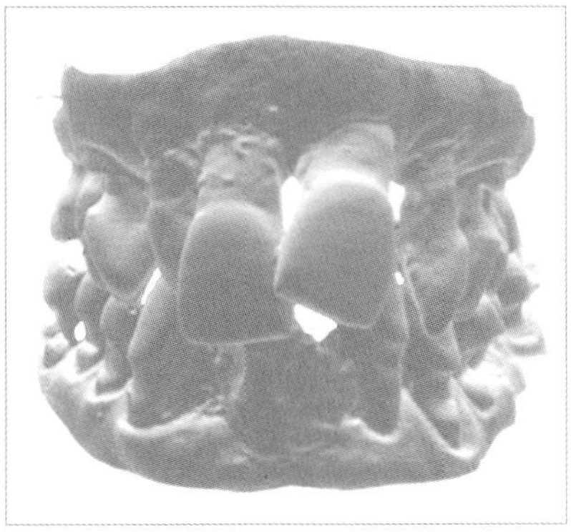

Figs 8 to 10 Pretreatment intraoral scans.

1. Extraction of all remaining teeth and immediate delivery of a temporary complete denture in the maxilla and mandible. After 2 to 3 months of healing, four implants would be placed in each arch, allowed to heal, and loaded with full-arch fixed dental prostheses (FDPs) according to an early or conventional protocol (6 to 8 weeks or longer).
2. Same as option 1, but with treatment performed one arch at a time.
3. Extraction of all remaining teeth and immediate placement of four implants in both the maxilla and mandible. The patient would receive immediate temporary complete denture to wear while the implants were allowed to heal undisturbed for 6 weeks to 3 months. The implants would then be loaded with full-arch FDPs (early or conventional).
4. Sequential treatment of one arch at a time, with extraction of the remaining teeth, immediate placement of four implants immediately loaded with provisional full-arch FDPs, first in the mandible and then in the maxilla.
5. Extraction of all remaining teeth, immediate placement of four implants in each arch and immediate loading of both arches simultaneously with a provisional full-arch FDP. After implant healing, CAD/CAM prototype prostheses would be provided. Following approval of their functional and esthetic performance, the definitive full-arch maxillary and mandibular zirconia FDPs would be delivered.

After all questions were answered and possible complications were discussed, the patient agreed to the following treatment:

- Removal of all remaining teeth.
- Immediate guided placement of four implants in both the maxilla and mandible
- Immediate restoration with CAD/CAM-designed and fabricated prototype full-arch screw-retained provisional full-arch FDP for both arches supported by SRA abutments.
- After another period of evaluation and consent to proceed, the definitive maxillary and mandibular definitive full-arch zirconia FDPs were to be delivered.

Factors influencing the patient's choice of treatment plan included his desire to minimize the number of surgical procedures, the treatment team's desire to limit the number of appointments requiring sedation or general anesthesia, the patient's preference for fixed options (including during the provisional phase), and the cost of treatment. The patient was advised that four successful implants in each arch were required to support the FDPs and that any implant failure would require replacement of the failed implant resulting in additional healing and treatment time. The experienced treatment team facilitated management according to the patient's preferences.

The decision was made to use a digital workflow that included fully guided (static) placement of all implants and CAD/CAM prototype prostheses to be converted to provisional full-arch FDPs. The patient was advised that the use of provisional full arch FDPs was dependent on adequate stability of the implants, which would be confirmed at placement. In the absence of adequate stability, delivery of the provisional full-arch RDP would be required. The Smile-In-A-Box protocol (Institut Straumann AG, Basel,

Switzerland) was selected to facilitate this approach. The patient was advised that after 3 months of healing with the provisional FDPs, secondary provisional prototype prostheses would be required for each arch. These prototypes would duplicate the planned occlusion and final contours of the final FDPs.

RISK ASSESSMENT ANALYSIS

The SAC risk analysis (Dawson and coworkers 2020) was utilized to determine the surgical and restorative risk for this patient.

The following tables illustrate the risk assessment for this patient. The risk was considered high for both the surgical and restorative phases of care. The team was considered to have a high level of experience and expertise and was capable of providing the care and preparing for and managing any complications that might arise.

The SAC Classification in Implant Dentistry, 2nd Edition
Anthony Dawson, Will Martin and Waldemar D. Polido
To view this material, you need to be an ITI Member.

Table 1 Medical modifying factors

Medical modifying factors			
	Low	**Medium**	**High**
ASA classification	ASA 1	ASA 2/3 Moderately compromised but can undergo procedure	ASA 4 and above Compromised health
Medication	No	Medications that can affect healing/procedure Low potency	Antiresorptive medications IV bisphosphonate
Growth status	Completed/mature	Incomplete Young adult/adolescent	Incomplete Young adolescent/child
Radiotherapy H&N	No	< 50 Gy > 5 years	> 50 Gy < 5 years

Table 2 Behavioral modifying factors

Behavioral modifying factors			
	Low	**Medium**	**High**
Oral hygiene	Good	Fair Can improve	Poor Uncontrolled
Compliance	Good Collaborative	Adequate Willing to collaborate	Inadequate Non-compliant
Smoking	Non-smoker	Light smoker ≤ 10- cigs/day)	Heavy smoker > 10 cigs/day
Expectations	Realistic	High but achievable	Unrealistic

Table 3 Site-related factors

Site related factors			
	Low	Medium	High
Periodontal status	Healthy No history of perio disease	History of perio disease Controlled/stable	Active perio disease
Access	Adequate	Limited	Inadequate
Nearby pathology	None	Can be managed Does not need treatment	Must be treated before
Previous surgery	None	Yes, but resulting in no or minimal bone and soft-tissue changes	Previous procedures Significant bone and soft-tissue changes

Table 4 Surgical complexity

Table 4.1 Site factors

Surgical complexity			
Site factors	Low	Medium	High
Timing of placement	Healed (late implant placement)	Partially healed (early implant placement)	Immediate placement
Grafting procedures	No adjunctive procedures	Simultaneous small hard- and/or soft-tissue augmentation	Need for large simultaneous small hard- and/or soft-tissue augmentation; need for staged hard- and/or soft-tissue procedures
Number of implants	One	Two to three	Four or more

Table 4.2 Anatomy

Surgical complexity			
Anatomy	Low	Medium	High
Bone volume – horizontal	Adequate	Deficient, but allowing simultaneous augmentation	Deficient, requiring a separate augmentation procedure prior to implant placement
Bone volume – vertical	Adequate	Small deficiency allowing implant placement Small deficiency allowing simultaneous augmentation Adequate for implant placement but requiring bone reduction	Deficient, requiring a separate vertical bone augmentation as a first step of a staged approach Deficient requiring vertical bone augmentation simultaneously with implant placement
Keratinized tissue	Sufficient (> 4 mm)	Minimal (2–4 mm)	Insufficient (< 2 mm)
Soft-tissue quality	No scars or inflammation	Presence of minimal scars/ no inflammation	Presence of scars and inflammation
Proximity to vital anatomical structures	No or minimal risk of involvement	Moderate risk of involvement	High risk of involvement

Table 4.3 Extractions

Surgical Complexity			
Extractions	**Low**	**Medium**	**High**
Radicular morphology/ interradicular bone	Uniradicular	Multiradicular divergent roots; Available interseptal bone allowing implant anchorage	Multiradicular convergent or wide roots, no available interseptal bone for implant anchorage
Alveolar and basal bone morphology	Sufficient bone height (> 4 mm) and width (> 2 mm) around apex of planned implant	Sufficient bone height (> 4 mm) but deficient bone width (< 2 mm) around apex of planned implant	Insufficient bone height (< 4 mm) for apical anchorage of planned implant
Thickness of facial bone wall	≥ 1 mm		< 1 mm
Anticipated residual defect after implant placement	No residual defect	Residual defect with implant position inside the alveolar bone envelope	Residual defect with implant position outside the alveolar bone envelope
Soft-tissue quality	Adequate keratinized tissue		Inadequate keratinized tissue
Soft-tissue quantity	Sufficient (no recession)		Insufficient (with recession)
Position in the arch	Not in the esthetic area		Esthetic area

Table 4.4 Edentulous surgical factors

Edentulous surgical factors			
	Low	**Medium**	**High**
Number of implants	2–3	4–6	> 6
Timing of placement	Healed ridge (type 4)	Early (type 2, 3)	Immediate (type 1)
Bone modification	None	Bone removal Horizontal bone augmentation	Vertical bone augmentation
Anatomical risk	None	Moderate atrophy but allowing implant placement with Narrow/Short implants OR Simultaneous grafts	Severe atrophy Requires staged grafts OR advanced alternatives (ultra-short, zygomatic)
Axial position	Parallel		Tilted

Table 5 Edentulous esthetic risk factors

Edentulous esthetic risk factors			
	Low	**Medium**	**High**
Arch	Mandible		Maxilla
Facial support (fixed)	Alveolar process provides adequate facial support	Minimal changes tolerated by the patient	Flange required for adequate facial support
Facial support (removable)	Flange provides adequate facial support	Minimal changes tolerated by the patient	Insufficient space for a flange
Labial support	Designed teeth position provides satisfactory labial support	Minimal changes tolerated by the patient	Designed teeth position provides unsatisfactory labial support
Upper lip length	Long upper lip (> 20 mm)		Short upper lip (< 20 mm)
Buccal corridor (atrophic ridge)	Removable prosthesis		Fixed prosthesis
Smile line	No display of the ridge(s) at full smile (Maxilla or Mandible)		Display of the ridge(s) at full smile (maxilla or mandible)
Maxillomandibular relationship	Class 1	Class II	Class III

Table 6 Restorative modifying factors

Table 6.1 Restorative factors

Restorative factors			
	Low	**Medium**	**High**
Prosthetic volume	Adequate. Space available for ideal anatomy of the restoration	Compromised. Can be resolved without adjunctive therapy	Inadequate. Adjunctive therapy will be needed to achieve a satisfactory result.
Interocclusal space	Adequate. Possible to create an anatomically and functionally correct planned restoration.	Compromised. Can be resolved without adjunctive therapy.	Inadequate. Adjunctive therapy will be necessary to achieve sufficient space for the planned restoration.
Volume and characteristics of the edentulous ridge	Adequate. No prosthetic soft-tissue replacement will be necessary.		Inadequate. Prosthetic replacement of soft tissue will be needed for esthetics or phonetics.

Table 6.2 Occlusal factors

Occlusal factors			
	Low	**Medium**	**High**
Occlusal scheme	User-defined occlusal scheme achievable		User-defined occlusal scheme not achievable
Involvement in occlusion	Minimal or no involvement		Implant restorations involved with guidance
Occlusal parafunction	Absent		Present

Table 6.3 Complexity

Complexity			
	Low	**Medium**	**High**
Access	Adequate		Inadequate
Interim prosthesis	None required	Tooth supported	Tissue or interim-implant supported
Implant-supported provisional restoration	None required	Required, reduced esthetic and/or functional demands	Required, elevated esthetic and/or functional demands
Number and location of implants	Single	Two (non-splinted)	> 2 (non-splinted) or ≥ 2 (splinted)
Loading protocols	Conventional/early		Immediate

Table 6.4 Complicating factors

Complicating factors			
	Low	**Medium**	**High**
Biological	Screw-retained with appropriate contours and biocompatible materials	Cemented single-unit restorations with appropriate contours and biocompatible materials	Cemented multi-unit reconstructions or restorations with contours inaccessible for maintenance procedures
Mechanical/technical	Absence of contributing factors	Presence of non-critical contributing factors	Presence of critical contributing factors
Maintenance	Low	Moderate	High

Summary of risk assessment

Surgical classification

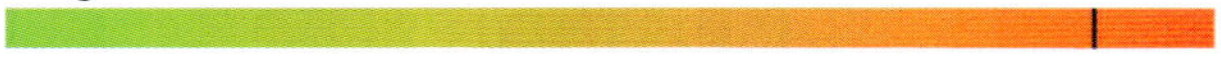

Prosthodontic classification

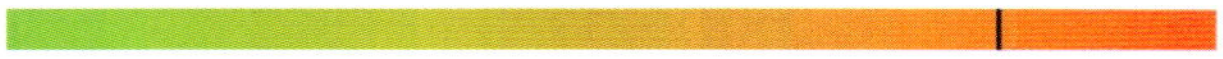

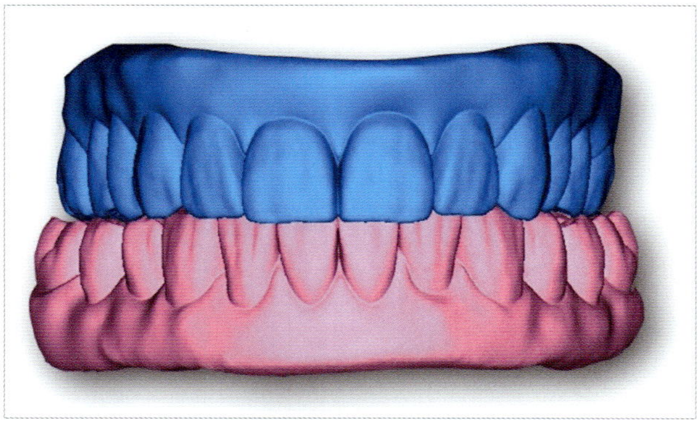

Fig 11 Virtual tooth arrangement and occlusion at the proposed vertical dimension.

VIRTUAL PLANNING

After evaluation and discussion of risks and potential complications with the patient, the patient agreed to the treatment plan.

A surgical plan was developed virtually using coDiagnostiX (Institut Straumann AG, Basel, Switzerland) and the services of Smile-in-a-Box. A full-face CBCT was uploaded and a virtual planning session was initiated. The proposed tooth set-up was identified using the patient's existing vertical dimension of occlusion and lip support as a reference (Fig 11). When developing the virtual tooth set-up, the denture base extensions were positioned below the lip to ensure that the

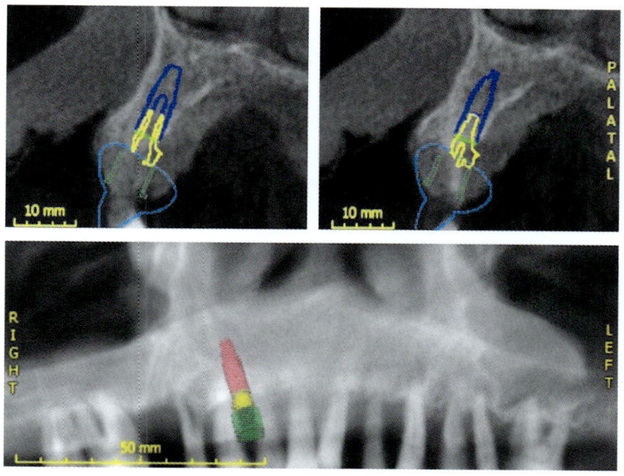

Fig 12 Planned implant position, site 12.

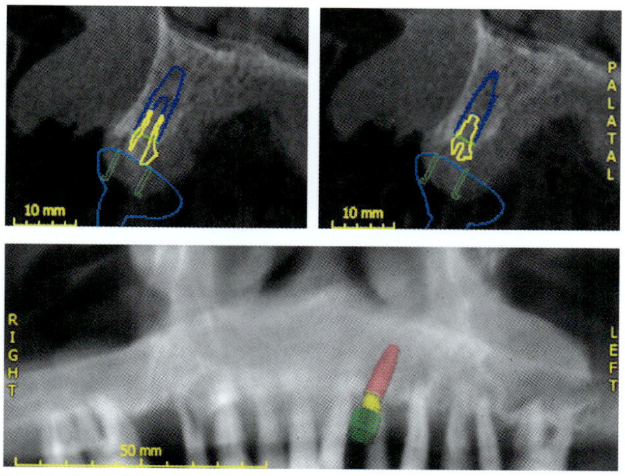

Fig 13 Planned implant position, site 22.

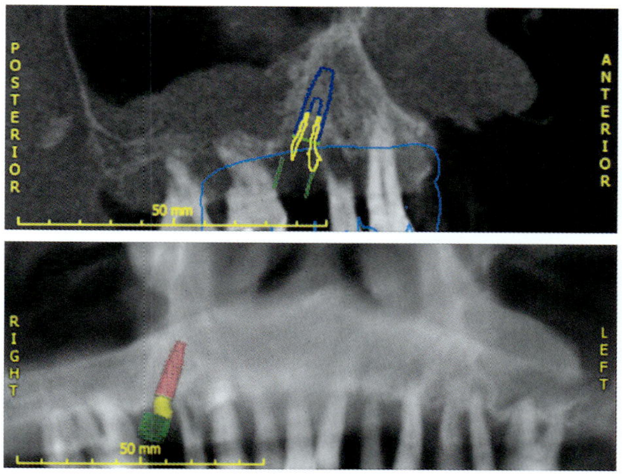

Fig 14 Planned implant position, site 15.

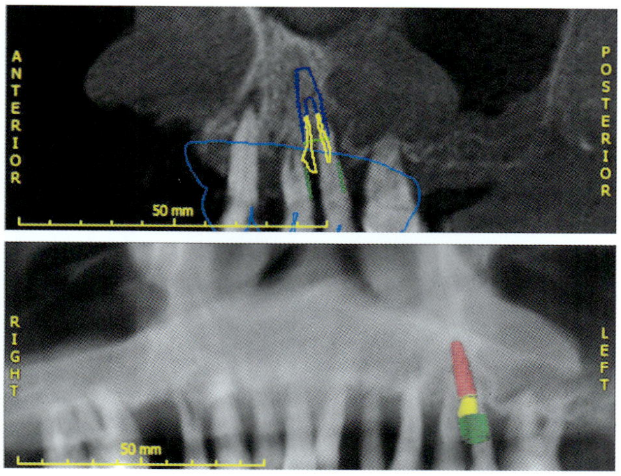

Fig 15 Planned implant position, site 25.

transition was not visible. The occlusion was planned based on the patient's class II skeletal characteristics and the size disparity between the arches.

The virtual tooth set-up was registered and merged with the CBCT data. Implant sites for both arches were then identified based on the patient's anatomy, expected ridge characteristics after extraction, and implant distribution based on the functional and esthetic requirements of the planned restorations.

Implant sites in the maxilla were identified bilaterally in the lateral incisor/canine regions (Figs 12 and 13) and in the second premolar regions (Figs 14 and 15). Implants at sites 15 and 25 were to be angled to avoid encroachment on the maxillary sinus, to eliminate the need for sinus grafting, and to improve the anteroposterior distribution of the implants. A small vertical reduction of the residual ridge was planned to provide adequate restorative space. Grafting of the gap between the implants and the facial bone was planned.

Implant sites in the mandible were identified bilaterally in lateral incisor/canine and first molar regions (Fig 16). The implants were to be axially inclined, as all sites were considered to have adequate bone volume. Adequate restorative volume was maintained along with an appropriate implant distribution. All implant positions were considered favorable because they were placed in the bone beyond the extraction sockets (Figs 17 to 20).

A series of templates were digitally designed to facilitate placement of the implants according to the virtual plan. Positioning templates were designed for each arch to facilitate the placement of horizontal pins for the development of bone reduction and drilling guides. The location of the horizontal pins ensured avoidance of the roots of the remaining teeth and did not compromise lip retraction and surgical access. The remaining teeth were used to place the positioning templates. The bone reduction and drilling guides were designed to be sequentially positioned using the horizontal pins.

Provisional maxillary and mandibular full-arch RDPs were fabricated to facilitate chairside conversion to fixed provisional FDPs once the primary stability of all implants was confirmed, and to be delivered as provisional RDPs if implant stability was not achieved.

IMPLANT SELECTION

All implants were positioned to utilize native bone beyond the extraction sites. In the maxilla, Straumann Bone Level Tapered (BLT) implants were selected to optimize primary stability and to address the need for angled abutments. The patient had sufficient bone volume to accommodate implants 4.1 mm in diameter and 12 mm in length to provide adequate primary stability. The implant depth was selected to provide space for proper seating and placement of screw-retained abutments (SRAs) and the planned prosthesis. The two distal implants were angled and planned to use of 17° angled SRAs.

In the mandible, all implants could be placed in a parallel (axially inclined) fashion. Hybrid design Straumann TLX implants were selected to maximize primary stability and to provide for a biologically and functionally reliable connection. The mandibular sites were considered to have sufficient bone width and height to accommodate implants 4.5 mm in diameter and 10 mm in length in the posterior regions, and 3.75 mm in diameter and 12 mm in length in the anterior regions.

SURGICAL PROCEDURES

Surgery was performed under intravenous deep sedation and local anesthesia on an outpatient basis, according to the patient's preference and his physical tolerance. In dosages calculated according to the patient's weight, midazolam, fentanyl and propofol were administered intravenously to ensure deep sedation. IV antibiotics (cefazolin 1 g) and corticosteroids (dexamethasone 8 mg) were administered preoperatively based on the patient's oral condition. Deep sedation, managed by a dental anesthesiologist in a hospital based clinic, was maintained throughout the surgical procedures and then reduced to light sedation for prosthesis placement and occlusion verification after implant stability was confirmed.

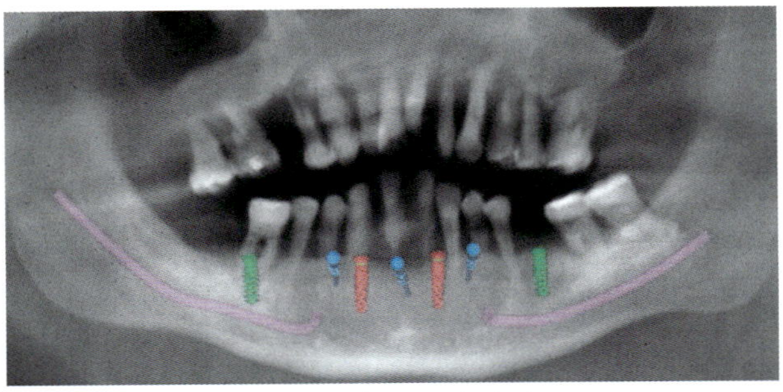

Fig 16 Proposed implant positions (panoramic view).

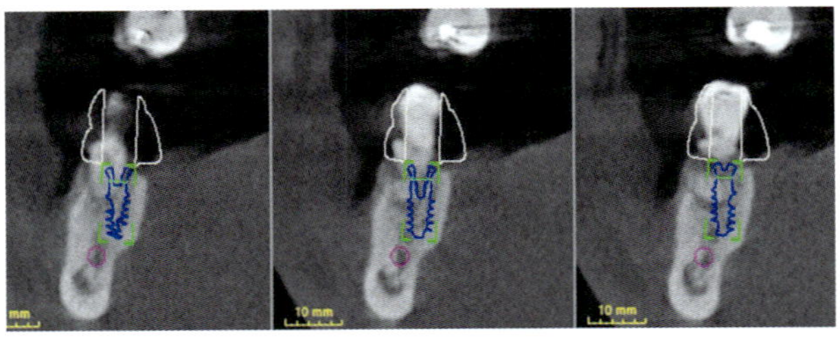

Fig 17 Planned implant position, site 46.

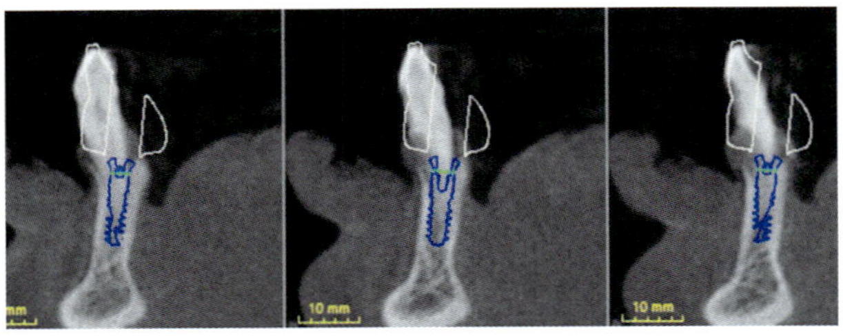

Fig 18 Planned implant position, site 43.

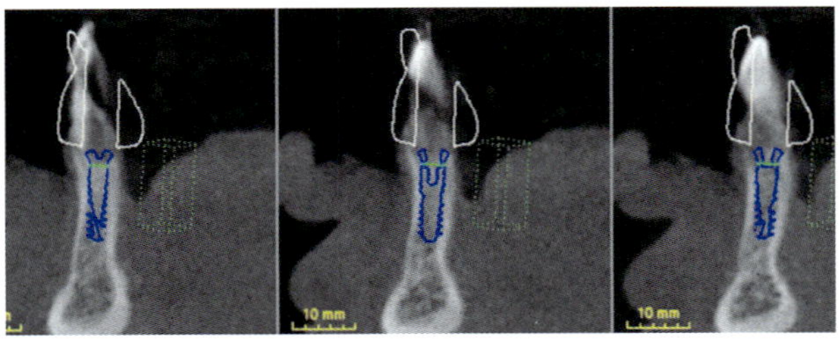

Fig 19 Planned implant position, site 33.

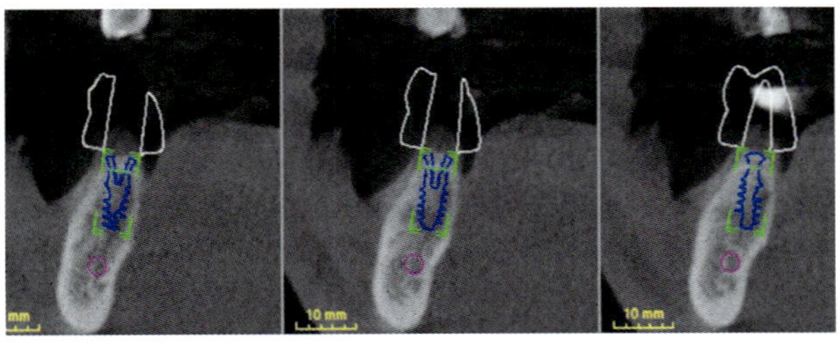

Fig 20 Planned implant position, site 36.

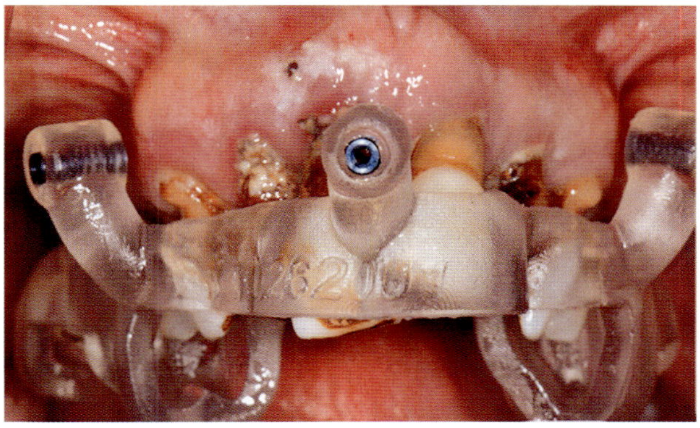

Fig 21 Template for positioning horizontal pins. Maxillary arch.

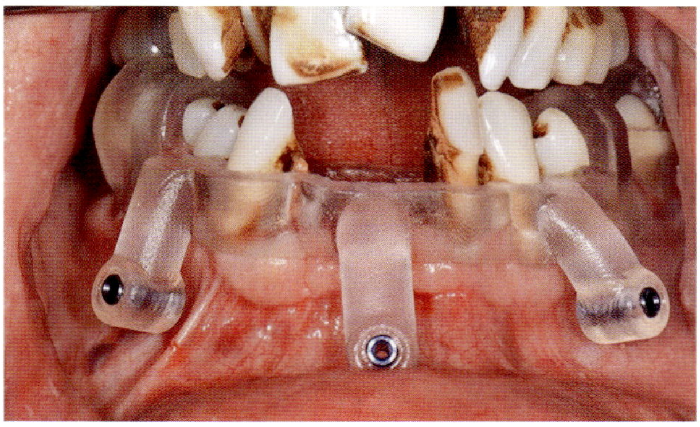

Fig 22 Template for positioning horizontal pins. Mandibular arch.

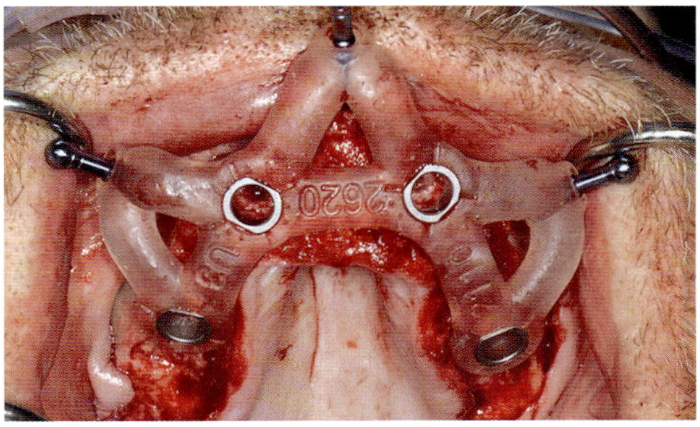

Fig 23 Maxillary implant positioning template.

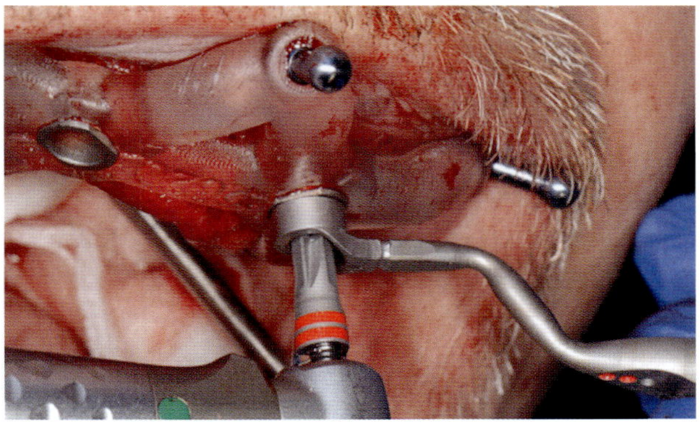

Fig 24 Surgical guide and twist drill.

The placement of the positioning templates on the remaining teeth was verified using visualization windows to assess template stability and intercuspation with the opposing dentition. The positioning templates were used to place horizontal pins in both arches (Figs 21 and 22).

Local anesthesia in the maxilla was achieved with infraorbital and posterior superior maxillary blocks (marcaine 0.5% with 1 : 200,000 adrenaline), combined with alveolar infiltration (articaine 4% with 1 : 100,000 adrenaline). This combination provides optimal duration and quality of local anesthesia, with excellent hemostatic control. In the mandible, inferior alveolar and lingual blocks were placed (Marcaine 0.5% with 1 : 200,000 adrenaline) again combined with alveolar infiltration (articaine 4% with 1 : 100,000 adrenaline).

Once the position of both positioning templates was deemed appropriate, holes were drilled to receive the horizontal pins. Preparation (drilling) was performed through the mucosa and bone under irrigation. In the mandible, the incisors were extracted to position the midline pin. Starting in the maxilla, a full-thickness mucoperiosteal flap was elevated to expose the alveolar and basal native bone. All teeth were extracted; the sockets were carefully curetted and all debris was removed. The bone reduction guide was positioned and stabilized with horizontal pins placed in the previously drilled holes. Excess bone was gently removed with a rongeur to the height indicated by the guide.

The reduction template was then removed and replaced by the drilling guide, which was stabilized using the same horizontal pins (Fig 23). Sequential drilling was performed using the drilling guides to develop osteotomies for all implant sites (Fig 24).

Following the manufacturer's recommendations, the drill sequence included 2.2 mm and 2.8 mm drills to the planned depth. The final twist drill (3.5 mm in diameter) stopped 5–6 mm short of the planned depth. This is an important aspect of the protocol designed to optimize primary stability for the BLT design, given that the apex of the 4.1 mm BLT is 2.7 mm wide.

Once the osteotomies were completed, the implants were placed in a fully guided fashion according to the virtual plan. Primary stability was achieved for each implant (45 Ncm of insertion torque). In addition, an implant stability quotient (ISQ) of greater than 70 was recorded for all implants. A

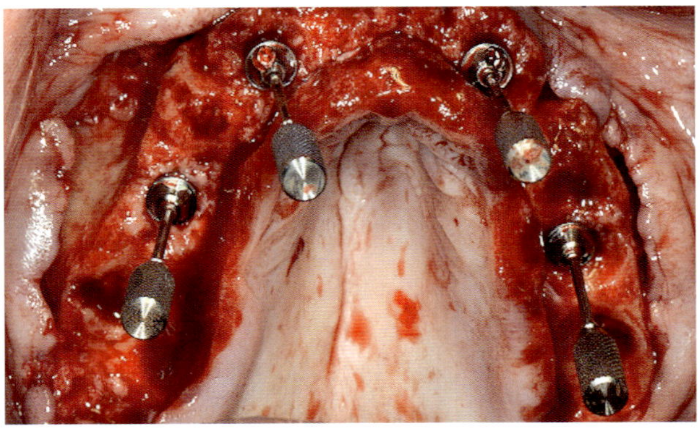

Fig 25 Maxillary implants and screw-retained abutments with inclination guides.

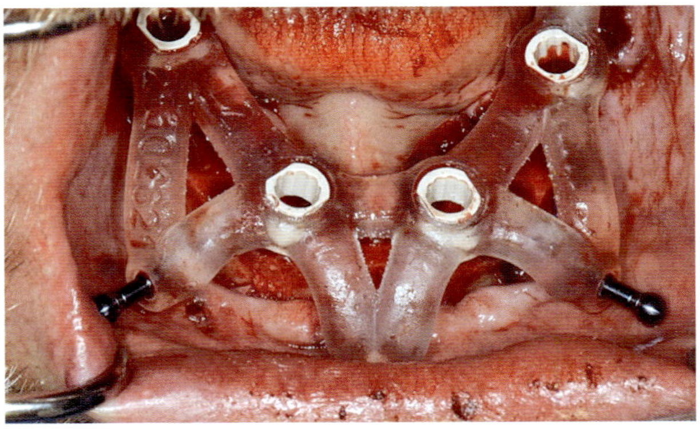

Fig 26 Mandibular drilling guide.

profile drill was used for the posterior (angled) implants to provide space for proper seating of the abutments. Screw-retained abutments (SRAs) were placed on all implants and the inclination confirmed before the abutments were tightened to 15 Ncm or more (Fig 25).

For the mandibular arch, a full-thickness mucoperiosteal flap was also elevated and the alveolar and native basal bone was exposed. As in the maxillary arch, all teeth were extracted and their sockets were curetted to remove all debris. The bone reduction guide was positioned and stabilized in the planned position using horizontal pins in the previously drilled holes. Excess bone was removed with rongeurs to the level indicated by the guide.

The drilling guide was positioned and stabilized using the same horizontal pins (Fig 26). Initially, the same drilling sequence as in the maxillary arch was followed for all implant sites, with the 2.2-mm and 2.8-mm drills used to the planned depth.

Because the two anterior implants were being placed in denser bone, the final twist drill used was 3.75 mm in diameter. This diameter was the same diameter as the implant being placed, and this drill was used to prepare the coronal 6 mm of the osteotomy. The apical region of the osteotomy was prepared to 2.8 mm to provide adequate primary stability. For the two posterior sites, the final twist drill was 3.75 mm in diameter and was used to the full depth as recommended for the placed implants (with diameters of 4.5 mm) (Fig 27).

Undersizing the osteotomy may be important to optimize primary stability. The thread design of the TLX implant creates its own path into the bone, allowing for improved primary stability. An insertion torque of 45 Ncm was obtained for all mandibular implants and an ISQ score of greater than 70 was also noted. The converted mandibular provisional restoration was planned to sit directly on the restorative platform using temporary cylinders.

Temporary cylinders were placed on the SRAs in the maxilla and the restorative platforms of the TLX implants in the mandible. The maxillary and mandibular surgical sites were protected with rubber dam stretched over the temporary cylinders and the SRAs or implant collars. The CAD/CAM provisional maxillary and mandibular prostheses were positioned with horizontal pins in the previously drilled holes. Intercuspation of the prostheses (occlusion) was also used to verify correct positioning (Fig 28).

All temporary cylinders were attached to the provisional prostheses using fast-setting acrylic resin. After complete polymerization, the provisional prostheses with the indexed temporary cylinders were removed. The rubber dam protecting the surgical wounds was also removed and protective caps were placed over the maxillary SRAs. Transmucosal healing abutments were placed on the mandibular TLX implants.

Minor horizontal defects around the implants and horizontal gaps between the implants and facial bone were grafted with deproteinized bovine bone mineral (DBBM + collagen) (Bio-Oss Collagen; Geistlich, Wolhusen, Switzerland). The same biomaterial was used in the extraction sites not used for implant placement to maintain ridge volume in the pontic areas. The reflected flaps were then repositioned and adapted with maximum preservation of healthy keratinized tissue adjacent to the implants. Sutures (Vicryl 4-0; Ethicon, Somerville, NJ, USA) were placed to close the tissues without tension.

The patient was then weaned from sedation without complication. Upon complete recovery, detailed postoperative instructions were given to both the patient and his companion. Postoperative antibiotics were prescribed (amoxicillin 875 mg plus clavulanic acid 125 mg) to be taken every

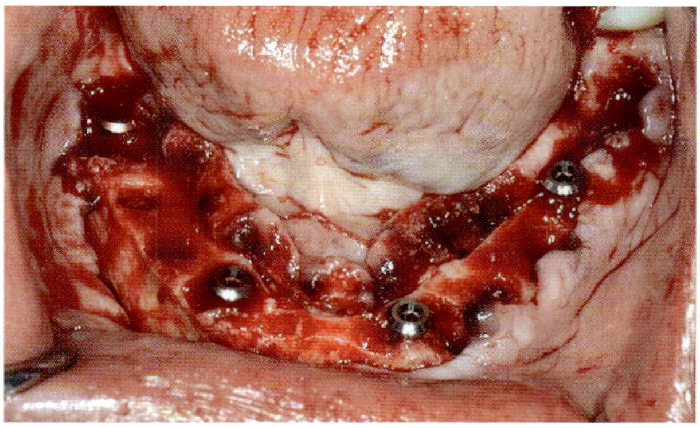

Fig 27 Mandibular implants in place.

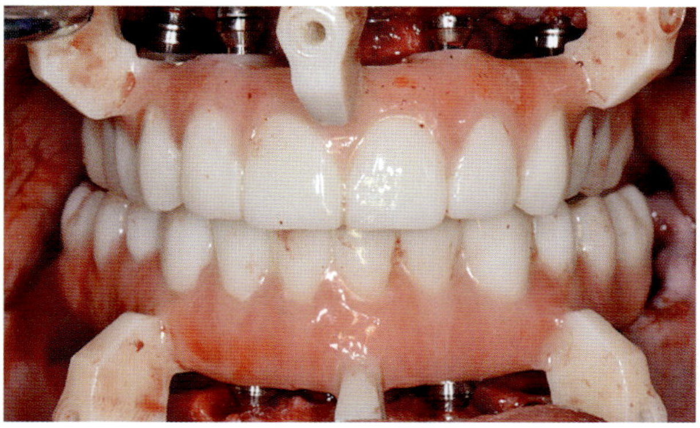

Fig 28 Stabilized and verified provisional restorations indexed at surgery.

8 hours for 1 week. For postoperative pain, ibuprofen was prescribed (600 mg every 8 hours), alternating with acetaminophen 500 mg every 6 hours as needed. A prescription for a stronger oral analgesic (acetaminophen 325 mg and hydrocodone 5 mg) was provided to be filled if postoperative pain was not adequately controlled. The patient was scheduled to return the following day for delivery of the finalized provisional prostheses. He tolerated all procedures well and was discharged.

PROSTHETIC PROCEDURES

Immediate restorative appointment: The next day (24 hours after surgery), the patient presented for delivery of the provisional prosthesis. He described persistent mild postoperative discomfort, which was adequately controlled with the prescribed medications (ibuprofen and acetaminophen). Local anesthesia was applied around all implants (lidocaine 2% with 1 : 100,000 adrenaline). The protective caps were removed from the maxillary SRAs and the maxillary provisional FDP seated and evaluated for passivity and tissue adaptation. The healing abutments were removed from the mandibular implants and the mandibular provisional FDP was seated and checked again for passivity and tissue adaptation. The occlusion was evaluated and minor adjustments were made. The patient approved the esthetic outcome and comfort. PTFE tape was placed in all access holes and sealed with composite resin to protect the screws. A panoramic radiograph was taken (Fig 29).

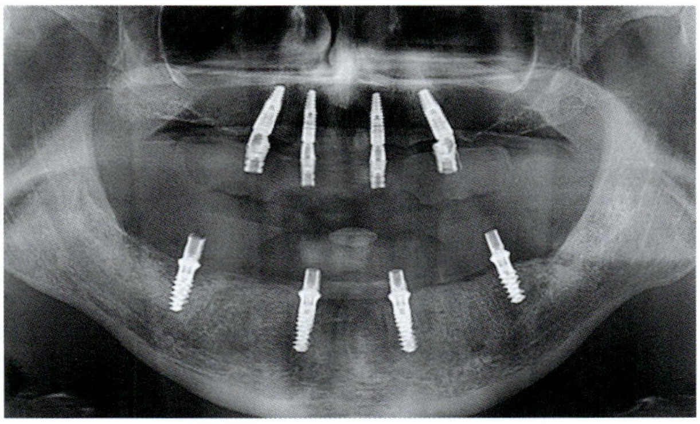

Fig 29 Panoramic radiograph after surgery and positioning of provisional prostheses.

Follow-up visits: The patient was seen again 10 days after the surgery and described continued uneventful healing. He was completely satisfied with the provisional prostheses, both functionally and esthetically. His occlusion was carefully evaluated and minor adjustments were made. The provisional FDPs were not removed. The patient's oral hygiene was considered excellent and was reinforced. Several sutures were present, and the patient was advised that these could be removed at the next follow-up visit. He was seen again 4 weeks after surgery. The remaining sutures were removed, and healing was excellent. The patient had no complaints and was meticulous in both oral hygiene and dietary management. He was scheduled to begin the definitive restorative phase after 8 weeks (i.e., 12 weeks after implant placement). This was considered adequate for healing of both the implants and the minor grafts.

Final restorative phase: The patient returned for continued treatment care 12 weeks after surgery. He was completely satisfied with both the esthetic and functional results. His oral hygiene remained impeccable, and he experienced no discomfort. The provisional FDPs were removed and the stability of each implant confirmed in addition to evaluation of the peri-implant soft tissue (Figs 30 and 31).

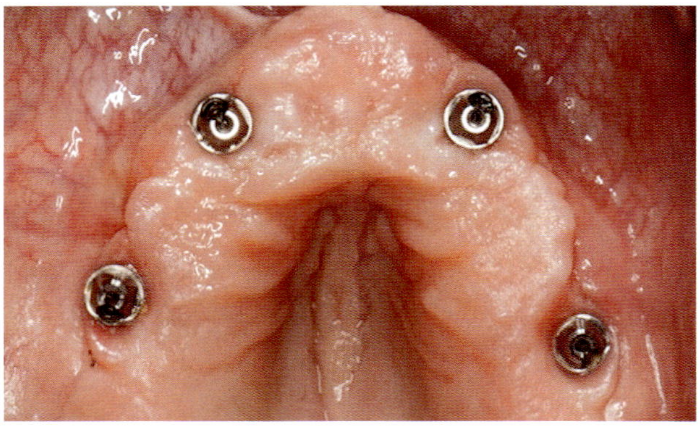
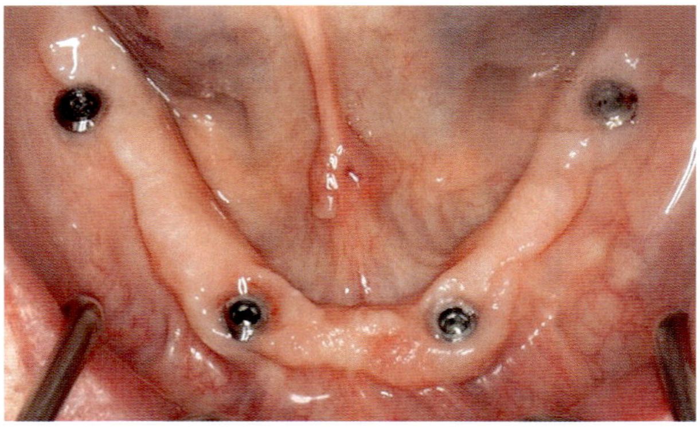

Figs 30 and 31 Maxillary and mandibular implants 12 weeks after placement.

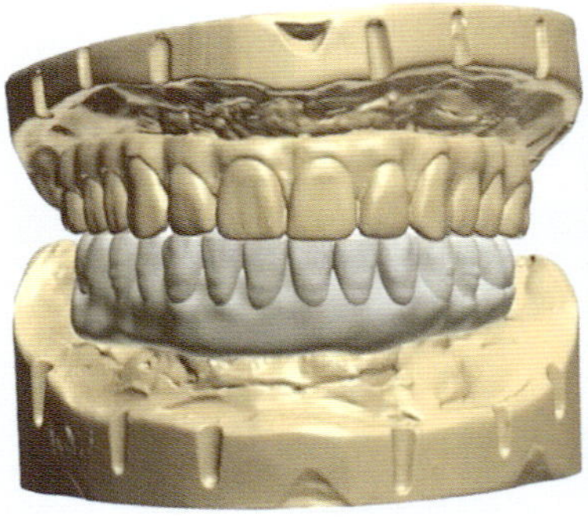

Fig 32 Anterior view. Prototype prosthesis design.

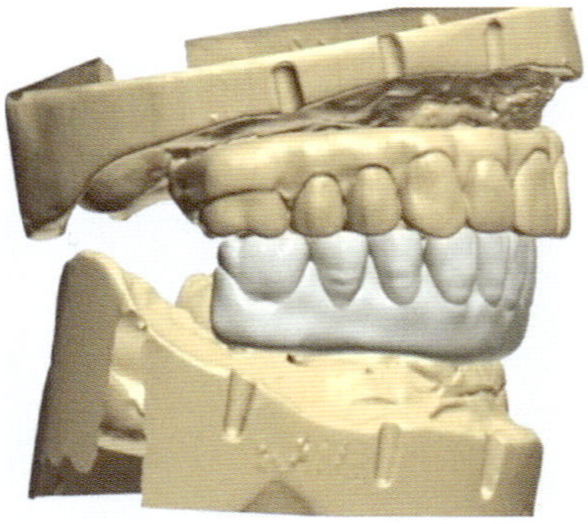
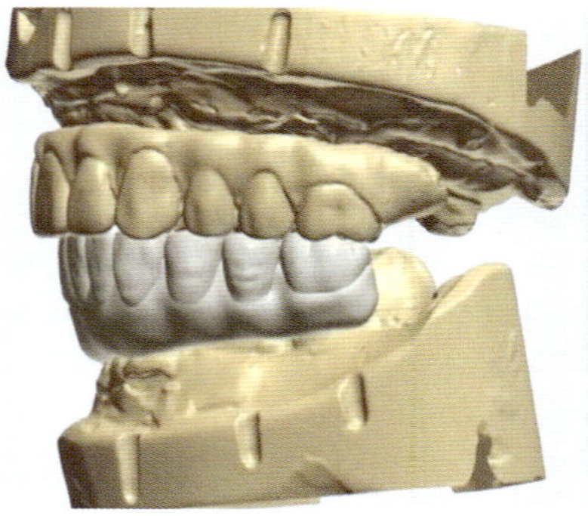

Figs 33 and 34 Right and left lateral views. Prototype prosthesis design.

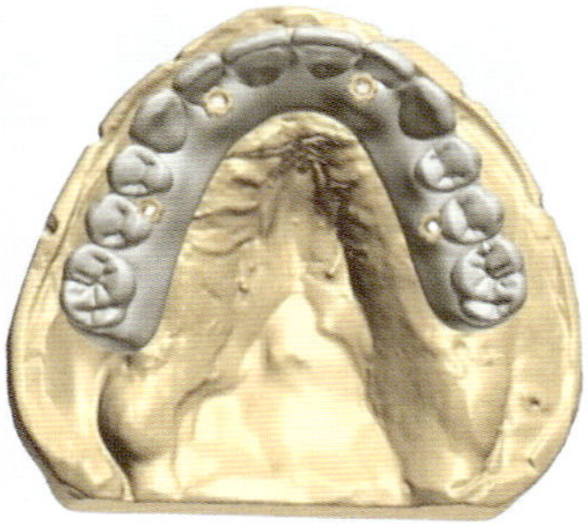
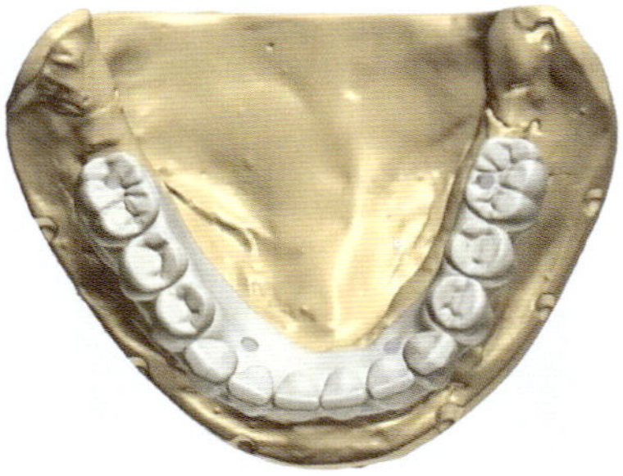

Figs 35 and 36 Maxillary and mand bular occlusal views. Prototype prosthesis design.

Final impressions were taken of both the maxillary and mandibular arches. The impression copings were splinted with a matrix made of dental floss and pattern resin. The matrix was sectioned and the relationship between the implants and overall passivity verified prior to taking the impressions. The impressions were poured in type 4 dental stone and articulated with the provisional FDPs, along with facebow records and bite records in centric relation. The articulated provisional FDPs (at the appropriate vertical dimension) were then scanned.

Definitive prototype prostheses were then digitally designed (Figs 32 to 36) that were intended to represent the final FDPs in terms of form, esthetics, and function (occlusal relationships).

The prototype prostheses were 3D-printed and bonded to provisional copings on the casts that had been used to scan the provisional prostheses. The occlusion was fir alized and the prototypes were characterized. The prototype prostheses were then evaluated intraorally for passivity and esthet-

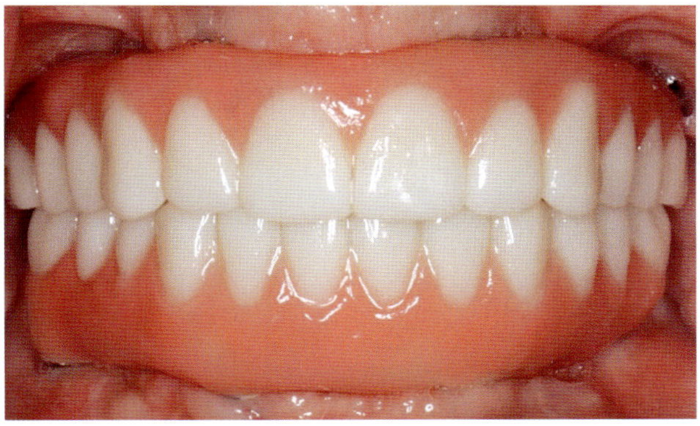

Fig 37 Anterior view. Prototype prostheses 9 months after implant placement.

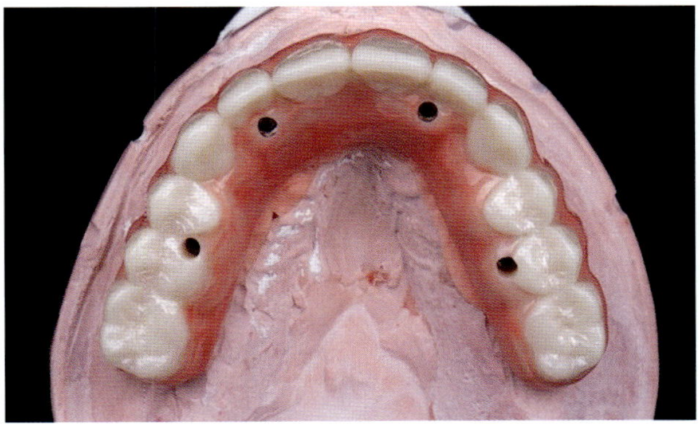

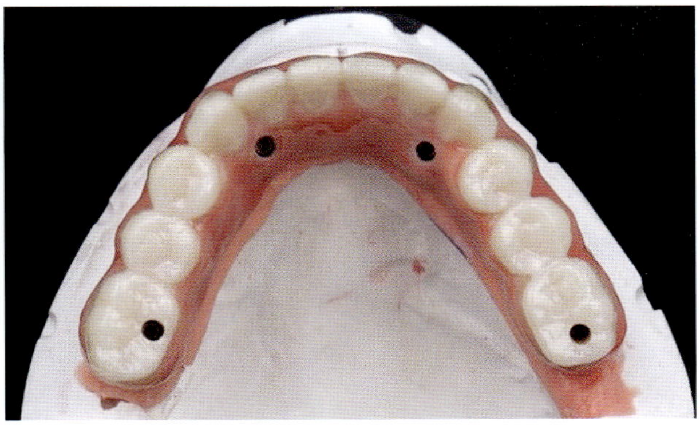

Figs 38 and 39 Occlusal views. Definitive zirconia full arch FDPs attached to copings on casts.

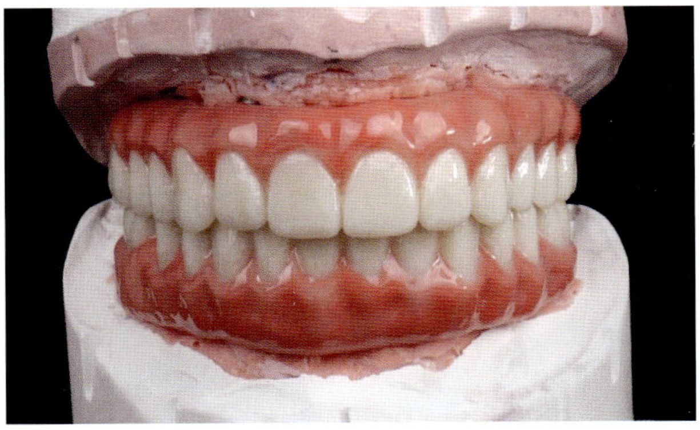

Fig 40 Anterior view. Definitive zirconia full arch FDPs attached to copings on casts.

ics and delivered upon approval. The patient was advised to maintain his oral hygiene regimen and was discharged. He returned for evaluation 9 months after implant placement and reported no concerns. He was completely satisfied with all aspects of the prostheses (Fig 37). It was decided to proceed with fabrication of the definitive full-arch zirconia FDPs in the maxilla and mandible.

The definitive zirconia FDPs were fabricated using the prototype design that had been evaluated and approved intraorally. The zirconia full arch FDPs were attached to metal copings on the previously checked casts and refined, adjusted, and finished (Figs 38 to 40).

The patient returned 11 months after implant placement for the delivery of the definitive FDPs. Each FDP was individually evaluated for fit, tissue adaptation, cleanability, and esthetics (Figs 41 and 21). After confirmation and approval by the patient, the two FDPs were inserted together and the occlusion carefully evaluated. After minor adjustments, the full

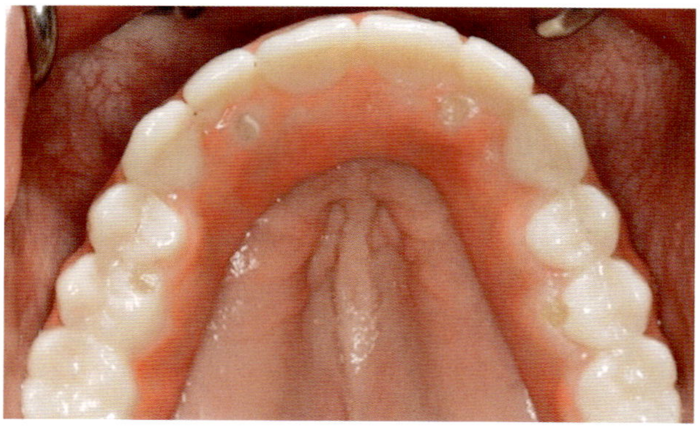
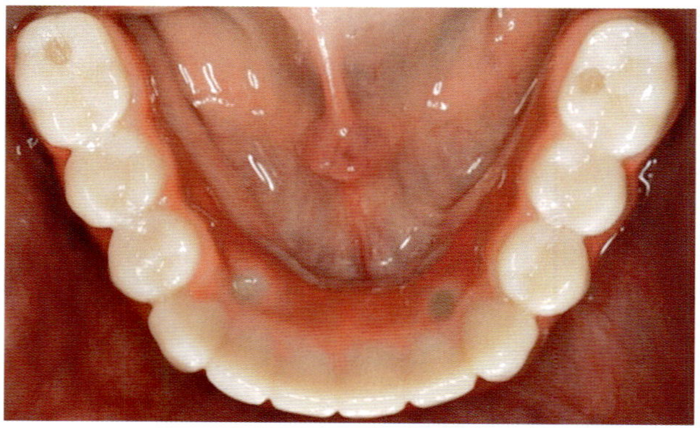

Figs 41 and 42 Occlusal view. Maxillary and mandibular definitive prostheses.

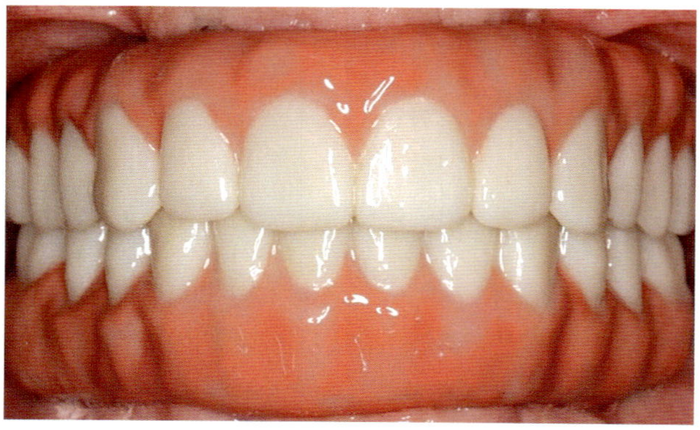

Fig 43 Anterior view. Definitive prostheses in maximum intercuspation.

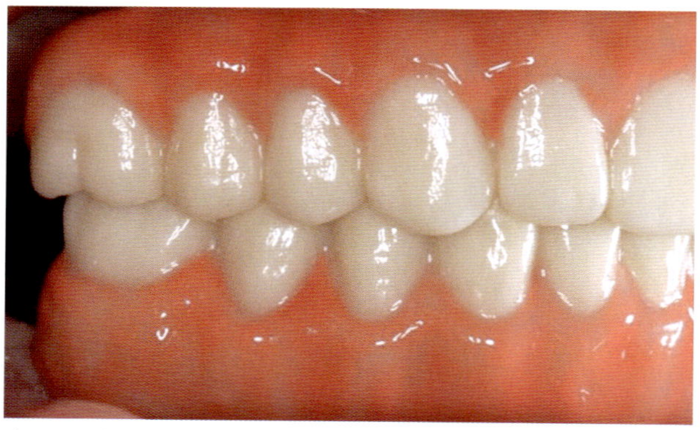
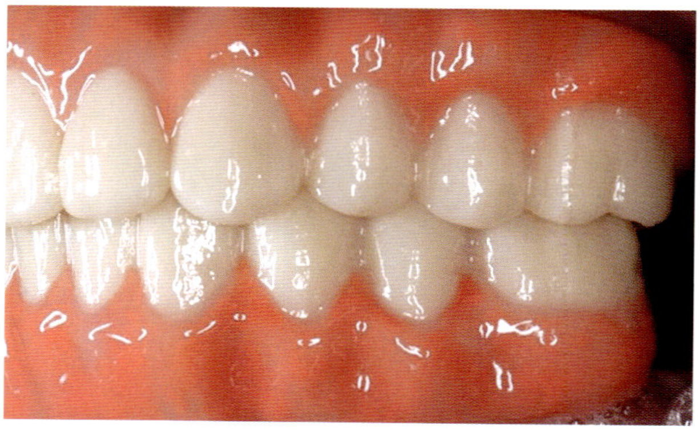

Figs 44 and 45 Right and left lateral views. Definitive prostheses in maximum intercuspation.

arch FDPs were removed and carefully polished, then reinserted and checked again for passivity and tissue adaptation (Figs 43 to 45). The patient felt completely comfortable with the final prostheses and was very pleased with the esthetic outcome (Figs 46 to 49).

FOLLOW-UP AND PATIENT SATISFACTION

This patient received definitive zirconia full-arch FDPs in both the maxilla and mandible. His treatment met all his concerns and requirements, and he has been followed for 2 years without any complications or concerns (Figs 50 to 52). Radiographic evaluation after 24 months confirmed the healthy state of the implant and FDPs (Fig 53).

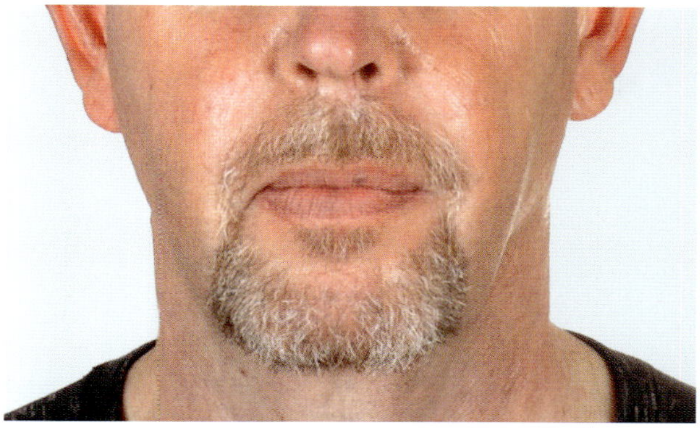
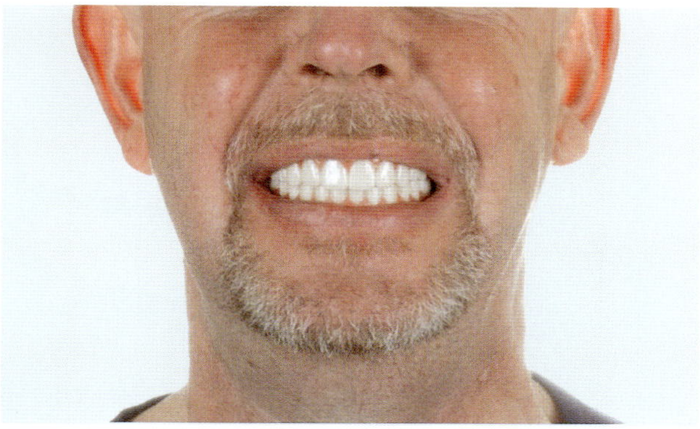

Figs 46 and 47 Anterior views. Resting and smiling. Definitive full arch FDPs.

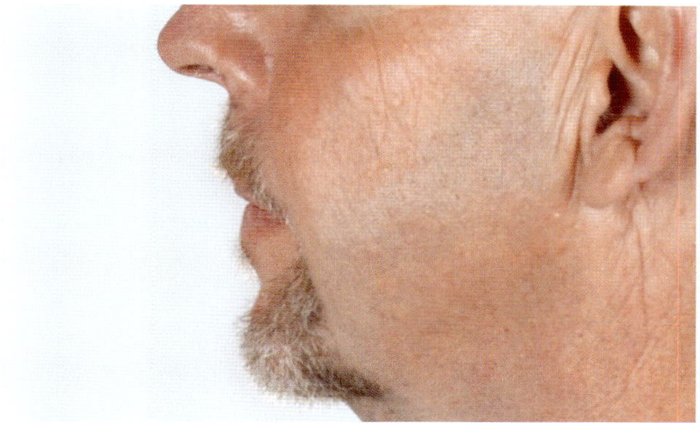
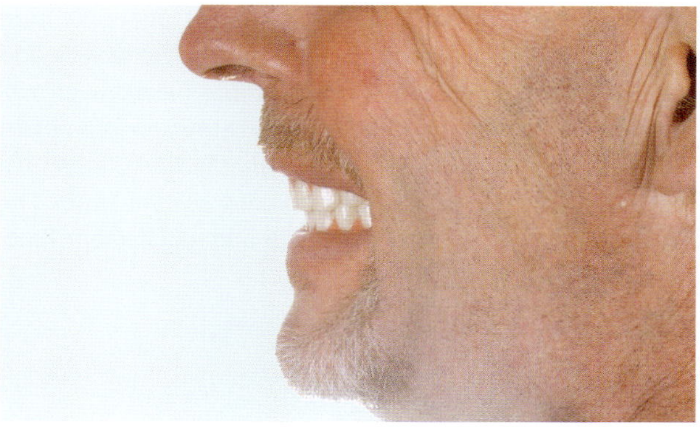

Figs 48 and 49 Lateral views. Resting and smiling. Definitive full arch FDPs.

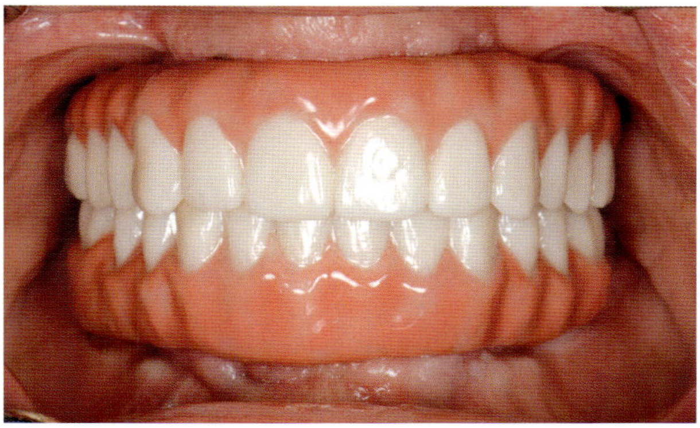

Fig 50 Anterior view. 24-month follow-up.

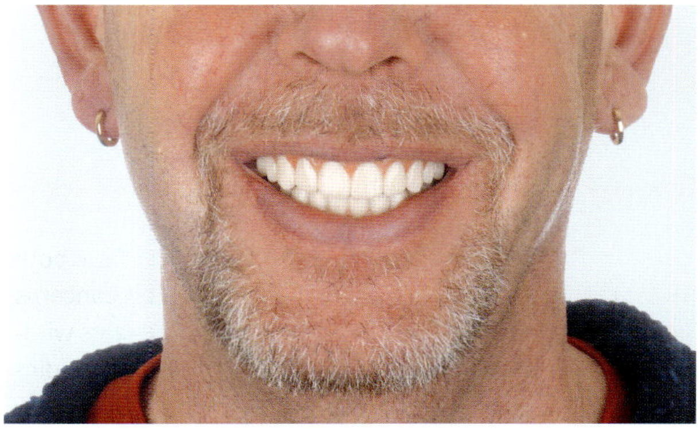
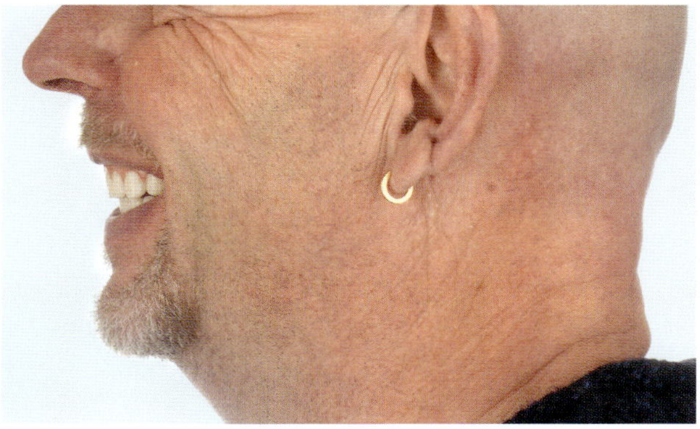

Figs 51 and 52 Anterior and lateral profile views. 24-month follow-up.

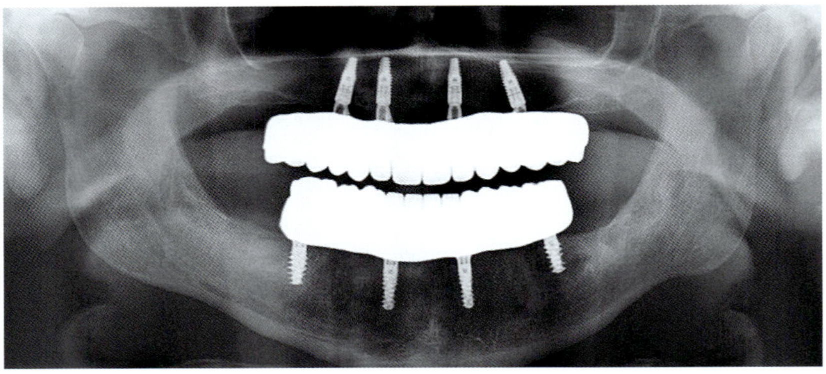

Fig 53 Panoramic radiograph. 24-month follow up.

The immediate placement and restoration of four implants in each arch, as well as the angled implants in the maxilla and the axially angled implants in the mandible, have proven successful over 24 months of follow-up, irrespective of implant inclination. The full arch FDPs are cleanable, and the zirconia material is excellent at minimizing biofilm accumulation. The prostheses have provided a reliable and satisfactory functional and esthetic outcome.

Use this code to watch a highlight video with the patient reporting on his satisfaction with the treatment.

Patients with severely atrophic maxilla

5.10 Treatment of the Atrophic Maxilla Using Two Standard Implants and Two Zygomatic Implants Immediately Loaded with a Fixed Restoration

P. Casentini, M. Chiapasco

PATIENT CHARACTERISTICS AND PATIENT PROFILE

A 65-year-old woman was referred to our clinic by another dentist she had recently visited and who had diagnosed a compromised and complex clinical and anatomical situation.

She complained of pain and difficulty when chewing, instability of her maxillary prosthesis, and unsatisfactory esthetics. She had received maxillary implants restored with partial fixed dental prostheses, but no stable clinical solution had been achieved. She expressed a preference for a fixed maxillary rehabilitation.

The patient did not smoke, was not taking any medication, and reported being in good general health.

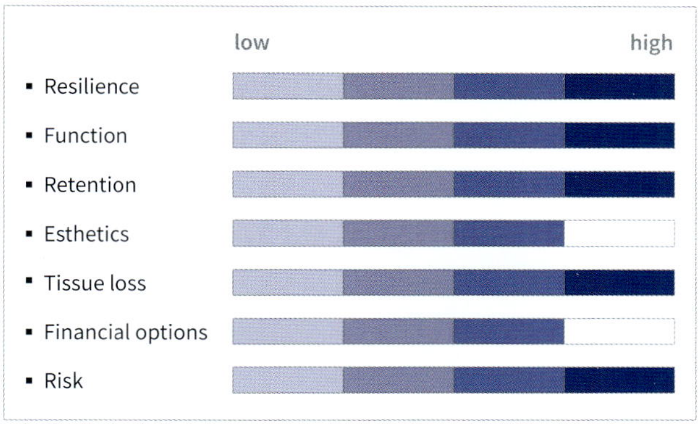

Fig 1 Patient profile.

Based on this information and the clinical and radiographic evaluation described below, the following patient profile (Fig 1) can be derived for this patient (for more information about patient profiles, see Chapters 2.1.3 and 3.6).

CLINICAL EVALUATION

The extraoral examination revealed mild lip incompetence at rest and an unsatisfactory smile due to tooth migration and inconsistent shades. The right lateral incisor was inclined laterally. There were discrepancies between the incisal margins and midline inclinations of the two central incisors (Figs 2 and 3).

Intraoral examination revealed the following clinical situation:

- In the maxilla, the residual dentition consisted of teeth 13 to 23. Teeth 13 and 23 served as the anterior abutments for two mixed tooth- and implant-supported posterior fixed bridges. The four incisors were splinted between them and to the posterior bridges with composite resin and a palatal metal wire. The occlusal view showed that tooth 23 had a fractured root and that all the teeth in the upper right quadrant had migrated buccally. Despite splinting, the posterior bridges and the remaining anterior teeth showed significant mobility. The posterior bridges contained gingiva-colored ceramics to compensate for the horizontal and vertical atrophy.
- In the mandible, the residual dentition consisted of teeth 44 to 33. Implant-supported fixed dental prostheses were present in the posterior regions of the mandible. There was no evidence of mobility or inflammation.
- Oral hygiene was considered adequate, and no pathologic probing depths were recorded on the remaining teeth, except for the fractured tooth 23. No probing depths were recorded around mandibular implants (Figs 4 and 5).

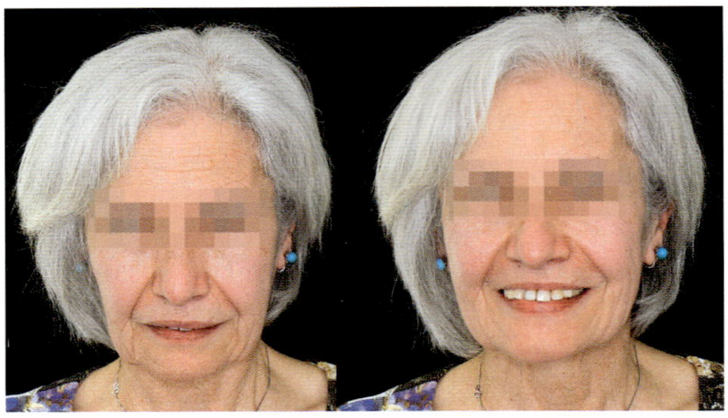

Figs 2 and 3 Extraoral view at baseline.

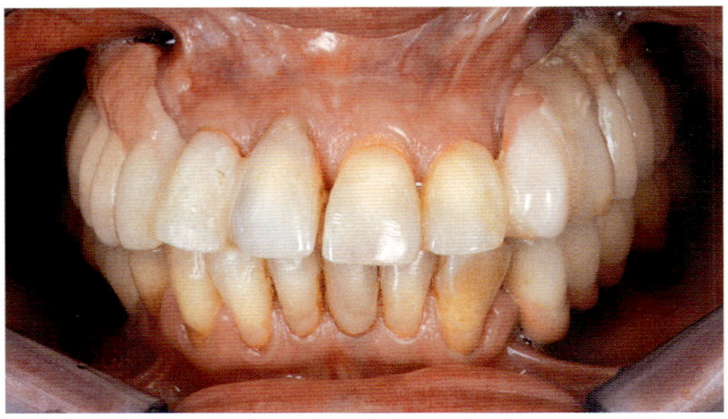

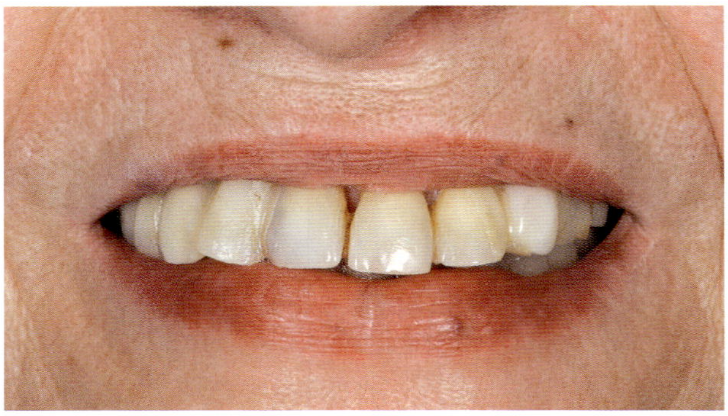

Fig 4 The patient's smile.

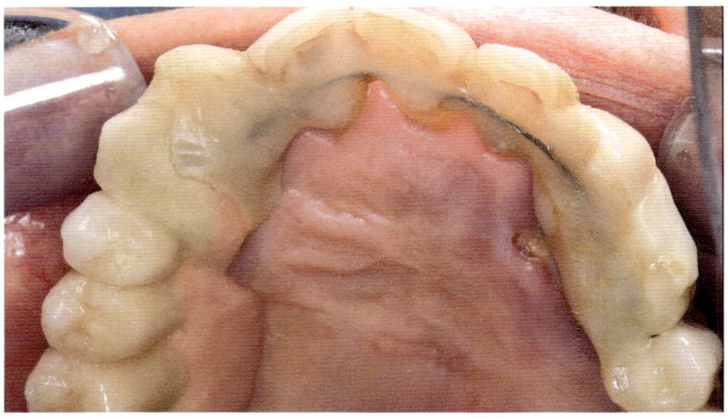

Fig 5 Intraoral situation at baseline.

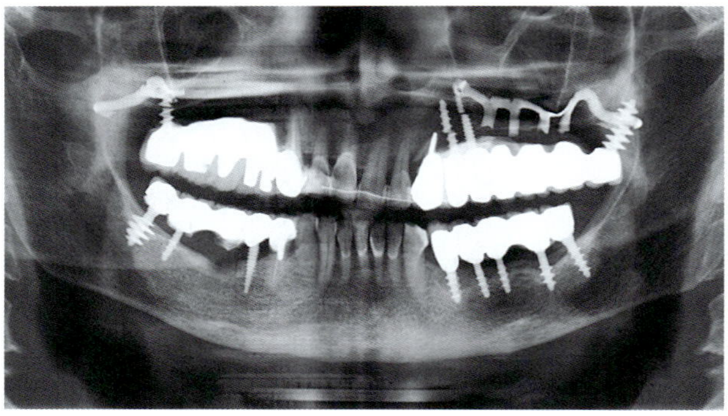

Fig 6 Panoramic radiograph at baseline.

PRELIMINARY RADIOGRAPHIC EXAMINATION

The patient provided a recent panoramic radiograph and a computed-tomography (CT) scan.

The panoramic radiograph showed multiple fractures of root-shaped implants in the left and right posterior maxilla and a significant degree of atrophy. Some fractured subperiosteal implants were stabilized with screws. In the left and right posterior mandible, the fixed dental prostheses were supported by implants of various shapes, but none of the implants appeared to be fractured. Normal levels of residual bone were maintained around the natural teeth, except for the fractured tooth 23 (Fig 6).

CT confirmed the presence of the fractured root-shaped implants (some of which penetrated the maxillary sinus), subperiosteal implants near the lateral sinus wall, and advanced atrophy, as well as complete bilateral resorption of the alveolar process in the posterior maxilla (Fig 7).

PRELIMINARY TREATMENT PLAN AND INITIAL SURGERY

Based on the clinical examination and the radiographic data, the following preliminary treatment plan was developed:

- Removal of the fractured implants and all subperiosteal implants in the maxilla
- Extraction of the fractured root of tooth 23

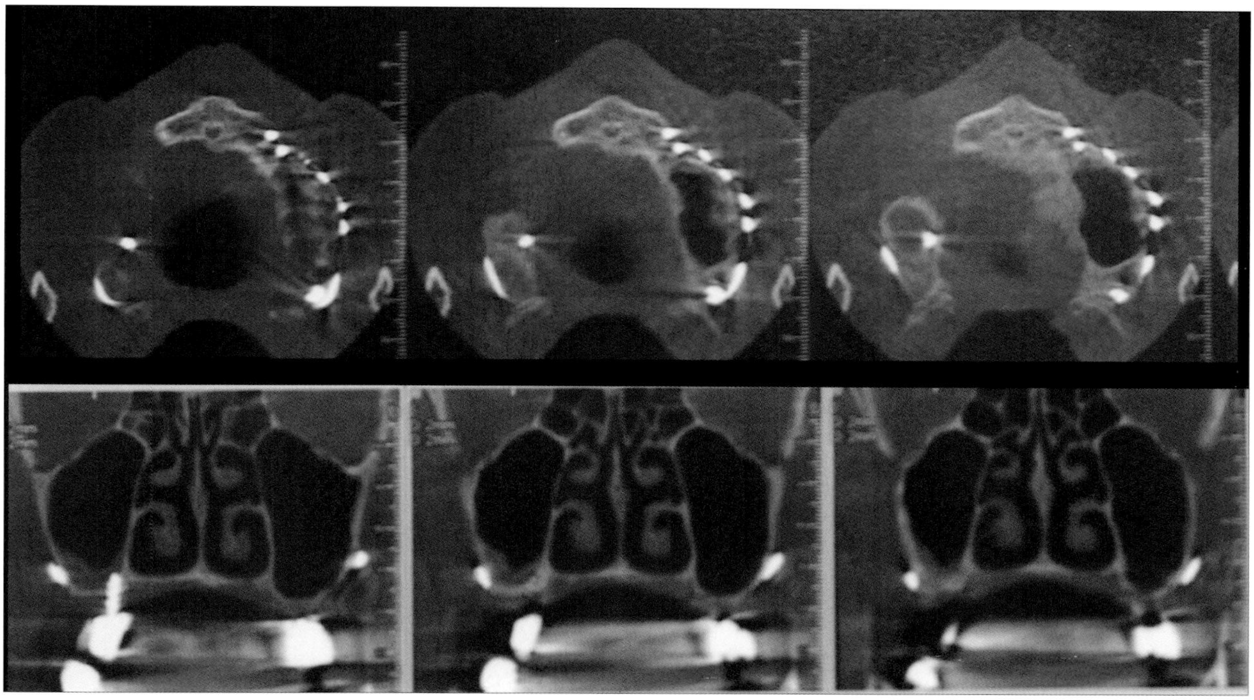

Fig 7 Initial CT scan.

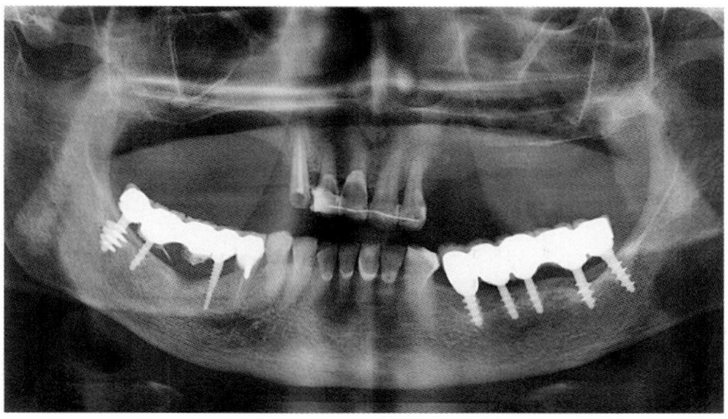

Fig 8 Panoramic radiograph after removal of the failed implants.

These preliminary procedures were considered mandatory before any type of definitive treatment plan could be determined. After preliminary healing, a removable provisional prosthesis was proposed to provide acceptable esthetics. The patient agreed to the treatment plan and provided written consent.

Given the anatomical complexity and the unfavorable position of the fractured implants, surgery was performed under general anesthesia. (Clinical documentation of the initial surgery is not available.)

The postoperative panoramic radiograph shows complete removal of the compromised maxillary implants (Fig 8).

PROVISIONAL REMOVABLE PROSTHESIS

After suture removal, digital impressions were taken with an intraoral scanner (IOS) (Trios-3; 3Shape, Copenhagen, Denmark) and a removable dental prosthesis supported by the remaining maxillary teeth was delivered. This temporary solution was well accepted by the patient, although its function was mainly esthetic (Figs 9 and 10).

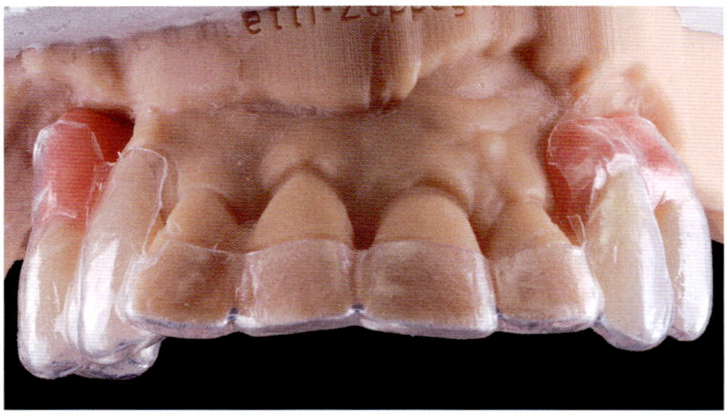

Fig 9 Provisional vacuum-formed retainer on the cast.

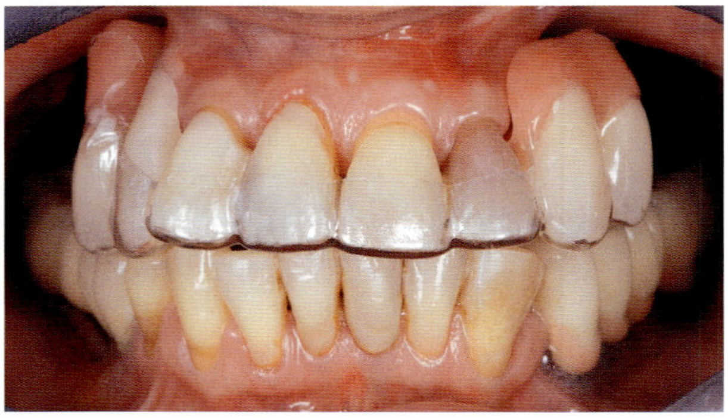

Fig 10 Intraoral situation with provisional removable prostheses.

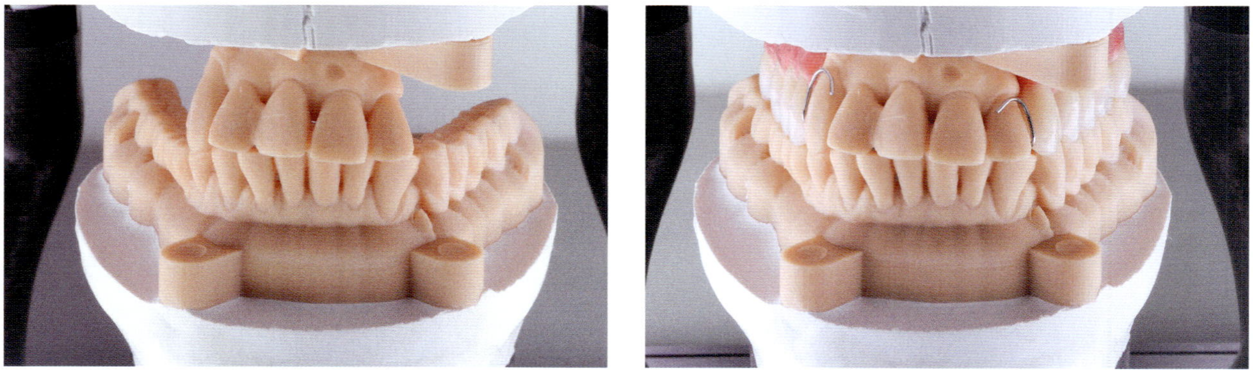

Figs 11 and 12 3D-printed models on the articulator with the diagnostic set-up.

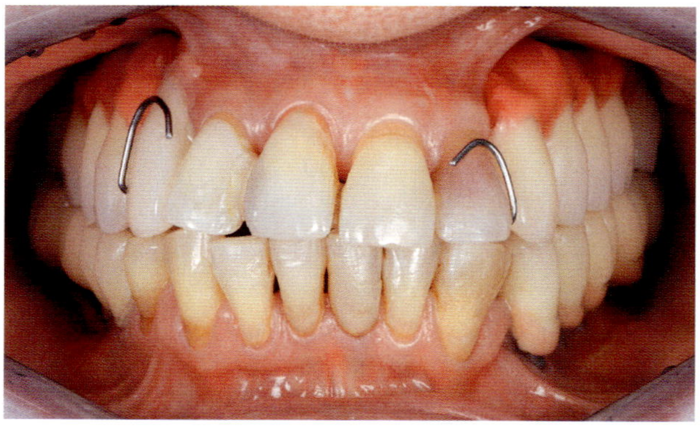

Fig 13 Intraoral situation with the diagnostic set-up.

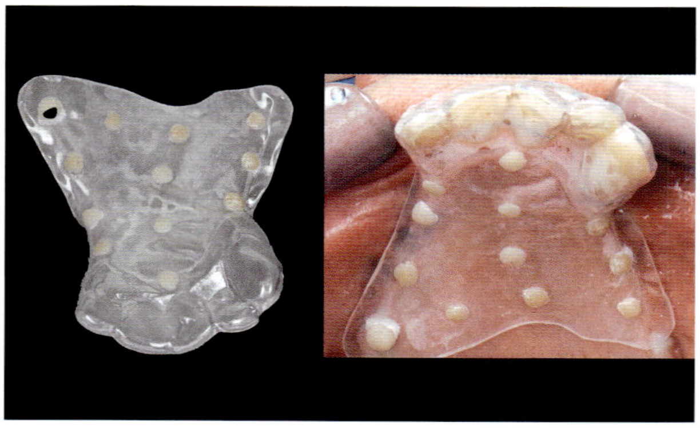

Fig 14 Radiographic template with radiopaque markers.

3-MONTH REEVALUATION AND DIGITAL DIAGNOSTIC WORKFLOW

The patient was reevaluated after 3 months. The maxillary soft tissue was found to be completely healed. New digital impressions of the two arches were taken with the IOS, and the dental technician was asked to produce 3D-printed models and fabricate a removable dental mock-up of the missing maxillary posterior teeth for a try-in in the patient's mouth (Figs 11 and 12).

The mock-up was then tried in in the oral cavity. A correct relationship with the opposing arch was confirmed (Fig 13). Based on the same printed model, the dental lab produced a vacuum-formed diagnostic guide in composite resin with radiopaque markers. The dental set-up and the diagnostic template were also scanned at the lab with a laboratory scanner to obtain STL files. A new CT was taken with the patient wearing the diagnostic guide (Fig 14).

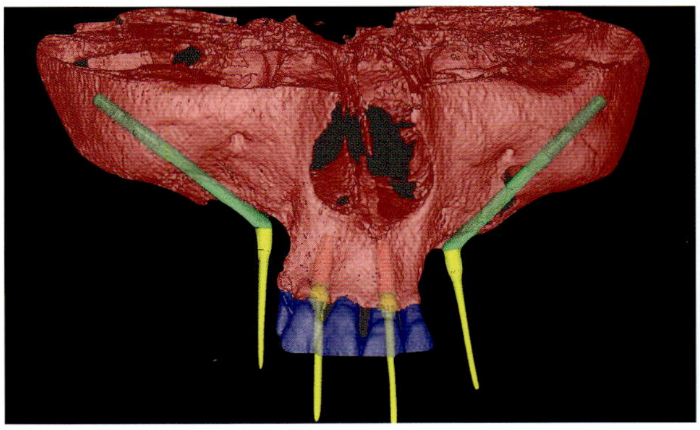

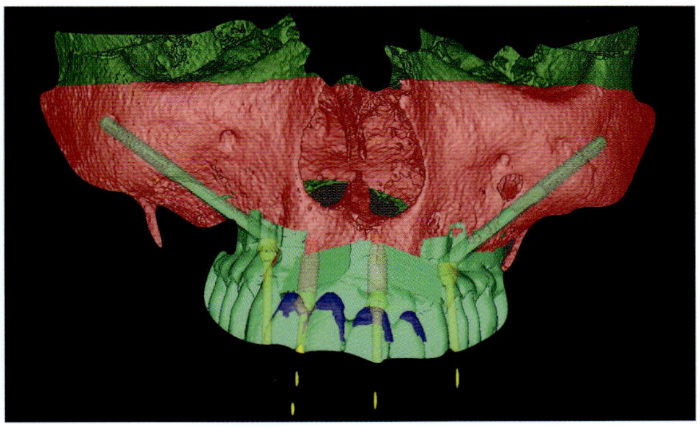

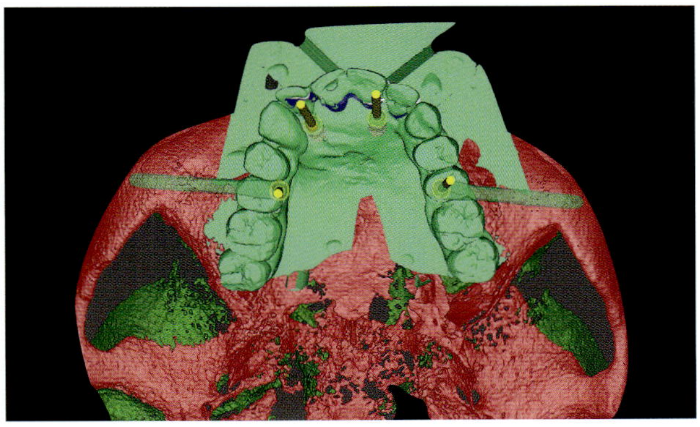

Figs 15 to 17 Prosthetically driven implant planning by the coDiagnostiX software after matching the DICOM and STL files.

The DICOM files (obtained from the new CT) and the STL files were then matched in a planning software (coDiagnostiX; Dental Wings, Montréal, Canada) to verify the relationship between the prosthetic volume and the residual bone volume.

The software simulated the placement of two standard implants in the anterior maxilla and two zygomatic implants in the zygomatic bone. Correct prosthetic emergence of the implants relative to the prosthetic volume was also verified (Figs 15 to 17). The software was also useful in defining the correct implant lengths.

FINAL TREATMENT PLAN

After evaluating the anatomical situation and the degree of atrophy, the option of placing two standard implants in the anterior maxilla in combination with two zygomatic implants was considered the best option for providing a fixed reconstruction.

The final treatment plan was developed accordingly. In the event that adequate primary implant stability was achieved, an immediately loaded provisional fixed dental prosthesis would be placed in the maxilla. After osseointegration of the implants, the definitive fixed prosthesis was to be realized.

The patient accepted the proposed treatment plan and gave her written consent.

ZYGOMATIC AND STANDARD IMPLANT PLACEMENT

Once the treatment plan was approved, the DICOM files were sent to a specialized laboratory for the fabrication of stereolithographic models. The placement of the zygomatic implants was simulated by the surgeon on the stereolithographic model using the company-provided sample implants (Zaga; Institut Straumann AG, Basel, Switzerland) (Figs 18 and 19).

The stereolithographic model was used for the simulated placement of the zygomatic implants to optimize their position relative to the surrounding anatomical structures, particularly the infraorbital nerve, the orbital cavity, and the infratemporal fossa.

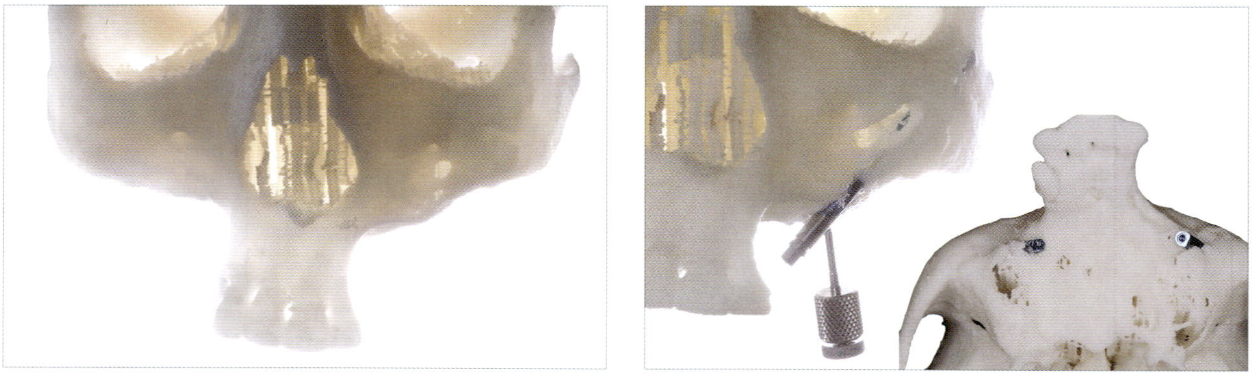

Figs 18 and 19 3D-printed stereolithographic model and simulation of zygomatic implant placement.

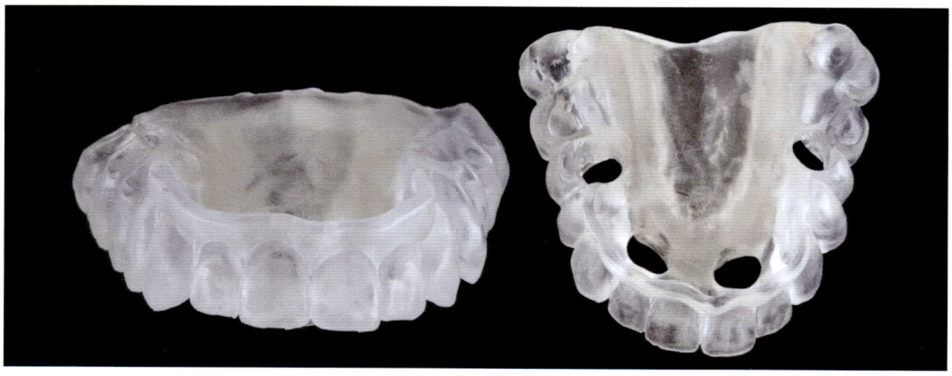

Fig 20 Transfer index.

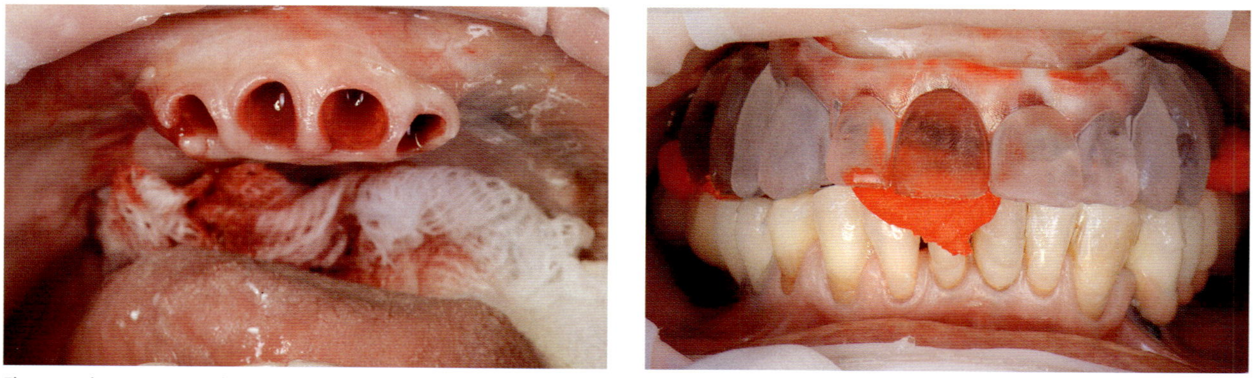

Figs 21 and 22 Extraction of the remaining teeth and relining of the index with autopolymerizing resin.

Due to the complexity of the procedure, the surgery was performed under general anesthesia. After the extraction of the remaining maxillary teeth and before the soft-tissue incisions and the elevation of a mucoperiosteal flap, a composite-resin transfer index was inserted and its position in relation to the mandibular arch was precisely defined by adding some autopolymerizing resin (Figs 20 to 22).

The transfer index was obtained from the previous set-up and was designed to transfer the implant position to the dental laboratory for fabrication of the prostheses for immediate loading. After a U-shaped incision along the maxillary arch, a full-thickness mucoperiosteal flap was elevated that connected the two tuberosities (Fig 23). A horizontal osteotomy/ostectomy of the residual alveolar process of the anterior maxilla was performed with a piezoelectric instrument (Piezosurgery; Mectron, Carasco, Italy) to reduce the discrepancy between the levels of the anterior and posterior implants (Fig 24). Two anterior implants (Bone Level Tapered, diameter 4.1 mm, length 12 mm; Institut Straumann

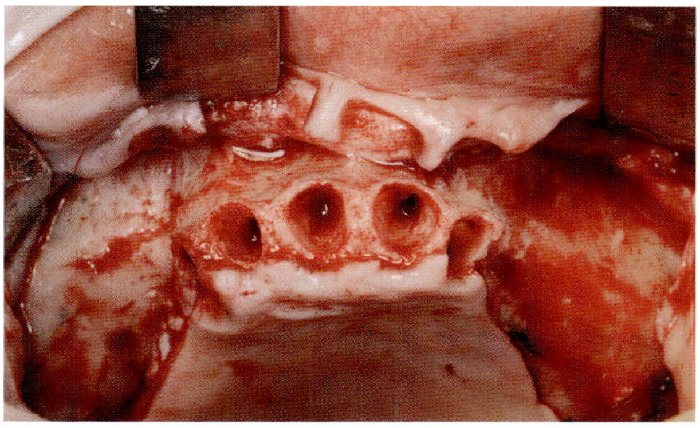

Fig 23 Elevation of a flap over the entire maxilla.

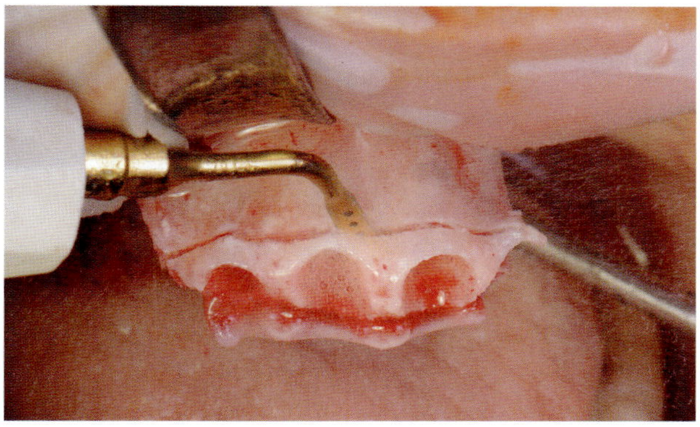

Fig 24 Surgical bone remodeling with a piezoelectric instrument.

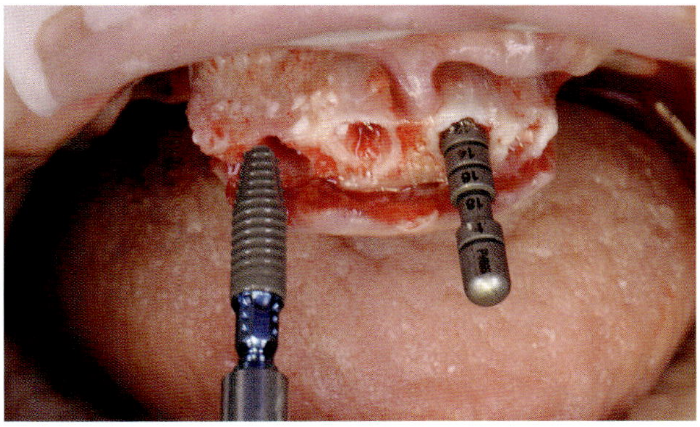

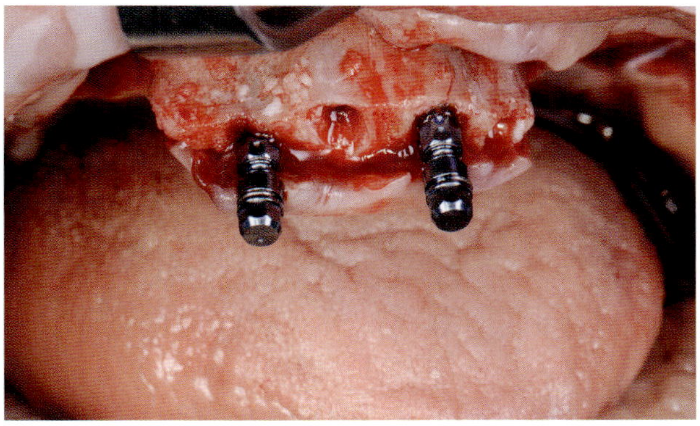

Figs 25 and 26 Placement of the anterior implants.

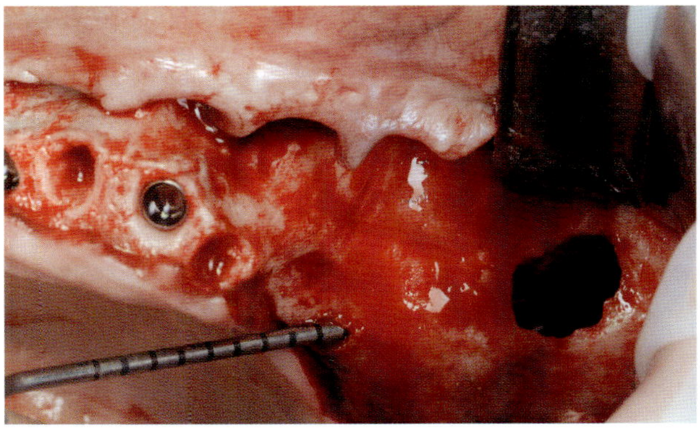

Fig 27 Final probing of the zygomatic implant sites prior to implant placement.

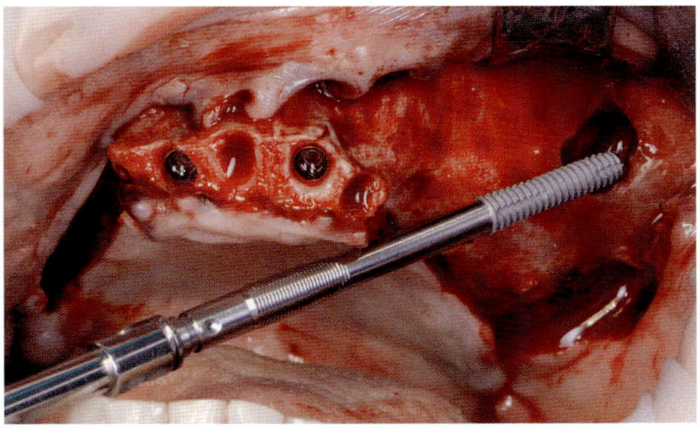

Fig 28 Intraoral view of the zygomatic implant before placement.

AG, Basel, Switzerland) were placed in the residual alveolar bone at sites 12 and 21 with insertion torques ≥ 30 Ncm (Figs 25 and 26).

Site preparation in the zygomatic process began after identification of the emergence of the infraorbital nerve, the inferior border of the orbital cavity, and the posterior wall of the zygomatic bone. A fenestration was also made in the lateral wall of the maxillary sinus; the Schneiderian membrane was elevated and preserved. This allowed preparation of the apical aspect of the zygomatic implant site with special drills through the sinus while preserving an intact membrane. The axis of the implant and its anchorage in the zygomatic bone were also optimized.

Before implant placement, the sites were measured and checked with a special probing instrument (Fig 27). The implants were positioned with a special manual driver (Fig 28). The manual insertion mode made it possible to determine precise final implant position with correct prosthetic axes

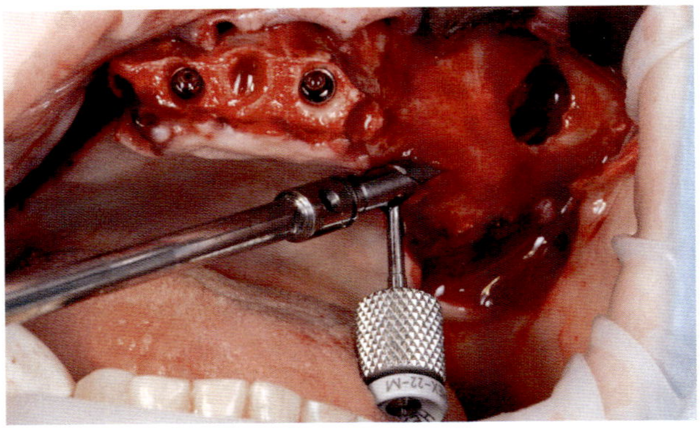

Fig 29 Prosthetic axis checked with the implant driver.

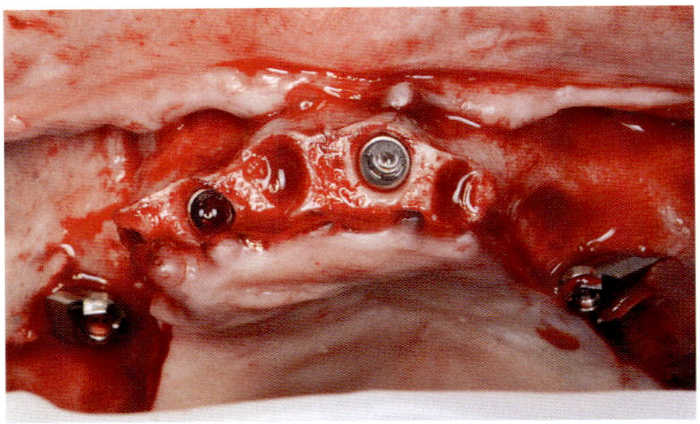

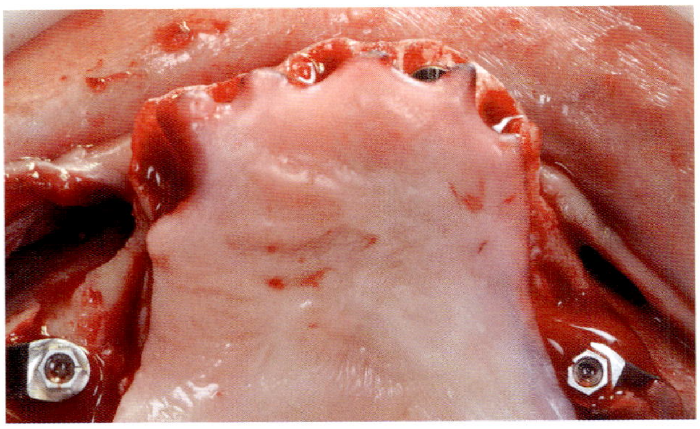

Figs 30 and 31 Frontal and occlusal views after implant placement.

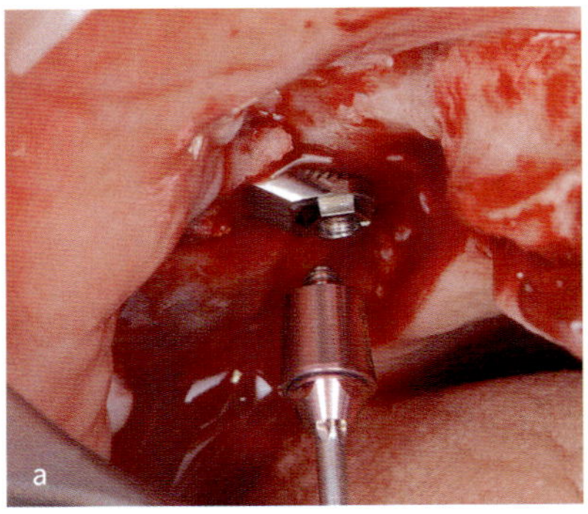

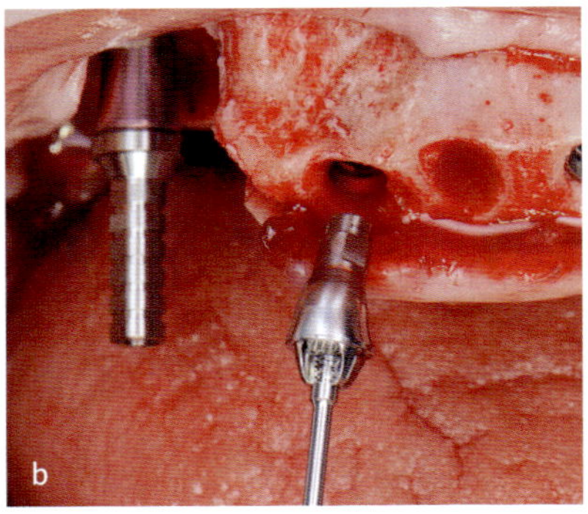

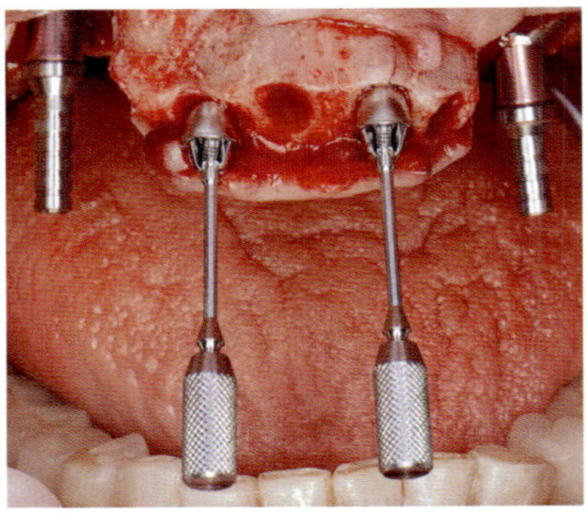

Figs 32a-b and 33 Positioning of the screw-retained abutments (SRA).

(Fig 29): both zygomatic implants achieved adequate primary stability (Figs 30 and 31). The mucoperiosteal flaps were sutured with single, interrupted sutures to achieve a hermetic closure.

After implant placement was completed, screw-retained abutments (SRA; Institut Straumann AG, Basel, Switzerland) were connected to the standard anterior implants and to the zygomatic implants and tightened to 30 Ncm. Two angled abutments (15°) were selected for the anterior implants (Figs 32a-b and 33). After insertion of the SRA, titanium copings were positioned and screwed in place. The flap was sutured and adapted to the emergence profile of the prosthetic components. After isolating the soft tissues with four pieces of rubber dam, the transfer index was repositioned and adapted to the position of the implants. Care was taken

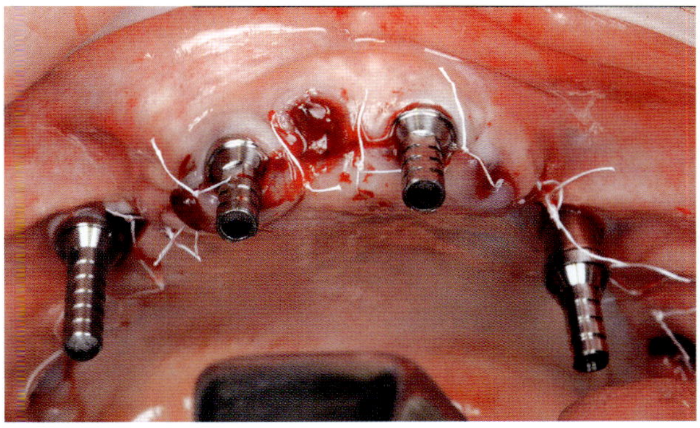

Fig 34 Final aspect of the surgical site after suturing and placement of titanium copings.

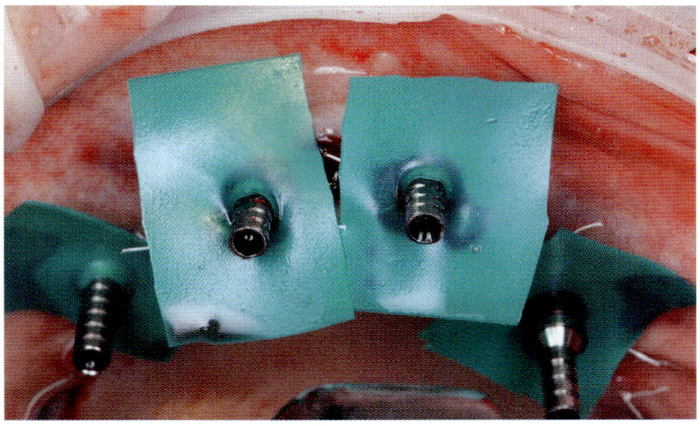

Fig 35 Isolation of the soft tissues by rubber dam.

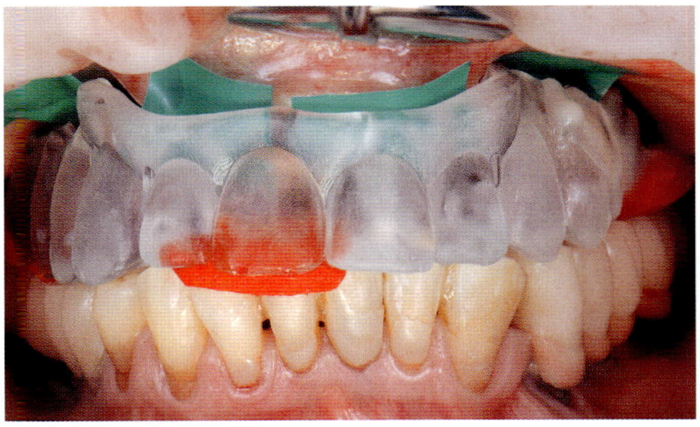

Fig 36 Indexing by bonding connecting the transfer index and titanium copings with autopolymerizing resin.

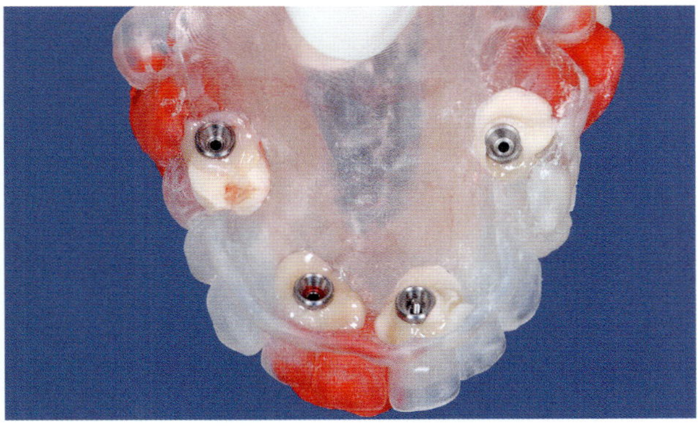

Fig 37 Removal of the transfer index after resin polymerization.

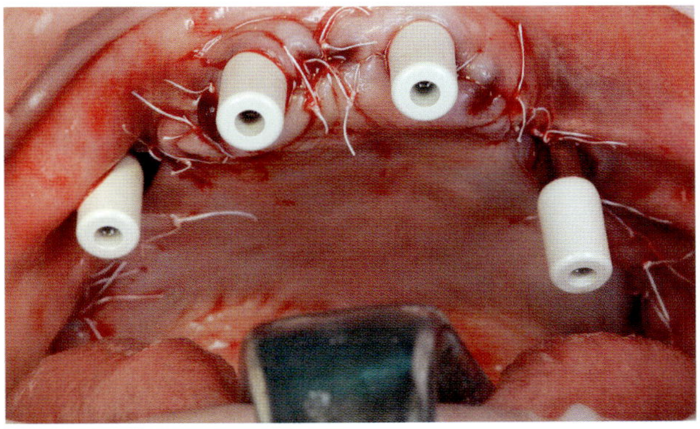

Fig 38 PEEK protective caps on the SRA.

to ensure that the index achieved the same initial position in relation to the opposing arch (Fig 34). Titanium copings were attached to the transfer index with a small amount of autopolymerizing resin (Figs 35 to 37). The transfer index served as an open impression tray and a bite registration index, providing to the laboratory with the necessary information to fabricate the provisional prostheses. Finally, PEEK protective caps were screwed onto the SRA (Fig 38).

Once the surgical and prosthetic procedures were completed, anesthesia was discontinued and the patient was discharged after 6 hours of observation. Postoperative instructions and medications included intermittent ice packs, a soft diet, antibiotic prophylaxis (amoxicillin and clavulanic acid, 1 g every 3 hours for 1 week), chlorhexidine 0.2% mouthwash (three times daily), and analgesics (ibuprofen, 600 mg three times daily as needed for pain).

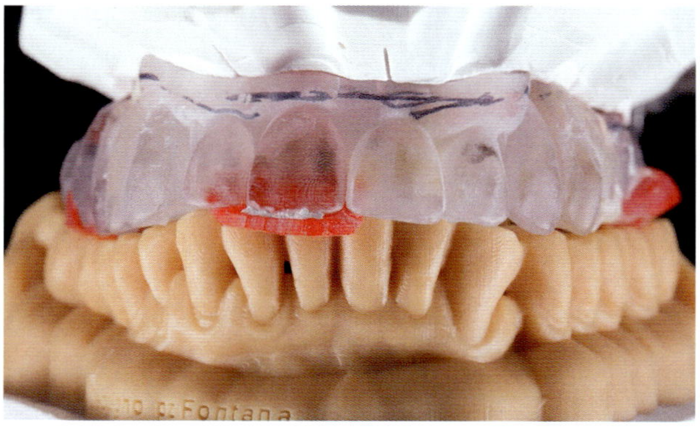

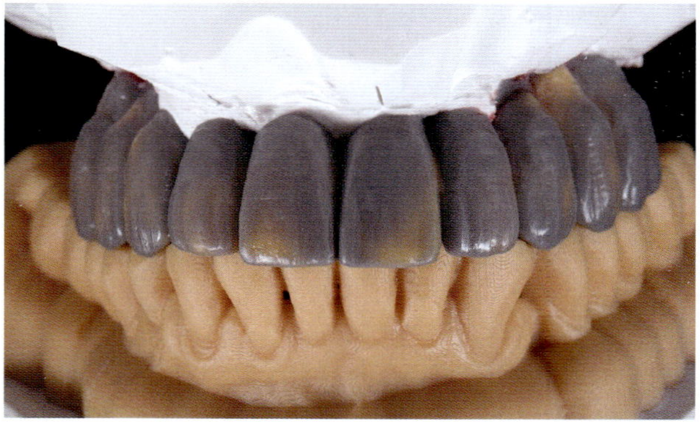

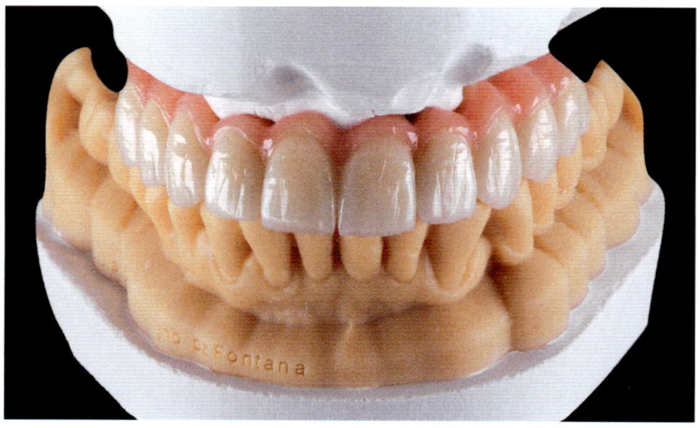

Figs 39 to 41 Laboratory procedures for the provisional screw-retained reconstruction.

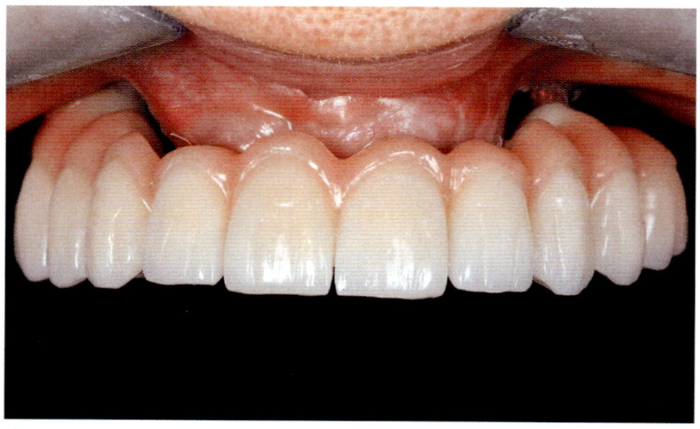

Fig 42 Intraoral aspect of the screw-retained provisional restoration after delivery.

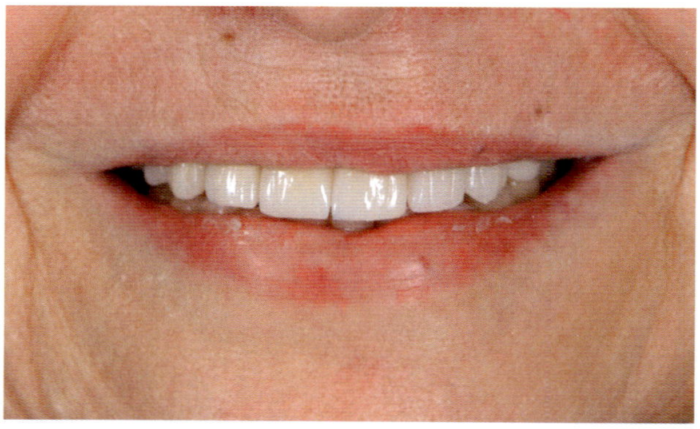

Fig 43 The patient's smile after delivery of the provisional screw-retained restoration.

FABRICATION AND DELIVERY OF THE PROVISIONAL PROSTHESIS

The transfer index allowed the laboratory to create stone casts showing the positions of the implants and the correct intermaxillary relationships. The screw-retained provisional full-arch prosthesis was then waxed up and realized in resin with a metal supporting framework (Figs 39 to 41).

The provisional prosthesis was delivered for immediate loading 5 days after surgery (Figs 42 and 43). It was connected to the SRA abutments without difficulty and torqued to 15 Ncm. The occlusion was checked and minor adjustments were performed. In particular, the presence of stable contacts with the opposite arch was verified. The screw access holes were sealed with PTFE tape and flowable composite. A panoramic radiograph confirmed the correct placement of the restoration (Fig 44).

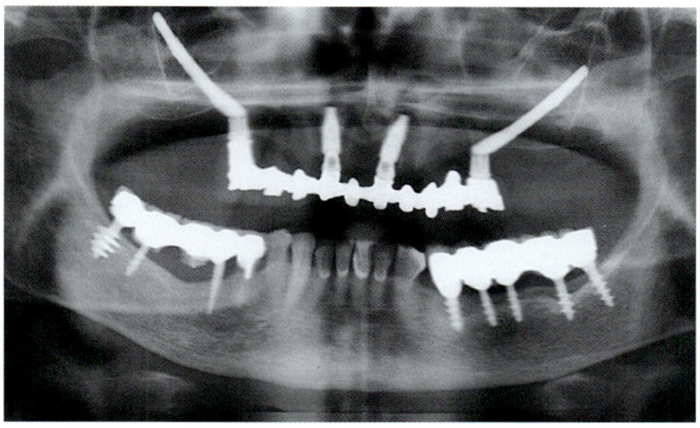

Fig 44 Panoramic radiograph after immediate loading.

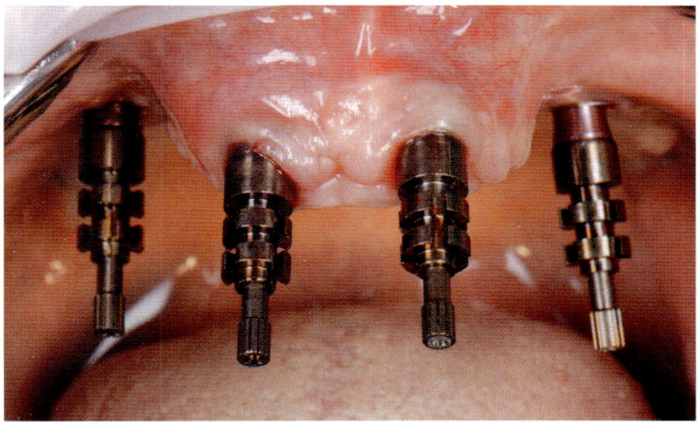

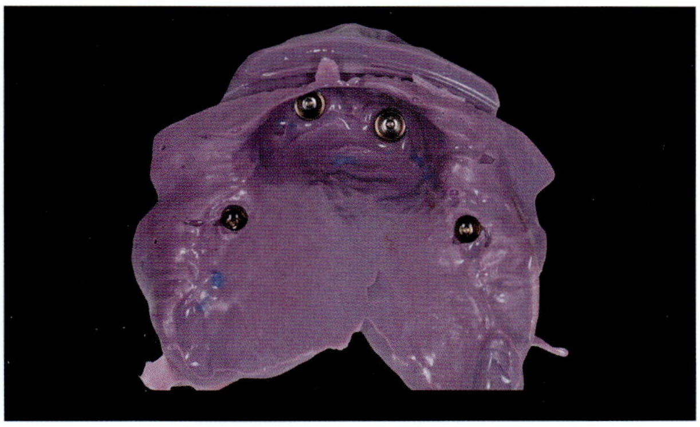

Figs 45 and 46 Open-tray polyether impression for the final reconstruction.

Although the surgery was complex and invasive, the patient reported only limited swelling and pain. She was recommended to maintain a soft diet for 12 weeks and to return for follow-up appointments every 4 weeks. The sutures were removed 2 weeks after surgery.

FABRICATION AND DELIVERY OF THE FINAL RESTORATION

After 4 months of tissue healing and implant osseointegration, the procedures for the final restoration could begin.

After removal of the provisional fixed prosthesis, the SRA abutments were disinfected with 1% chlorhexidine gel. Metal transfer copings were connected to the SRA abutments and an open-tray polyether impression (Impregum; 3M Espe, Seefeld, Germany) was taken (Figs 45 and 46).

The dental laboratory fabricated a master cast, the accuracy of which was validated using a stone verification index (Figs 47a-b and 48). It is indeed important to verify an exact match with the master cast in the oral cavity before the CAD/CAM metal framework is created. If the stone verification index can be screwed onto the implants in the oral cavity without tension and without breaking, the model can be considered accurate. If the stone verification index breaks, it should be fixed with autopolymerizing resin and the master model should be modified. To define the interarch relationships, the provisional was used for a chairside cross-mount procedure after facebow registration (Figs 49 and 50a-c).

The dental laboratory designed and fabricated a CAD/CAM screw-retained titanium framework at an external milling center (Createch, Mendaro, Spain) (Fig 51). The framework was waxed up and veneered with an injectable composite resin (Figs 52 to 54a-b). The design of the final restoration included one cantilever unit on each side and sufficient space for oral hygiene with cleanable convex surfaces.

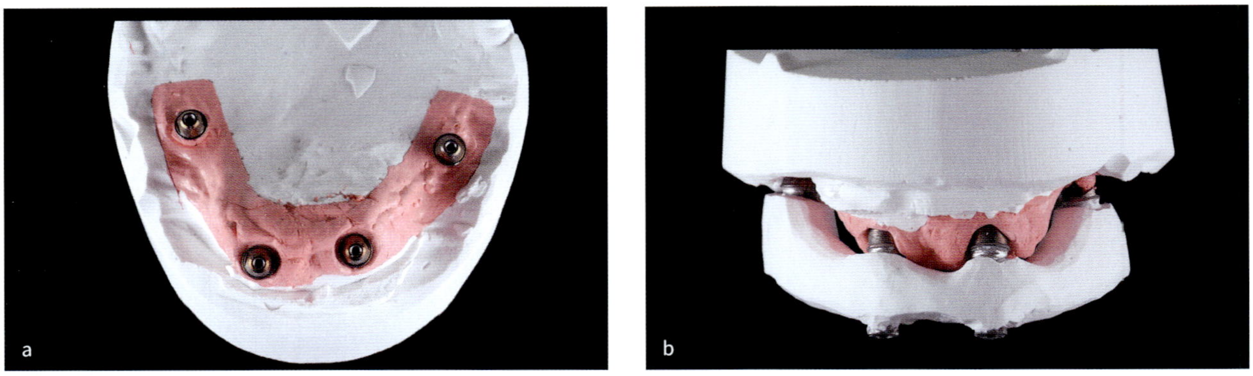

Fig 47a-b Master cast and stone verification index for the final reconstruction.

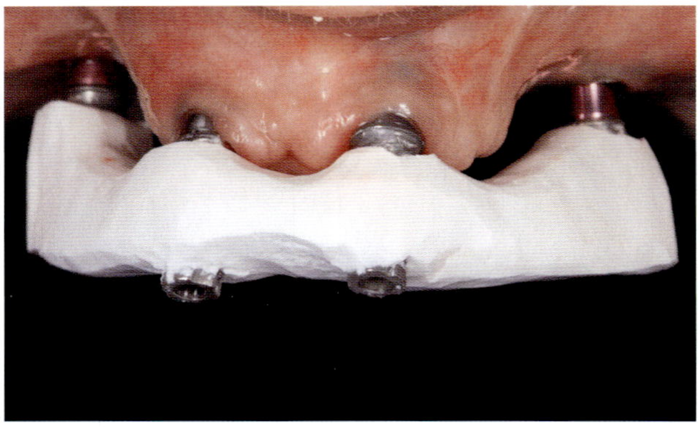

Fig 48 Stone verification index screwed onto the implants.

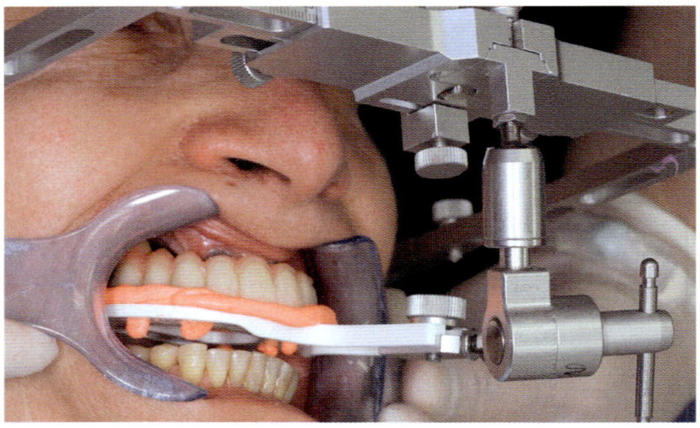

Fig 49 Facebow registration.

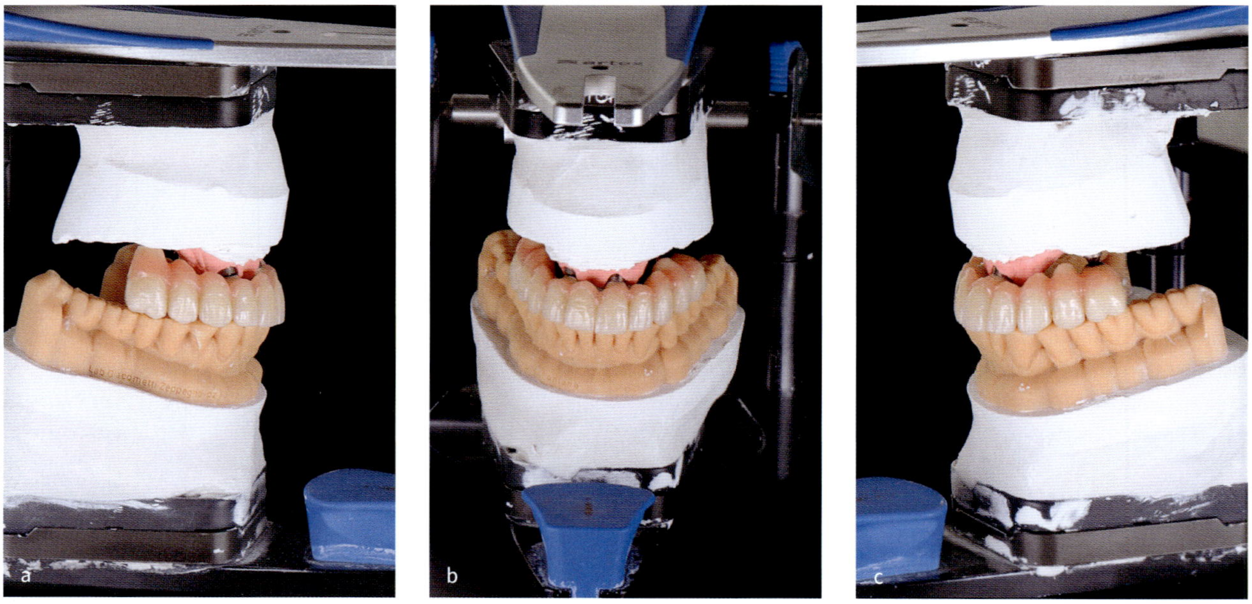

Fig 50a-c Models on the articulator after chairside cross-mounting with the provisional reconstruction.

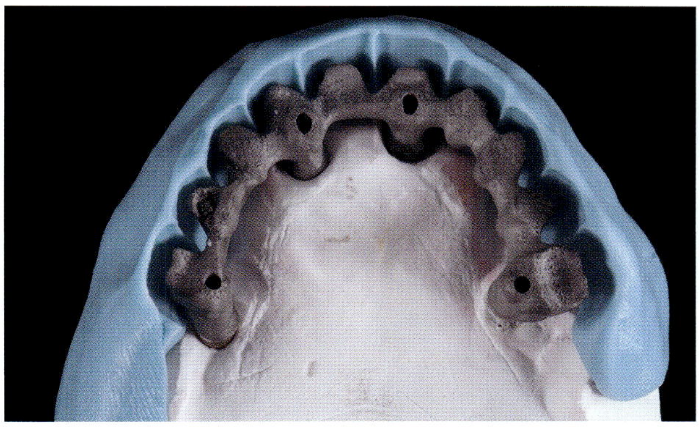

Fig 51 CAD/CAM titanium framework on the cast.

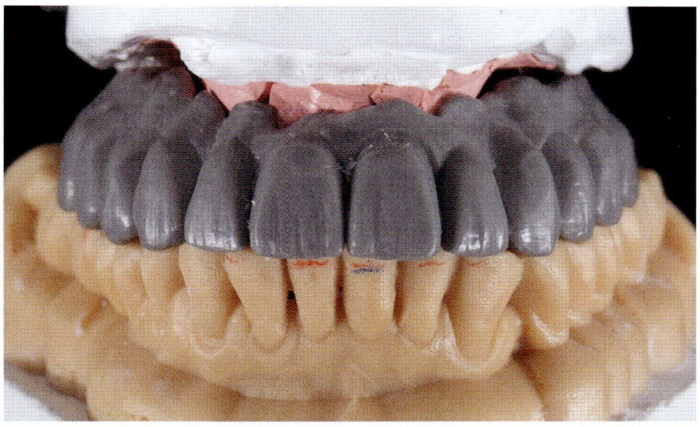

Fig 52 Wax-up of the final reconstruction.

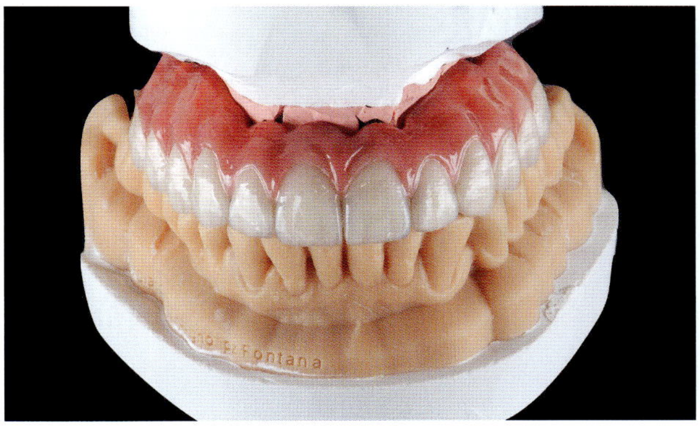

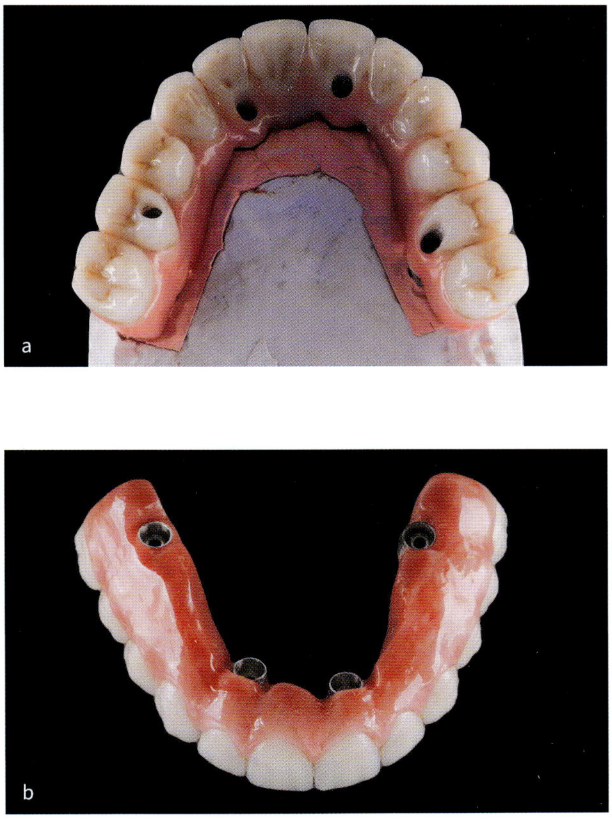

Figs 53 and 54a-b Final restoration before delivery.

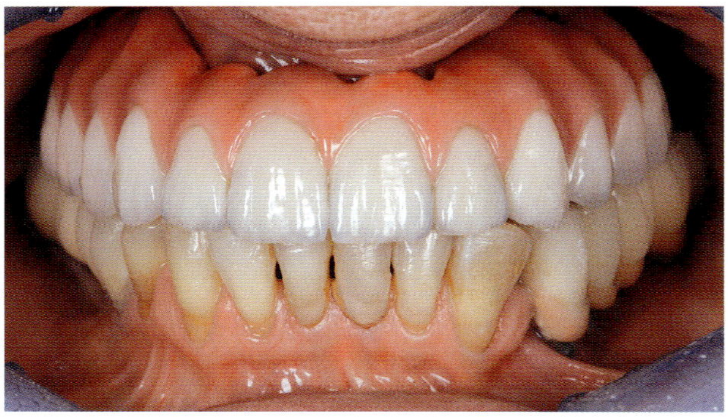

Fig 55 Intraoral view after the delivery of the restoration.

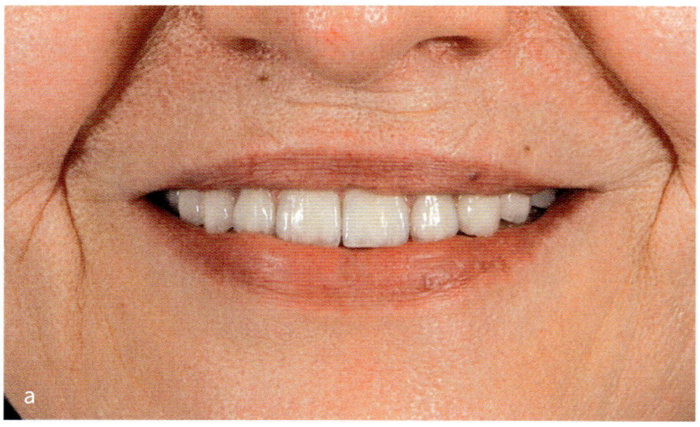

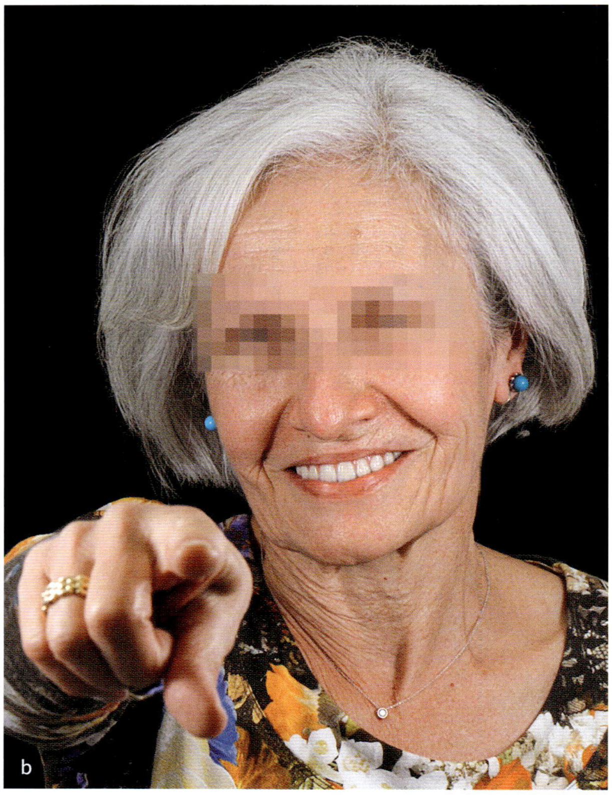

Fig 56a-b Extraoral view after the treatment.

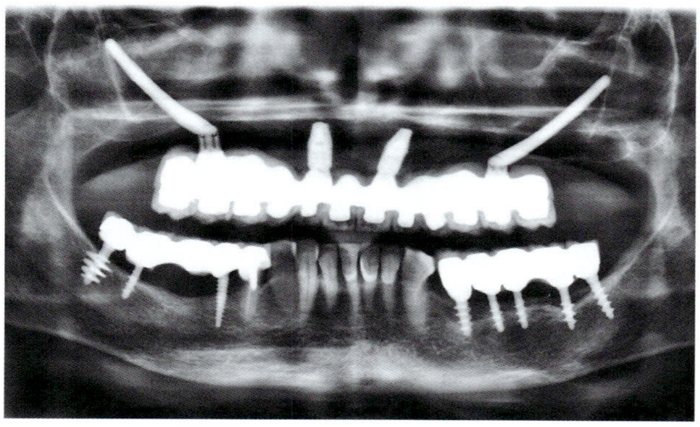

Fig 57 Panoramic radiograph after delivery of the restoration.

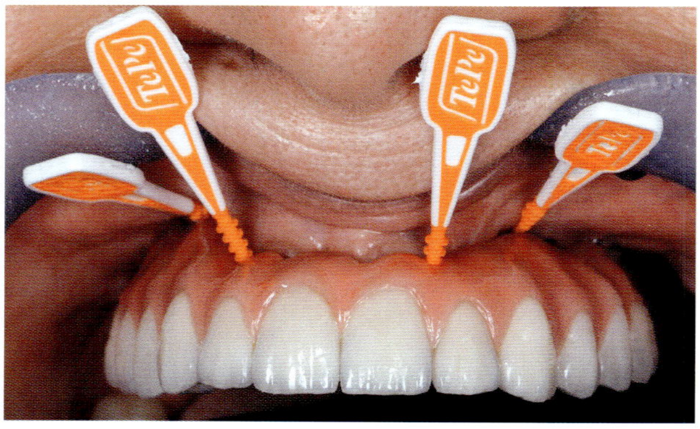

Fig 58 Instructions for the use of interproximal brushes and dental floss.

After removal of the provisional, peri-implant probing depths were recorded to facilitate monitoring. The patient approved the esthetic appearance of the prosthetic restoration, which was tightened to a torque of 15 Ncm. The occlusion was checked and slightly adjusted. The access holes were sealed with PTFE tape and a flowable composite (Figs 55 and 56a-b).

A panoramic radiograph confirmed the exact placement of the restoration (Fig 57).

The patient was given specific oral hygiene instructions, including brushing instructions and guidance on the use of interproximal brushes (Fig 58).

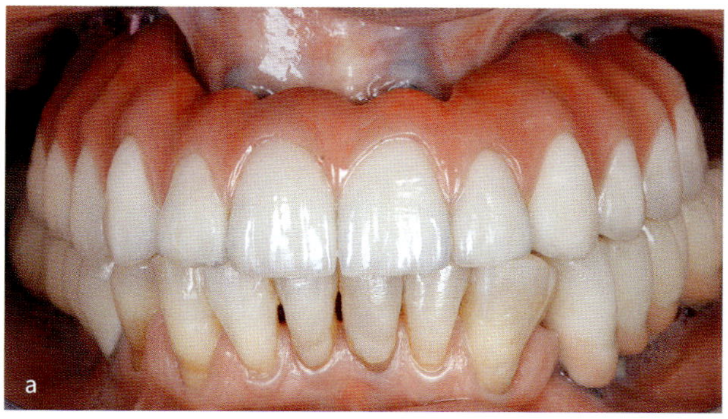

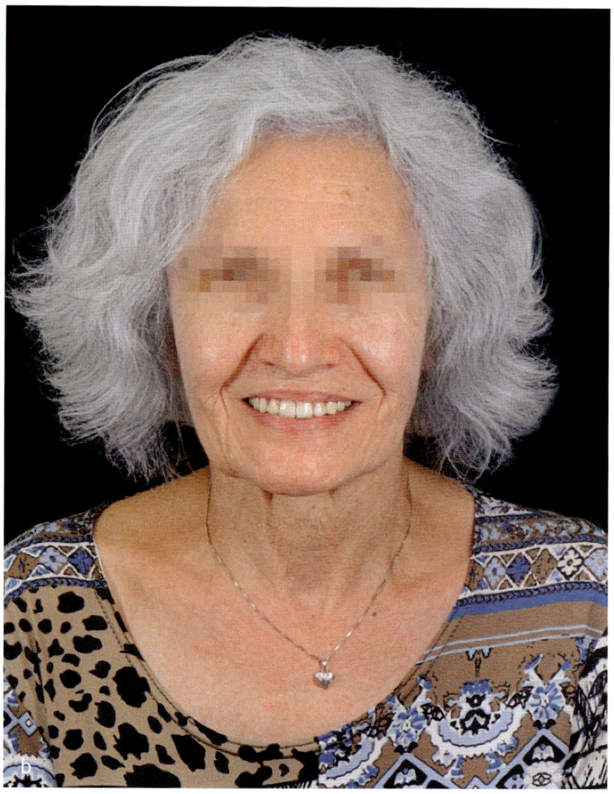

FOLLOW-UP AND PATIENT SATISFACTION

After delivery of the final restoration, the patient was enrolled in a periodic recall system and returned every 4 months for professional tooth cleaning. She continued to demonstrate good oral hygiene.

At 2 years after loading, the prosthesis showed a favorable esthetic appearance and a stable clinical and radiographic situation as well as a precise fit of the prosthetic framework. The patient reported complete satisfaction with the treatment outcome (Figs 59a-b and 60).

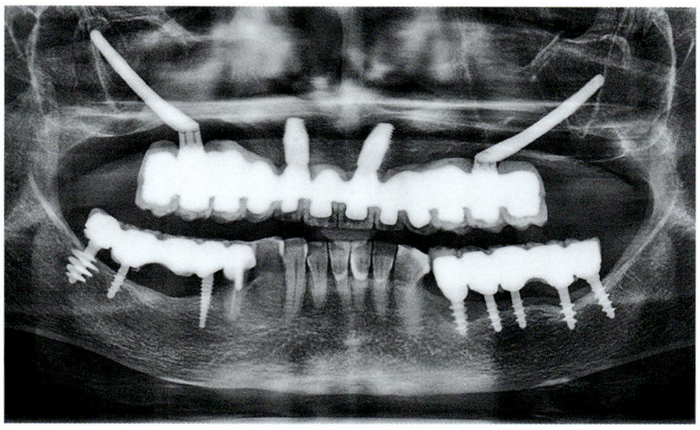

Fig 59a-b and 60 Clinical and radiographic control 2 years after loading.

DISCUSSION

Zygomatic implants to support a fixed dental prosthesis can be considered when other, more conventional treatment modalities are not indicated. In the present case, zygomatic implants were used because no other treatment options were available to achieve a fixed reconstruction.

An advanced degree of atrophy in the posterior maxilla and the presence of scar tissue are indeed contraindications to other reconstructive solutions. Theoretically, an alternative treatment could be represented by bilateral sinus floor and subsequent implants. Actually, bilateral sinus floor elevation and subsequent implants in very atrophic cases does not offer significant advantages and increase the cost of treatment. It is also necessary to consider the need to provide in such an atrophic case, a removable temporary prosthesis for at least 9 months, during sinus graft and then implant integration.

The use of zygomatic implants to support a fixed reconstruction has been well documented, with limited complication rates (Brennand Roper and coworkers 2023; Polido and coworkers 2023).

The 3D position of zygomatic implants, although essentially determined by the anatomy of the zygomatic bone, should also be prosthetically guided to ensure an appropriately designed prosthetic restoration.

Implant-planning software represents a significant advance because it allows verification of the correct position of the implants in the zygomatic bone (avoiding damage to the adjacent anatomical structures) and the planned prosthetic rehabilitation. However, although software can assist in planning the positions of zygomatic implants, the realization of a computer-designed surgical guide remains a challenge.

This limitation can be partially overcome by simulating the implant positions on a 3D-printed stereolithographic model that helps identify anatomical landmarks for precise implant placement in the zygomatic bone. Because zygomatic implants are placed in close proximity to important anatomical structures such as the orbital cavity, the infraorbital nerve, and the infratemporal cavity, incorrect positioning can result in serious complications (Chrcanovic and coworkers 2016). For this reason, zygomatic implants should only be used by highly specialized and skilled surgeons with in-depth knowledge of the facial anatomy.

Since zygomatic implants are used to support a dental prosthesis, the presence of the restorative specialist and, if possible, of the dental technician during the surgical procedure is highly recommended to achieve prosthetically driven 3D implant positions. In particular, this team approach is mandatory when immediate loading of the implants is planned, as in the case reported here, since the prosthetic procedures will begin immediately after implant placement.

Because a fixed restoration supported by zygomatic implants should be limited to highly atrophic cases, there will always be a degree of prosthetic compromise in this type of reconstruction.

The prosthetic design will include a significant amount of pink restorative material to compensate for the horizontal and vertical maxillary atrophy. Similarly, oral hygiene may be difficult, and the cleanability of the prostheses should be facilitated by an appropriate design.

To avoid biological complications around zygomatic implants, oral hygiene should be carefully monitored, and an overdenture option should be considered if the patient's cleaning efforts are inadequate.

If peri-implantitis occurs, there is always a risk of concurrent sinusitis. Due to the dimensions of this type of implant, any contamination of the implant surface can reach the orbital cavity and the superficial layers of cutaneous tissue that cover the zygomatic bone, with an accompanying risk of osteitis and cutaneous fistulas.

ACKNOWLEDGMENTS

Laboratory procedures

Alessandro Giacometti – Genova, Italy

6 Conclusions

S. Wolfart, B. Al-Nawas

Despite considerable progress in dental health worldwide, significant disparities remain, particularly between high-income and low- and middle-income countries. In Western industrialized countries, the prevalence of edentulism has declined sharply, reflecting improvements in access to care and public health policies. However, the burden of tooth loss remains high in many low- and middle-income countries, with 23% of adults aged 60 years and older worldwide being edentulous. At the same time, the demands of these patients for dental restorations and a good oral health-related quality of life have increased significantly.

Dental implants for older and medically compromised patients present unique challenges and increasing demands, particularly for elderly individuals who require high-level masticatory function. These patients often face physiological limitations due to systemic health conditions, bone density loss, or compromised immune systems that can affect implant integration and longevity.

At the same time, many older patients are seeking solutions that offer superior functional and esthetic results. Innovations in digital planning and implantology have significantly improved the safety and precision of treatment, enabling better clinical decision-making and customization of implant solutions. This technology enables clinicians to design customized, patient-specific treatment plans that minimize surgical invasiveness and reduce patient burden, making implant procedures more feasible even for those with compromised health.

In addition, by leveraging the diverse range of dental technologies and expertise available in different countries, state-of-the-art prosthetic and surgical solutions can be implemented, ultimately improving patient outcomes and satisfaction. In the future, this trend toward personalized, minimally invasive care is likely to expand, providing more accessible and durable implant options for older patients with varying health conditions and expectations.

Both fixed, implant-supported dental protheses and removable, implant-supported dentures can improve the function and quality of life compared to complete dentures. Fixed and removable dentures can be recommended to maximize stability, retention, and comfort. Other relevant factors such as speech, esthetic concerns, prosthetic space requirements, cost, stability, retention, maintenance requirements, and manual skills must also be considered when making a clinical decision. The patient's ability to manage the denture and maintain plaque control should be assessed on an ongoing basis (Schimmel and coworkers 2023).

Patients with teeth that are not worth retaining are of particular concern. In these cases, immediate implant placement and immediate restoration allow patients to receive an implant-supported prosthesis without ever having been truly edentulous.

The complex decision-making process for the best possible treatment in the individual patient case is further supported in this ITI Treatment Guide by the introduction of the *patient profile*. This decision-making process is structured by matching the patient profile with appropriate surgical and prosthetic treatment options. In the case presentations, the decision-making processes and the resulting treatment concepts are developed and explained step by step using the patient as an example.

In general, a hybrid workflow (a mixture of analog and digital treatment steps) is used to implement the treatment plan. The ratio of analog to digital techniques varies considerably depending on the clinician and the treatment concept. Most clinical cases have a follow-up of at least 3 years, which provides insight into the good medium-term efficacy and functional efficiency of the different treatment modalities.

The current scientific literature and the clinical cases presented show that implant-prosthetic treatment of the edentulous jaw can significantly improve the oral health-related quality of life of patients. To illustrate this, the clinical cases are linked to patient interviews that vividly illustrate the success of treatment from the patient's perspective.

7 References

References have been listed in the order of (1) the first or only author's last name and (2) the year of publication. Identical short references are distinguished in the text by lowercase letters, which if used are given in parentheses at the end of the respective entry in this list of references.

Digital Object Identifier (DOI) names have been added to the individual references wherever they were available with reasonable effort, to allow readers to check the respective references quickly. For more information, refer to https://www.doi.org. When entering a DOI name in the search field on that site, make sure not to enter the leading "doi:" or the trailing period. You may also access a reference by pointing your browser to https://doi.org/<DOI name>, where <DOI name> should be replaced with the actual DOI name without the leading "doi:" or the trailing period (e.g., "10.1000/xyz123").

Abouleish AE, Vinta SR, Shabot SM, et al. Improving agreement of ASA physical status class between pre-anesthesia screening and day of surgery by adding institutional-specific and ASA-approved examples: a quality improvement project. Perioper Med (Lond). **2020** Nov 19; 9(1): 34. doi: 10.1186/s13741-020-00162-4.

Ahlgren F, Størksen K, Tornes K. A study of 25 zygomatic dental implants with 11 to 49 months' follow-up after loading. Int J Oral Maxillofac Implants. 2006 May–Jun; 21(3): 421–425.

AIWH (Australian Institute of Health and Welfare). Dental health of adults and older adults. **2016**.

Albaker AM. The oral health-related quality of life in edentulous patients treated with conventional complete dentures. Gerodontol. **2013** Mar; 30(1): 61–66. doi: 10.1111/j.1741-2358.2012.00645.x.

Al-Nawas B, Lambert F, Andersen SWM, et al. Group 3 ITI Consensus Report: Materials and antiresorptive drug-associated outcomes in implant dentistry. Clin Oral Implants Res. **2023**; 34 Suppl 26: 169–176. doi: 10.1111/clr.14135.

Andreiotelli M, Att W, Strub JR. Prosthodontic complications with implant overdentures: a systematic literature review. Int J Prosthodont. **2010** May–Jun; 23(3): 195–203.

Aparicio C. A proposed classification for zygomatic implant patient based on the zygoma anatomy guided approach (ZAGA): a cross-sectional survey. Eur J Oral Implantol. **2011** Autumn; 4(3): 269–275.

Aparicio C, López-Piriz R, Albrektsson T. ORIS Criteria of success for the zygoma-related rehabilitation: the (revisited) zygoma success code. Int J Oral Maxillofac Implants. **2020** Mar/Apr; 35(2): 366–378. doi: 10.11607/jomi.7488.

Aparicio C, Polido WD, Zarrinkelk HM. The zygoma anatomy-guided approach for placement of zygomatic implants. Atlas Oral Maxillofac Surg Clin North Am. **2021** Sep; 29(2): 203–231. doi: 10.1016/j.cxom.2021.05.004.

Apaza Alccayhuaman KA, Soto-Peñaloza D, Nakajima Y, Papageorgiou SN, Botticelli D, Lang NP. Biological and technical complications of tilted implants in comparison with straight implants supporting fixed dental prostheses. A systematic review and meta-analysis. Clin Oral Implants Res. **2018** Oct; 29 Suppl 18: 295–308. doi: 10.1111/clr.13279.

Assaf A, Daas M, Boittin A, Eid N, Postaire M. Prosthetic maintenance of different mandibular implant overdentures: A systematic review. J Prosthet Dent. **2017** Aug; 118(2): 144–152.e5 doi: 10.1016/j.prosdent.2016.10.037.

Assunção WG, Barão VA, Delben JA, Gomes EA, Tabata LF. A comparison of patient satisfaction between treatment with conventional complete dentures and overdentures in the elderly: a literature review. Gerodontology. **2010** Jun; 27(2): 154–162. doi: 10.1111/j.1741-2358.2009.00299.x.

Att W, Witkowski S, Strub J. Digital workflow in reconstructive dentistry. Berlin: Quintessence Publishing. **2019**. ISBN: 978-1-78698-025-0.

Bakshi M, Tarnow D, Bittner N. Changes in ridge dimension with pontics immediately placed at extraction sites: A pilot study. Int J Periodontics Restorative Dent. **2018** Jul–Aug; 38(4): 541–547.

Barkarmo S, Longhorn D, Leer K, et al. Biofilm formation on polyetheretherketone and titanium surfaces. Clin Exp Dent Res. **2019** Jun 13; 5(4): 427–437. doi: 10.1002/cre2.205.

Barnett K, Mercer SW, Norbury M, Watt G, Wyke S, Guthrie B. Epidemiology of multimorbidity and implications for health care, research, and medical education: a cross-sectional study. Lancet. **2012** Jul 7; 380(9836): 37–43. doi: 10.1016/S0140-6736(12)60240-2.

Berglundh T, Armitage G, Araújo MG, et al. Peri-implant diseases and conditions: Consensus report of workgroup 4 of the 2017 World Workshop on the Classification of Periodontal and Peri-Implant Diseases and Conditions. J Clin Periodontol. **2018** Jun; 45 Suppl 20: S286–S291. doi: 10.1111/jcpe.12957.

Bernauer SA, Zitzmann NU, Joda T. The complete digital workflow in fixed prosthodontics updated: a systematic review. Healthcare (Basel). **2023** Feb 25; 11(5): 679. doi: 10.3390/healthcare11050679.

Bishti S, Tuna T, Rittich A, Wolfart S. Patient-reported outcome measures (PROMs) of implant-supported reconstructions using digital workflows: A systematic review and meta-analysis. Clin Oral Implants Res. **2021** Oct; 32 Suppl 21: 318–335. doi: 10.1111/clr.13846.

Boboeva O, Kwon TG, Kim JW, Lee ST, Choi SY. Comparing factors affecting dental-implant loss between age groups: A retrospective cohort study. Clin Implant Dent Relat Res. **2021** Apr; 23(2): 208–215. doi: 10.1111/cid.12967.

Borges GA, Barbin T, Dini C, et al. Patient-reported outcome measures and clinical assessment of implant-supported overdentures and fixed prostheses in mandibular edentulous patients: A systematic review and meta-analysis. J Prosthet Dent. **2022** Apr; 127(4): 565–577. doi: 10.1016/j.prosdent.2020.11.005.

Bouhy A, Lamy M, Altaep Y, Lambert F. Maxillary implant overdenture retained by four unsplinted attachments and opposed by a natural or fixed dentition: Five-year clinical outcomes. A prospective case series. Clin Oral Implants Res. **2023** Apr; 34(4): 285–296. doi: 10.1111/clr.14033.

Boven GC, Raghoebar GM, Vissink A, Meijer HJ. Improving masticatory performance, bite force, nutritional state and patient's satisfaction with implant overdentures: a systematic review of the literature. J Oral Rehabil. **2015** Mar; 42(3): 220–233. doi: 10.1111/joor.12241.

Boven GC, Slot JWA, Raghoebar GM, Vissink A, Meijer HJA. Maxillary implant-supported overdentures opposed by (partial) natural dentitions: a 5-year prospective case series study. J Oral Rehabil. **2017** Dec; 44(12): 988–995. doi: 10.1111/joor.12557.

Boven GC, Meijer HJA, Vissink A, Raghoebar GM. Maxillary implant overdentures retained by use of bars or Locator attachments: 1-year findings from a randomized controlled trial. J Prosthodont Res. **2020** Jan; 64(1): 26–33. doi: 10.1016/j.jpor.2019.04.013.

Brandt S, Winter A, Weigl P, Brandt J, Romanos G, Lauer HC. Conical zirconia telescoping into electroformed gold: A retrospective study of prostheses supported by teeth and/or implants. Clin Implant Dent Relat Res. **2019** Apr; 21(2): 317–323. doi: 10.1111/cid.12739.

Brennan M, Houston F, O'Sullivan M, O'Connell B. Patient satisfaction and oral health-related quality of life outcomes of implant overdentures and fixed complete dentures. Int J Oral Maxillofac Implants. **2010** Jul–Aug; 25(4): 791–800.

Brennand Roper M, Vissink A, Dudding T, et al. Long-term treatment outcomes with zygomatic implants: a systematic review and meta-analysis. Int J Implant Dent. **2023** Jul 5; 9(1): 21. doi: 10.1186/s40729-023-00479-x.

Bryant SR, Walton JN, MacEntee MI. A 5-year randomized trial to compare 1 or 2 implants for implant overdentures. J Dent Res. **2015** Jan; 94(1): 36–43. doi: 10.1177/0022034514554224.

Bueno-Samper A, Hernández-Aliaga M, Calvo-Guirado JL. The implant-supported milled bar overdenture: a literature review. Med Oral Patol Oral Cir Bucal. **2010** Mar 1; 15(2): e375–378. doi: 10.4317/medoral.15.e375.

Burns DR, Unger JW, Coffey JP, Waldrop TC, Elswick RK, Jr. Randomized, prospective, clinical evaluation of prosthodontic modalities for mandibular implant overdenture treatment. J Prosthet Dent. **2011** Jul; 106(1): 12–22. doi: 10.1016/S0022-3913(11)60088-7.

Caramês JMM, Vieira FA, Caramês GB, Pinto AC, Francisco HCO, Marques D. Guided bone regeneration in the edentulous atrophic maxilla using deproteinized bovine bone mineral (DBBM) combined with platelet-rich fibrin (PRF) – a prospective study. J Clin Med. **2022** Feb; 11(3): 894. doi: 10.3390/jcm11030894.

Cawood JI, Howell RA. A classification of the edentulous jaws. Int J Oral Maxillofac Surg. **1988** Aug; 17(4): 232–236. doi: 10.1016/s0901-5027(88)80047-x.

CDC (Centers for Disease Control and Prevention). National Center for Health Statistics. **2015;** https://www.cdc.gov/nchs/data/hus/hus15.pdf [accessed 2024 Oct 9]

Çehreli MC, Karasoy D, Kökat AM, Akça K, Eckert SE. Systematic review of prosthetic maintenance requirements for implant-supported overdentures. Int J Oral Maxillofac Implant. **2010** Jan-Feb; 25(1): 163–180.

Chaar MS, Naguib AA, Abd Alsamad AM, Ahmed DF, Abdel Nabi N, Kern M. Vascular and neurosensory evaluation in relation to lingual canal anatomy after mandibular midline implant installation in edentulous patients. Clin Oral Investig. **2022** Mar; 26(3): 3311–3323. doi: 10.1007/s00784-021-04312-w.

Chen J, Cai M, Yang J, Aldhohrah T, Wang Y. Immediate versus early or conventional loading dental implants with fixed prostheses: A systematic review and meta-analysis of randomized controlled clinical trials. J Prosthet Dent. **2019** Dec; 122(6): 516–536. doi: 10.1016/j.prosdent.2019.05.013.

Chmielewski K, Ryncarz W, Yüksel O, et al. Image analysis of immediate full-arch prosthetic rehabilitations guided by a digital workflow: assessment of the discrepancy between planning and execution. Int J Implant Dent. **2019** Jul 15; 5(1): 26. doi: 10.1186/s40729-019-0179-1.

Chrcanovic BR, Albrektsson T, Wennerberg A. Survival and complications of zygomatic implants: an updated systematic review. J Oral Maxillofac Surg. **2016** Oct; 74(10): 1949–1964. doi: 10.1016/j.joms.2016.06.166.

Cordaro L, Torsello F, Ercoli C, Gallucci G. Transition from failing dentition to a fixed implant-supported restoration: a staged approach. Int J Periodontics Restorative Dent. **2007** Oct; 27(5): 481–487.

Cordaro L, Terheyden H. Ridge Augmentation Procedures in Implant Patients: A Staged Approach. In: Chen S, Buser D, Wismeijer D (eds). ITI Treatment Guide, Volume 7. Berlin: Quintessence Publishing, **2014**. ISBN: 978-3-86867-217-6.

Cordioli G, Majzoub Z, Castagna S. Mandibular overdentures anchored to single implants: a five-year prospective study. J Prosthet Dent. **1997** Aug; 78(2): 159–165. doi: 10.1016/s0022-3913(97)70120-3.

Cune M, Burgers M, van Kampen F, de Putter C, van der Bilt A. Mandibular overdentures retained by two implants: 10-year results from a crossover clinical trial comparing ball-socket and bar-clip attachments. Int J Prosthodont. **2010** Jul-Aug; 23(4): 310–317.

Dawson A, Chen S, Buser D, Cordaro L, Martin W, Belser U. The SAC Classification in Implant Dentistry. Berlin: Quintessence Publishing; **2009**. ISBN: 978-1-85097-188-7.

Dawson A, Martin W, Polido W (eds). The SAC Classification in Implant Dentistry. Second edition. Berlin: Quintessence Publishing; **2022**. ISBN: 978-1-78698-110-3.

De Bruyn H, Raes S, Ostman PO, Cosyn J. Immediate loading in partially and completely edentulous jaws: a review of the literature with clinical guidelines. Periodontol 2000. **2014** Oct; 66(1): 153–187. doi: 10.1111/prd.12040.

De Bruyn H, Raes S, Matthys C, Cosyn J. The current use of patient-centered/reported outcomes in implant dentistry: a systematic review. Clin Oral Implants Res. **2015** Sep; 26 Suppl 11: 45–56. doi: 10.1111/clr.12634.

de Resende GP, Jordão LMR, de Souza JAC, Schimmel M, Leles CR. Single versus two-implant mandibular overdentures using early-loaded titanium-zirconium implants with hydrophilic surface and ball attachments: 1-year randomized clinical trial. Clin Oral Implants Res. **2021** Mar; 32(3): 359–368. doi: 10.1111/clr.13707.

de Souza RF, Jabbar AA, Jafarpour D, et al. Single-implant overdentures retained by a novel attachment: A mixed methods crossover randomized clinical trial. JDR Clin Trans Res. **2022** Sep 20: 23800844221124083. doi: 10.1177/23800844221124083.

De Souza AB, Papaspyridakos P, Weber HP, Vazouras K, Matarazzo F. Effect of dental implant therapy on the preservation of orofacial tissues: A systematic review and meta-analysis. Clin Oral Implants Res. **2023** Sep; 34 Suppl 26: 240–256. doi: 10.1111/clr.14106.

Del Fabbro M, Pozzi A, Romeo D, de Araújo Nobre M, Agliardi E. Outcomes of fixed full-arch rehabilitations supported by tilted and axially placed implants: a systematic review and meta-analysis. Int J Oral Maxillofac Implants. **2022** Sep–Oct; 37(5): 1003–1025. doi: 10.11607/jomi.9710.

Derks J, Håkansson J, Wennström JL, Tomasi C, Larsson M, Berglundh T. Effectiveness of implant therapy analyzed in a Swedish population: early and late implant loss. J Dent Res. **2015** Mar; 94(3 Suppl): 44S–51S. 10.1177/0022034514563077.

Derksen W, Joda T, Chantler J, et al. Group 2 ITI Consensus Report: Technological developments in implant prosthetics. Clin Oral Implants Res. **2023** Sep; 34 Suppl 26: 104–111. doi: 10.1111/clr.14148.

Di Francesco F, De Marco G, Gironi Carnevale UA, Lanza M, Lanza A. The number of implants required to support a maxillary overdenture: a systematic review and meta-analysis. J Prosthodont Res. **2019** Jan; 63(1): 15–24. doi: 10.1016/j.jpor.2018.08.006.

Diedrichs G, Rosenhain P. Galvano-Außenteleskope in der direkten Technik. [Galvano-outer telescope by direct technique.] Quintessenz. **1991** Jan; 42(1): 49–56.

Donos N, Asche NV, Akbar AN, et al. Impact of timing of dental implant placement and loading: Summary and consensus statements of group 1—The 6th EAO Consensus Conference 2021. Clin Oral Implants Res. **2021** Oct; 32 Suppl 21: 85–92. doi: 10.1111/clr.13809.

Eccellente T, Piombino M, Piattelli A, D'Alimonte E, Perrotti V, Lezzi G. Immediate loading of dental implants in the edentulous maxilla. Quintessence Int. **2011** Apr; 42(4): 281–289.

Eerdekens L, Schols M, Coelst L, Quirynen M, Naert I. A 5-year prospective study on cone-anchored implants in the edentulous maxilla. Clin Implant Dent Relat Res. **2015** Oct; 17 Suppl 2: e621–e632. doi: 10.1111/cid.12295.

Egido Moreno S, Ayuso Montero R, Schemel Suárez M, et al. Evaluation of the quality of life and satisfaction in patients using complete dentures versus mandibular overdentures. Systematic review and meta-analysis. Clin Exp Dent Res. **2021 Apr**; 7(2): 231–241. doi: 10.1002/cre2.347.

Engels J, Schubert O, Güth JF, et al. Wear behavior of different double-crown systems. Clin Oral Investig. **2013** Mar; 17(2): 503–510. doi: 10.1007/s00784-012-0746-9.

Enkling N, Moazzin R, Geers G, Kokoschka S, Abou-Ayash S, Schimmel M. Clinical outcomes and bone-level alterations around one-piece mini dental implants retaining mandibular overdentures: 5-year follow-up of a prospective cohort study. Clin Oral Implants Res. **2020** Jun; 31(6): 549–556. doi: 10.1111/clr.13591.

Feine JS, Carlsson GE, Awad MA, et al. The McGill consensus statement on overdentures. Mandibular two-implant overdentures as first choice standard of care for edentulous patients. Gerodontol. **2002** Jul; 19(1): 3–4.

Feine JS, Abou-Ayash S, Al Mardini M, et al. Group 3 ITI Consensus Report: Patient-reported outcome measures associated with implant dentistry. Clin Oral Implants Res. **2018** Oct; 29 Suppl 16: 270–275. doi: 10.1111/clr.13299.

Flanagan D, Fisher A, Ciardiello C, et al. A theoretical iteration for predicting the feasibility for immediate functional dental implant loading. J Oral Implantol. **2021** Aug 1; 47(4): 310–317. doi: 10.1563/aaid-joi-D-20-00194.

Fobbe H, Rammelsberg P, Lorenzo Bermejo J, Kappel S. The up-to-11-year survival and success of implants and abutment teeth under solely implant-supported and combined tooth-implant-supported double crown-retained removable dentures. Clin Oral Implants Res. **2019** Nov; 30(11): 1134–1141. doi: 10.1111/clr.13527.

Fonteyne E, Van Doorne L, Becue L, Matthys C, Bronckhorst E, De Bruyn H. Speech evaluation during maxillary mini-dental implant overdenture treatment: A prospective study. J Oral Rehabil. **2019** Dec; 46(12): 1151–1160. doi: 10.1111/joor.12852.

Friedrichsen M, Dirksen D, Runte C. In vitro measurement of the retention force of two stud attachment systems during cyclic load. J Prosthodont. **2023** Feb. doi: 10.1111/jopr.13665. Online ahead of print.

Fu L, Liu G, Wu X, Zhu Z, Sun H, Xia H. Patient-reported outcome measures of edentulous patients restored with single-implant mandibular overdentures: A systematic review. J Oral Rehabil. **2021** Jan; 48(1): 81–94. doi: 10.1111/joor.13103.

Gallucci G, Morton D, Weber HP. Loading protocols for dental implants in edentulous patients. Int J Oral Maxillofac Implants. **2009**; 24: 132–146.

Gallucci GO, Benic GI, Eckert SE, Papaspyridakos P, Schimmel M, Schrott A, Weber HP. Consensus statements and clinical recommendations for implant loading protocols. Int J Oral Maxillofac Implants. **2014**; 29 Suppl: 287–290. doi: 10.11607/jomi.2013.g4.

Gallucci GO, Avrampou M, Taylor JC, Elpers J, Thalji G, Cooper LF. Maxillary implant-supported fixed prosthesis: a survey of reviews and key variables for treatment planning. Int J Oral Maxillofac Implants. **2016**; 31 Suppl: s192–s197. doi: 10.11607/jomi.16suppl.g5.3.

GBD 2017 Oral Disorders Collaborators; Bernabe E, Marcenes W, Hernandez CR, et al. Global, regional, and national levels and trends in burden of oral conditions from 1990 to 2017: a systematic analysis for the global burden of disease 2017 study. J Dent Res. **2020** Apr; 99(4): 362–373. doi: 10.1177/0022034520908533.

Gonçalves GSY, de Magalhães KMF, Rocha EP, Dos Santos PH, Assunção WG. Oral health-related quality of life and satisfaction in edentulous patients rehabilitated with implant-supported full dentures all-on-four concept: a systematic review. Clin Oral Investig. **2022** Jan; 26(1): 83–94. doi: 10.1007/s00784-021-04213-y.

Gotfredsen K, Hosseini M, Rimborg S, Özhayat E. Patient's perception of timing concepts in implant dentistry: A systematic review. Clin Oral Implants Res. **2021** Oct; 32 Suppl 21: 67–84. doi: 10.1111/clr.13861.

Gross D. Ethik in der Zahnmedizin. Ein praxisorientiertes Lehrbuch mit 20 kommentierten klinischen Fällen. [Ethics in dentistry. A practice-oriented textbook with 20 commented clinical cases.] Berlin: Quintessenz Publishing; **2012**. ISBN 978-3-86867-104-9.

Guarda GB, Correr AB, Gonçalves LS, et al. Effects of surface treatments, thermocycling, and cyclic loading on the bond strength of a resin cement bonded to a lithium disilicate glass ceramic. Oper Dent. **2013** Mar–Apr; 38(2): 208–217. doi: 10.2341/11-076-L.

Hahnel S, Wieser A, Lang R, Rosentritt M. Biofilm formation on the surface of modern implant abutment materials. Clin Oral Implants Res. **2015** Nov; 26(11): 1297–1301. doi: 10.1111/clr.12454.

Hartmann R, Bandeira ACFM, Araújo SC, Brägger U, Schimmel M, Leles CR. A parallel 3-group randomised clinical trial comparing different implant treatment options for the edentulous mandible: 1-year effects on dental patient-reported outcomes and chewing function. J Oral Rehabil. **2020** Oct; 47(10): 1264–1277. doi: 10.1111/joor.13070.

Hauck KE, Trentin MS, Skiba THI, Shibli JA, De Carli JP. Clinical and satisfaction outcomes of using one or two dental implants for mandibular overdentures: preliminary short-term follow-up of a randomized clinical trial. Int J Implant Dent. **2021** Feb 11; 7(1): 10. doi: 10.1186/s40729-020-00286-8.

Heimes D, Becker P, Pabst A, et al. How does dental implant macrogeometry affect primary implant stability? A narrative review. Int J Implant Dent. **2023** Jul 5; 9(1): 20. doi: 10.1186/s40729-023-00485-z.

Heitz-Mayfield LJA, Salvi GE, Mombelli A, et al. Supportive peri-implant therapy following anti-infective surgical peri-implantitis treatment: 5-year survival and success. Clin Oral Implants Res. **2018** Jan; 29(1): 1–6. doi: 10.1111/clr.12910.

Heitz-Mayfield LJ, Aaboe M, Araújo M, et al. Group 4 ITI Consensus Report: Risks and biologic complications associated with implant dentistry. Clin Oral Implants Res. **2018** Oct; 29 Suppl 16: 351–358. doi: 10.1111/clr.13307.

Heitz-Mayfield LJA, Heitz F, Lang NP. Implant Disease Risk Assessment IDRA—a tool for preventing peri-implant disease. Clin Oral Implants Res. **2020** Apr; 31(4): 397–403. doi: 10.1111/clr.13585.

Heydecke G, Boudrias P, Awad MA, De Albuquerque RF, Lund JP, Feine JS. Within-subject comparisons of maxillary fixed and removable implant prostheses: Patient satisfaction and choice of prosthesis. Clin Oral Implants Res. **2003** Feb; 14(1): 125–130. doi: 10.1034/j.1600-0501.2003.140117.x.

Heydecke G, Zwahlen M, Nicol A, et al. What is the optimal number of implants for fixed reconstructions: a systematic review. Clin Oral Implants Res. **2012** Oct; 23 Suppl 6: 217–228. doi: 10.1111/j.1600-0501.2012.02548.x.

Jamjoom FZ, Aldghim A, Aldibasi O, Yilmaz B. Impact of intraoral scanner, scanning strategy, and scanned arch on the scan accuracy of edentulous arches: an in vitro study. J Prosthet Dent. **2024** Jun; 131(6): 1218

Jin HY, Teng MH, Wang ZJ, et al. Comparative evaluation of BioHPP and titanium as a framework veneered with composite resin for implant-supported fixed dental prostheses. J Prosthet Dent. **2019** Oct; 122(4): 383–388. doi: 10.1016/j.prosdent.2019.03.003.

Joda T, Zarone F, Ferrari M. The complete digital workflow in fixed prosthodontics: a systematic review. BMC Oral Health. **2017** Sep 19; 17(1): 124. doi: 10.1186/s12903-017-0415-0.

Jokstad A, Ganeles J. Systematic review of clinical and patient-reported outcomes following oral rehabilitation on dental implants with a tapered compared to a non-tapered implant design. Clin Oral Implants Res. **2018** Oct; 29 Suppl 16: 41–54. doi: 10.1111/clr.13128.

Jordan AR, Micheelis W, eds. Fünfte Deutsche Mundgesundheitsstudie (DMS V). (IDZ) IdDZ, ed; No. Material enreihe Band 35. Köln: Deutscher Zahnärzte Verlag DÄV; **2016.** ISBN 978-3-7691-0020-4.

Jordan AR, Meyer-Lückel H, Kuhr K, Sasunna D, Bekes K, Schiffner U. Karieserfahrung und Versorgung in Deutschland: Ergebnisse der 6. Deutschen Mundgesundheitsstudie (DMS • 6). DZZ **2025** Apr;80(2):90–100.

Jung RE, Al-Nawas B, Araújo M, et al. Group 1 ITI Consensus Report: The influence of implant length and design and medications on clinical and patient-reported outcomes. Clin Oral Implants Res. **2018** Oct; 29 Suppl 16: 69–77. doi: 10.1111/clr.13342.

Kamperos G, Zambara I, Petsinis V, Zambaras D. The impact of buccal bone defects and immediate placement on the esthetic outcome of maxillary anterior single-tooth implants. J Oral Implantol. **2016** Aug; 42(4): 337–341. doi: 10.1563/aaid-joi-D-16-00004.

Kassolis JD, Scheper M, Jham B, Reynolds MA. Histopathologic findings in bone from edentulous alveolar ridges: a role in osteonecrosis of the jaws? Bone. **2010** Jul; 47(1): 127–130. doi: 10.1016/j.bone.2010.04.588.

Katsuyama H, Storgård Jensen S. Sinus Floor Elevation Procedures. In: Chen S, Buser D, Wismeijer D (eds). ITI Treatment Guide, Volume 5. Berlin: Quintessence Publishing, **2011**. ISBN: 978-3-938947-18-0.

Kern JS, Kern T, Wolfart S, Heussen N. A systematic review and meta-analysis of removable and fixed implant-supported prostheses in edentulous jaws: post-loading implant loss. Clin Oral Implants Res. **2016** Feb; 27(2): 174–195. doi: 10.1111/clr.12531.

Kern M, Att W, Fritzer E, et al. Survival and complications of single dental implants in the edentulous mandible following immediate or delayed loading: A randomized controlled clinical trial. J Dent Res. **2018** Feb; 97(2): 163–170. doi: 10.1177/0022034517736063.

Kern M, Wolfart S, Heydecke G, Witkowski S, Türp JC, Strub JR. Curriculum Prothetik III. Kombinierte und abnehmbare Prothetik | Implantologie | Nachsorge | Lebensqualität. 5th, revised ed. Berlin: Quintessence Publishing; **2022**. ISBN 978-3-86867-575-7.

Khaohoen A, Powcharoen W, Sornsuwan T, Chaijareenont P, Rungsiyakull C, Rungsiyakull P. Accuracy of implant placement with computer-aided static, dynamic, and robot-assisted surgery: a systematic review and meta-analysis of clinical trials. BMC Oral Health. **2024** Mar 21; 24(1): 359. doi: 10.1186/s12903-024-04033-y.

Kim HY, Lee JY, Shin SW, Bryant SR. Attachment systems for mandibular implant overdentures: a systematic review. J Adv Prosthodont. **2012** Nov; 4(4): 197–203. doi: 10.4047/jap.2012.4.4.197.

Kim HJ, Karasan D, Park K, Kwon HB, Han JS, Lee JH. Abutment margin levels and residual cement occurrence in cement-retained implant restorations: An observational study. Clin Oral Implants Res. **2023**; 34(1): 33–41.

Kuoppala R, Näpänkangas R, Raustia A. Quality of life of patients treated with implant-supported mandibular overdentures evaluated with the oral health impact profile (OHIP-14): a survey of 58 patients. J Oral Maxillofac Res. **2013** Jul 1; 4(2): e4. doi: 10.5037/jomr.2013.4204.

La Monaca G, Pranno N, Annibali S, Di Carlo S, Pompa G, Cristalli MP. Immediate flapless full-arch rehabilitation of edentulous jaws on 4 or 6 implants according to the prosthetic-driven planning and guided implant surgery: a retrospective study on clinical and radiographic outcomes up to 10 years of follow-up. Clin Implant Dent Relat Res. **2022** Dec; 24(6): 831–844. doi: 10.1111/cid.13134.

Landes CA, Paffrath C, Koehler C, Thai VD, Stübinger S, Sader R, Lauer HC, Piwowarczyk A. Zygoma implants for midfacial prosthetic rehabilitation using telescopes: 9-year follow-up. Int J Prosthodont. **2009** Jan–Feb; 22(1): 20–32.

Lang NP, Zitzmann NU, Working Group 3 of the VEWoP. Clinical research in implant dentistry: evaluation of implant-supported restorations, aesthetic and patient-reported outcomes. J Clin Periodontol. **2012** Feb; 39 Suppl 12: 133–138. doi: 10.1111/j.1600-051X.2011.01842.x.

Leles CR, Dias DR, Nogueira TE, McKenna G, Schimmel M, Jordão LMR. Impact of patient characteristics on edentulous subjects' preferences for prosthodontic rehabilitation with implants. Clin Oral Implants Res. **2019** Mar; 30(3): 285–292. doi: 10.1111/clr.13414.

Leles CR, de Paula MS, Curado TFF, et al. Flapped versus flapless surgery and delayed versus immediate loading for a four mini implant mandibular overdenture: A RCT on post-surgical symptoms and short-term clinical outcomes. Clin Oral Implants Res. **2022** Sep; 33(9): 953–964. doi: 10.1111/clr.13974.

Lemos CAA, Verri FR, Cruz RS, Gomes JML, Dos Santos DM, Goiato MC, Pellizzer EP. Comparison between flapless and open-flap implant placement: a systematic review and meta-analysis. Int J Oral Maxillofac Surg. **2020** Sep; 49(9): 1220–1231. doi: 10.1016/j.ijom.2018.04.002.

Lin GH, Chan HL, Wang HL. The significance of keratinized mucosa on implant health: a systematic review. J Periodontol. **2013** Dec; 84(12): 1755–1767. doi: 10.1902/jop.2013.120688.

Lo Russo L. Edentulous scan strategy – designed for optimal scan experience of edentulous patients with 3Shape TRIOS. A 3Shape publication. **2020**; https://www.3shape.com/en/news/2020/get-your-edentulous-intraoral-scanning-protocol.

Maló P, de Araújo Nobre M, Lopes A, Ferro A, Gravito I. Immediate loading of implants placed in patients with untreated periodontal disease: a 5-year prospective cohort study. Eur J Oral Implantol. **2014** Autumn; 7(3): 295–304.

Maló P, de Araújo Nobre M, Lopes A, Ferro A, Nunes M. The All-on-4 concept for full-arch rehabilitation of the edentulous maxillae: A longitudinal study with 5–13 years of follow-up. Clin Implant Dent Relat Res. **2019** Aug; 21(4): 538–549. doi: 10.1111/cid.12771.

Maló P, de Araújo Nobre M, Lopes A, Ferro A, Botto J. The All-on-4 treatment concept for the rehabilitation of the completely edentulous mandible: A longitudinal study with 10 to 18 years of follow-up. Clin Implant Dent Relat Res. **2019** Aug; 21(4): 565–577. doi: 10.1111/cid.12769.

McGrath C, Lam O, Lang N. An evidence-based review of patient-reported outcome measures in dental implant research among dentate subjects. J Clin Periodontol. **2012** Feb; 39 Suppl 12: 193–201. doi: 10.1111/j.1600-051X.2011.01841.x.

McKenna GJ, Gjengedal H, Harkin J, Holland N, Moore C, Srinivasan M. Effect of autogenous bone graft site on dental implant survival and donor site complications: a systematic review and meta-analysis. J Evid Based Dent Pract. **2022** Sep; 22(3): 101731. doi: 10.1016/j.jebdp.2022.101731.

Mehl C, Harder S, Shahriari A, Steiner M, Kern M. Influence of abutment height and thermocycling on retrievability of cemented implant-supported crowns. Int J Oral Maxillofac Implants. **2012** Sep–Oct; 27(5): 1106–1115.

Meijer HJ, Raghoebar GM, Batenburg RH, Visser A, Vissink A. Mandibular overdentures supported by two or four endosseous implants: a 10-year clinical trial. Clin Oral Implants Res. **2009** Jul; 20(7): 722–728. doi: 10.1111/j.1600-0501.2009.01710.x.

Menees TS, Lawson NC, Beck PR, Burgess JO. Influence of particle abrasion or hydrofluoric acid etching on lithium disilicate flexural strength. J Prosthet Dent. **2014** Nov; 112(5): 1164–1170. doi: 10.1016/j.prosdent.2014.04.021.

Mertens C, Steveling HG. Implant-supported fixed prostheses in the edentulous maxilla: 8-year prospective results. Clin Oral Implants Res. **2011** May; 22(5): 464–472. doi: 10.1111/j.1600-0501.2010.02028.x.

Messias A, Karasan D, Nicolau P, Pjetursson BE, Guerra F. Rehabilitation of full-arch edentulism with fixed or removable dentures retained by root-form dental implants: A systematic review of outcomes and outcome measures used in clinical research in the last 10 years. J Clin Periodontol. **2023** May; 50 Suppl 25: 38–54. doi: 10.1111/jcpe.13616.

Micheelis W, Schiffner U, eds. Vierte Deutsche Mundgesundheitsstudie (DMS IV). Ergebnisse zu oralen Erkrankungsprävalenzen, Risikogruppen und zum zahnärztlichen Versorgungsgrad in Deutschland 2005. (IDZ) IdDZ, ed; Materialienreihe Band 31. Köln: Deutscher Zahnärzte Verlag DÄV; **2006.** ISBN 978-3-934280-94-6.

Mijiritsky E, Ben Zaken H, Shacham M, Cinar IC, Tore C, Nagy K, Ganz SD. Variety of surgical guides and protocols for bone reduction prior to implant placement: a narrative review. Int J Environ Res Public Health. **2021** Feb 27; 18(5): 2341. doi: 10.3390/ijerph18052341.

Miller SC. Textbook of periodontia (oral medicine). Philadelphia: Blakiston's Son, **1938**.

Misch CE. Bone density: a key determinant for treatment planning. (Chapter 11.) In: Misch CE (ed.) Dental implant prosthetics (2nd ed.). St. Louis, MO: Elsevier Mosby, **2015**. ISBN 978-0-323-07845-0.

Mishra SK, Chowdhary R. Patient's oral health-related quality of life and satisfaction with implant supported overdentures—a systematic review. J Oral Biol Craniofac Res. **2019** Oct–Dec; 9(4): 340–346. doi: 10.1016/j.jobcr.2019.07.004.

Mori G, Oda Y, Sakamoto K, Ito T, Yajima Y. Clinical evaluation of full-arch screw-retained implant-supported fixed prostheses and full-arch telescopic-retained implant-supported fixed prostheses: A 5–12 year follow-up retrospective study. Clin Oral Implants Res. **2019** Mar; 30(3): 197–205. doi: 10.1111/clr.13406.

Morton D, Chen ST, Martin WC, Levine RA, Buser D. Consensus statement and recommended clinical procedures regarding optimizing esthetic outcomes in implant dentistry. Int J Oral Maxillofacial Implants. **2014**; 29 (Suppl): 216–220. doi: 10.11607/jomi.2013.g3.

Morton D, Gallucci G, Lin WS, et al. Group 2 ITI Consensus Report: Prosthodontics and implant dentistry. Clin Oral Implants Res. **2018** Oct; 29 Suppl 16: 215–223. doi: 10.1111/clr.13298.

Mosnegutu A, Wismeijer D, Geraets W. Implant-supported mandibular overdentures can minimize mandibular bone resorption in edentulous patients: results of a long-term radiologic evaluation. Int J Oral Maxillofac Implants. **2015** Nov–Dec; 30(6): 1378–1386. doi: 10.11607/jomi.4009.

Müller F, Barter S. Implant Therapy in the Geriatric Patient. In: Wismeijer D, Chen S, Buser D (eds). ITI Treatment Guide, Volume 9. Berlin: Quintessence Publishing, **2016**. ISBN: 978-3-86867-311-1.

Naert I, Alsaadi G, Quirynen M. Prosthetic aspects and patient satisfaction with two-implant-retained mandibular overdentures: a 10-year randomized clinical study. Int J Prosthodont. **2004** Jul-Aug; 17(4): 401–410.

Naert I, Alsaadi G, van Steenberghe D, Quirynen M. A 10-year randomized clinical trial on the influence of splinted and unsplinted oral implants retaining mandibular overdentures: peri-implant outcome. Int J Oral Maxillofac Implant. **2004** Sep–Oct; 19(5): 695–702.

Nevins M. Periodontal prosthesis reconsidered. Int J Prosthodont **1993**; 6: 209–217. doi: 10.11607/prd.3496.

Nomiyama LM, Matumoto EK, Corrêa MG, et al. Comparison between flapless-guided and conventional surgery for implant placement: a 12-month randomized clinical trial. Clin Oral Investig. **2023** Apr;27(4): 1665–1679. doi: 10.1007/s00784-022-04793-3. Erratum in: Clin Oral Investig. **2023** Jun; 27(6): 3285. doi: 10.1007/s00784-023-05045-8.

Okawa M, Yamazaki R, Yamamoto K. Clinical application of the plane system. In: Duarte S (ed.), Quintessence of Dental Technology 2019. (QDT Yearbook vol. 42.) **2019**. 81–104. ISBN: 978-0-86715-816-8.

Papaspyridakos P, Chen CJ, Chuang SK, Weber HP, Gallucci GO. A systematic review of biologic and technical complications with fixed implant rehabilitations for edentulous patients. Int J Oral Maxillofac Implant. **2012** Jan-Feb; 27(1): 102–110.

Papaspyridakos P, Mokti M, Chen CJ, Benic GI, Gallucci GO, Chronopoulos V. Implant and prosthodontic survival rates with implant fixed complete dental prostheses in the edentulous mandible after at least 5 years: a systematic review. Clin Implant Dent Relat Res. **2014** Oct; 16(5): 705–717. doi: 10.1111/cid.12036. (**a**)

Papaspyridakos P, Chen CJ, Chuang SK, Weber HP. Implant loading protocols for edentulous patients with fixed prostheses: a systematic review and meta-analysis. Int J Oral Maxillofac Implants. **2014**; 29 Suppl: 256–270. doi: 10.11607/jomi.2014suppl.g4.3. (**b**)

Paratelli A, Perrone G, Ortega R, Gómez-Polo M. Polyetheretherketone in implant prosthodontics: A scoping review. Int J Prosthodont. **2020** Nov–Dec; 33(6): 671–679. doi: 10.11607/ijp.6649.

Park JH, Shin SW, Lee JY. Bar versus ball attachments for maxillary four-implant retained overdentures: a randomized controlled trial. Clin Oral Implants Res. **2019** Nov; 30(11): 1076–1084. doi: 10.1111/clr.13521.

Passia N, Kern M. The single midline implant in the edentulous mandible-current status of clinical trials. J Clin Med. **2023** May 31; 12(11): 3773. doi: 10.3390/jcm12113773.

Passia N, Abou-Ayash S, Reissmann DR, et al. Single mandibular implant study (SMIS) — masticatory performance — results from a randomized clinical trial using two different loading protocols. J Dent. **2017** Oct; 65: 64–69. doi: 10.1016/j.jdent.2017.07.005.

Passia N, Att W, Freitag-Wolf S, et al. Single mandibular implant study (SMIS)—denture satisfaction in the elderly. J Oral Rehabil. **2017** Mar; 44(3): 213–219. doi: 10.1111/joor.12473.

Passia N, Wolfart S, Kern M. Ten-year clinical outcome of single implant-retained mandibular overdentures—a prospective pilot study. J Dent. **2019** Mar; 82: 63–65. doi: 10.1016/j.jdent.2019.01.006.

Passia N, Oberbillig F, Goulioumis V, Naumova EA, Kern M, Arnold W. Three-dimensional reconstruction of the genial spinal canal. Clin Anat. **2020** Oct; 33(7): 1102–1108. doi: 10.1002/ca.23512.

Passia N, Chaar MS, Krummel A, et al. Influence of the number of implants in the edentulous mandible on chewing efficacy and oral health-related quality of life—A within-subject design study. Clin Oral Implants Res. **2022** Oct; 33(10): 1030–1037. doi: 10.1111/clr.13984.

Pawlowski J, Beczinski J, Stege H, et al. Bridging the gaps: management of lichen planus subtypes in a joint dermatology-oral surgery clinic. Clin Exp Dermatol. **2023** Dec 19; 49(1): 18–25. doi: 10.1093/ced/llad335.

Payne AG, Alsabeeha NH, Atieh MA, Esposito M, Ma S, Anas El-Wegoud M. Interventions for replacing missing teeth: attachment systems for implant overdentures in edentulous jaws. Cochrane Database Syst Rev. **2018** Oct 11; 10(10): CD008001. doi: 10.1002/14651858.CD008001.pub2.

Pieralli S, Kohal RJ, Rabel K, von Stein-Lausnitz M, Vach K, Spies BC. Clinical outcomes of partial and full-arch all-ceramic implant-supported fixed dental prostheses. A systematic review and meta-analysis. Clin Oral Implants Res. **2018** Oct; 29 Suppl 18: 224–236. doi: 10.1111/clr.13345.

Pieri F, Aldini NN, Fini M, Marchetti C, Corinaldesi G. Immediate functional loading of dental implants supporting a bar-retained maxillary overdenture: preliminary 12-month results. J Periodontol. **2009** Nov; 80(11): 1883–1893. doi: 10.1902/jop.2009.090227.

Pitts N, Amaechi B, Niederman R, et al. Global oral health inequalities: dental caries task group—research agenda. Adv Dent Res. **2011** May; 23(2): 211–220. doi: 10.1177/0022034511402016.

Pjetursson BE, Sailer I, Latyshev A, Rabel K, Kohal RJ, Karasan D. A systematic review and meta-analysis evaluating the survival, the failure, and the complication rates of veneered and monolithic all-ceramic implant-supported single crowns. Clin Oral Implants Res. **2021** Oct; 32 Suppl 21: 254–288. doi: 10.1111/clr.13863.

Poli PP, Manfredini M, Maiorana C, Salina FE, Beretta M. Correlation between accuracy in computer-guided implantology and peri-implant tissue stability: a prospective clinical and radiological pilot study. J Clin Med. **2023** Aug 3; 12(15): 5098. doi: 10.3390/jcm12155098.

Polido WD, Aghaloo T, Emmett TW, Taylor TD, Morton D. Number of implants placed for complete-arch fixed prostheses: A systematic review and meta-analysis. Clin Oral Implants Res. **2018** Oct; 29 Suppl 16: 154–183. doi: 10.1111/clr.13312.

Polido WD, Machado-Fernandez A, Lin WS, Aghaloo T. Indications for zygomatic implants: a systematic review. Int J Implant Dent. **2023** Jul 1; 9(1): 17. doi: 10.1186/s40729-023-00480-4.

Pommer B, Mailath-Pokorny G, Haas R, Busenlechner D, Fürhauser R, Watzek G. Patients' preferences towards minimally invasive treatment alternatives for implant rehabilitation of edentulous jaws. Eur J Oral Implantol. **2014** Summer; 7 Suppl 2: S91–S109.

Prasad S, Faverani LP, Santiago Junior JF, Sukotjo C, Yuan JC. Attachment systems for mandibular implant-supported overdentures: a systematic review and meta-analysis of randomized controlled trials. J Prosthet Dent. **2024** Aug; 132(2): 354–368. doi: 10.1016/j.prosdent.2022.08.004.

Raghoebar GM, Vissink A, Reintsema H, Batenburg RH. Bone grafting of the floor of the maxillary sinus for the placement of endosseous implants. Br J Oral Maxillofac Surg. **1997** Apr; 35(2): 119–125. doi: 10.1016/s0266-4356(97)90687-2.

Raghoebar GM, Meijer HJ, Slot W, Slater JJ, Vissink A. A systematic review of implant-supported overdentures in the edentulous maxilla, compared to the mandible: how many implants? Eur J Oral Implantol. **2014**; 7 Suppl 2: S191–S201.

Raghoebar GM, Onclin P, Boven GC, Vissink A, Meijer HJA. Long-term effectiveness of maxillary sinus floor augmentation: A systematic review and meta-analysis. J Clin Periodontol. **2019** Jun; 46 Suppl 21: 307–318. doi: 10.1111/jcpe.13055.

Rammelsberg P, Bernhart G, Lorenzo Bermejo J, Schmitter M, Schwarz S. Prognosis of implants and abutment teeth under combined tooth-implant-supported and solely implant-supported double-crown-retained removable dental prostheses. Clin Oral Implants Res. **2014** Jul; 25(7): 813–818. doi: 10.1111/clr.12197.

Ravidà A, Vera RM, Saleh M, et al. The correlation between history of periodontitis according to staging and grading and the prevalence/severity of peri-implantitis in patients enrolled in maintenance therapy. J Periodontol. **2021** Nov; 92(11): 1522–1535. doi: 10.1002/JPER.21-0012.

Raymond CWW, John SPL, Islam I. The role of finite element analysis in studying potential failure of mandibular reconstruction methods. In: Radostina P (ed). Perusal of the finite element method. Rijeka: IntechOpen; **2016**: Ch. 8.

Rentsch-Kollar A, Huber S, Mericske-Stern R. Mandibular implant overdentures followed for over 10 years: patient compliance and prosthetic maintenance. Int J Prosthodont. **2010** Mar–Apr; 23(2): 91–98.

Richter EJ. Prothetik im Unterkiefer. In-vivo-Messungen zur Unterkieferdeformation und Konsequenzen für implantatverankerte Suprastrukturen. ["Prostheses in the mandible. The in-vivo measurements of mandibular deformation and the consequences for implant-anchored suprastructures."]. Schweiz Monatsschr Zahnmed. **1999**; 109(2): 116–134.

Rinke S, Buergers R, Ziebolz D, Roediger M. Clinical outcome of double crown-retained implant overdentures with zirconia primary crowns. J Adv Prosthodont. **2015** Aug; 7(4): 329–337. doi: 10.4047/jap.2015.7.4.329.

Roccuzzo M, Grasso G, Dalmasso P. Keratinized mucosa around implants in partially edentulous posterior mandible: 10-year results of a prospective comparative study. Clin Oral Implants Res. **2016** Apr; 27(4): 491–496. doi: 10.1111/clr.12563.

Roccuzzo M, Bonino F, Gaudioso L, Zwahlen M, Meijer HJ. What is the optimal number of implants for removable reconstructions? A systematic review on implant-supported overdentures. Clin Oral Implants Res. **2012** Oct; 23 Suppl 6: 229–237. doi: 10.1111/j.1600-0501.2012.02544.x.

Römer P, Heimes D, Pabst A, Becker P, Thiem DGE, Kämmerer PW. Bleeding disorders in implant dentistry: a narrative review and a treatment guide. Int J Implant Dent. **2022** Apr 16; 8(1): 20. doi: 10.1186/s40729-022-00418-2.

Rosentritt M, Preis V, Behr M, Sereno N, Kolbeck C. Shear bond strength between veneering composite and PEEK after different surface modifications. Clin Oral Investig. **2015** Apr; 19(3): 739–744. doi: 10.1007/s00784-014-1294-2.

Saavedra G, Ariki EK, Federico CD, et al. Effect of acid neutralization and mechanical cycling on the microtensile bond strength of glass-ceramic inlays. Oper Dent. **2009** Mar–Apr; 34(2): 211–216. doi: 10.2341/08-68.

Sadowsky SJ, Zitzmann NU. Protocols for the maxillary implant overdenture: a systematic review. Int J Oral Maxillofac Implants. **2016**; 31 Suppl: s182–s191. doi: 10.11607/jomi.16suppl.g5.2.

Sailer I, Mühlemann S, Zwahlen M, Hämmerle CH, Schneider D. Cemented and screw-retained implant reconstructions: a systematic review of the survival and complication rates. Clin Oral Implants Res. **2012** Oct; 23 Suppl 6: 163–201. doi: 10.1111/j.1600-0501.2012.02538.x.

Salvi GE, Brown CE, Fujihashi K, et al. Inflammatory mediators of the terminal dentition in adult and early onset periodontitis. J Periodontal Res. **1998** May; 33(4): 212–225. doi: 10.1111/j.1600-0765.1998.tb02193.x.

Sanz M, Schwarz F, Herrera D, et al. Importance of keratinized mucosa around dental implants: Consensus report of group 1 of the DGI/SEPA/Osteology Workshop. Clin Oral Implants Res. **2022** Jun; 33 Suppl 23: 47–55. doi: 10.1111/clr.13956.

Schenk N, Bukvic H, Schimmel M, Abou-Ayash S, Enkling N. One-piece mini dental implant-retained mandibular overdentures: 10-year clinical and radiological outcomes of a non-comparative longitudinal observational study. J Funct Biomater. **2024** Apr 11; 15(4): 99. doi: 10.3390/jfb15040099.

Scherer MD, Ingel AP, Rathi N. Flapped or flapless surgery for narrow-diameter implant placement for overdentures: advantages, disadvantages, indications, and clinical rationale. Int J Periodontics Restorative Dent. **2014**; 34 Suppl 3: s89–95. doi: 10.11607/prd.1581.

Schiegnitz E, Al-Nawas B. Narrow-diameter implants: A systematic review and meta-analysis. Clin Oral Implants Res. **2018** Oct; 29 Suppl 16: 21–40. doi: 10.1111/clr.13272.

Schimmel M, Srinivasan M, Herrmann F, Müller F. Loading protocols for implant-supported overdentures in the edentulous jaw: a systematic review and meta-analysis. Int J Oral Maxillofac Implants. **2014**; 29: 271–286. doi: 10.11607/jomi.2014suppl.g4.4.

Schimmel M, Walther M, Al-Haj Husain N, Igarashi K, Wittneben J, Abou-Ayash S. Retention forces between primary and secondary CAD/CAM manufactured telescopic crowns: an in vitro comparison of common material combinations. Clin Oral Investig. **2021** Nov; 25(11): 6297–6307. doi: 10.1007/s00784-021-03928-2.

Schimmel M, Araujo M, Abou-Ayash S, et al. Group 4 ITI Consensus Report: Patient benefits following implant treatment in partially and fully edentulous patients. Clin Oral Implants Res. **2023** Sep; 34 Suppl 26: 257–265. doi: 10.1111/clr.14145.

Schlee M, Esposito M. Aesthetic and patient preference using a bone substitute to preserve extraction sockets under pontics. A cross-sectional survey. Eur J Oral Implantol. **2009** Autumn; 2(3): 209–217.

Schrott AR, Jimenez M, Hwang JW, Fiorellini J, Weber HP. Five-year evaluation of the influence of keratinized mucosa on peri-implant soft-tissue health and stability around implants supporting full-arch mandibular fixed prostheses. Clin Oral Implants Res. **2009** Oct; 20(10): 1170–1177. doi: 10.1111/j.1600-0501.2009.01795.x.

Schubert O, Reitmaier J, Schweiger J, Erdelt K, Güth JF. Retentive force of PEEK secondary crowns on zirconia primary crowns over time. Clin Oral Investig. 2019 May; 23(5): 2331–2338. doi: 10.1007/s00784-018-2657-x.

Schwarz S, Bernhart G, Hassel AJ, Rammelsberg P. Survival of double-crown-retained dentures either tooth-implant or solely implant-supported: an 8-year retrospective study. Clin Implant Dent Relat Res. **2014** Aug; 16(4): 618–625. doi: 10.1111/cid.12023.

Schwindling FS, Deisenhofer UK, Séché AC, Lehmann F, Rammelsberg P, Stober T. Randomized trial investigating zirconia electroplated telescopic retainers: quality of life outcomes. Clin Oral Investig. **2017** May; 21(4): 1157–1163. doi: 10.1007/s00784-016-1869-1. (**a**)

Schwindling FS, Lehmann F, Terebesi S, Corcodel N, Zenthöfer A, Rammelsberg P, Stober T. Electroplated telescopic retainers with zirconia primary crowns: 3-year results from a randomized clinical trial. Clin Oral Investig. **2017** Dec; 21(9): 2653–2660. doi: 10.1007/s00784-017-2067-5. (**b**)

Serino G, Strom C. Peri-implantitis in partially edentulous patients: association with inadequate plaque control. Clin Oral Implants Res. **2009** Jan; 20(2): 169–174. doi: 10.1111/clr.14015.

Sharka R, Abed H, Hector M. Oral health-related quality of life and satisfaction of edentulous patients using conventional complete dentures and implant-retained overdentures: An umbrella systematic review. Gerodontology. **2019** Sep; 36(3): 195–204. doi: 10.1111/ger.12399.

Slot W, Raghoebar GM, van Dijk G, Meijer HJ. Attachment of clips in a bar-retained maxillary implant overdenture: a clinical report. J Prosthet Dent. **2012** Jun; 107(6): 353–357. doi: 10.1016/S0022-3913(12)60088-2.

Slot W, Raghoebar GM, Vissink A, Meijer HJ. Maxillary overdentures supported by four or six implants in the anterior region; 1-year results from a randomized controlled trial. J Clin Periodontol. **2013** Mar; 40(3): 303–310. doi: 10.1111/jcpe.12051.

Slot W, Raghoebar GM, Cune MS, Vissink A, Meijer HJ. Maxillary overdentures supported by four or six implants in the anterior region: 5-year results from a randomized controlled trial. J Clin Periodontol. **2016** Dec; 43(12): 1180–1187. doi: 10.1111/jcpe.12625.

Slot W, Raghoebar GM, Cune MS, Vissink A, Meijer HJA. Four or six implants in the maxillary posterior region to support an overdenture: 5-year results from a randomized controlled trial. Clin Oral Implants Res. **2019** Feb; 30(2): 169–177. doi: 10.1111/clr.13403.

Slot W, Raghoebar GM, Cune MS, Vissink A, Meijer HJA. Maxillary bar overdentures on four or six posterior implants: 10-year results from a randomized clinical trial. Clin Oral Implants Res. **2022** Nov; 33(11): 1147–1156. doi: 10.1111/clr.13997.

Slot W, Raghoebar GM, Cune MS, Vissink A, Meijer HJA. Maxillary overdentures supported by four or six implants in the anterior region: 10-year randomized controlled trial results. J Clin Periodontol. **2023** Jan; 50(1): 36–44. doi: 10.1111/jcpe.13726.

Srinivasan M, Kamnoedboon P, Angst L, Müller F. Oral function in completely edentulous patients rehabilitated with implant-supported dental prostheses: a systematic review and meta-analysis. Clin Oral Implants Res. **2023** Sep; 34 Suppl 26: 196–239. doi: 10.1111/clr.14068.

Stefanini M, Barootchi S, Sangiorgi M, et al. Do soft tissue augmentation techniques provide stable and favorable peri-implant conditions in the medium and long term? A systematic review. Clin Oral Implants Res. **2023** Sep; 34 Suppl 26: 28–42. doi: 10.1111/clr.14150.

Stoker GT, Wismeijer D. Immediate loading of two implants with a mandibular implant-retained overdenture: a new treatment protocol. Clin Implant Dent Relat Res. **2011** Dec; 13(4): 255–261. doi: 10.1111/j.1708-8208.2009.00210.x.

Tahmaseb A, Wu V, Wismeijer D, Coucke W, Evans C. The accuracy of static computer-aided implant surgery: a systematic review and meta-analysis. Clin Oral Implants Res. **2018** Oct; 29 Suppl 16: 416–435. doi: 10.1111/clr.13346.

Tallgren A. The continuing reduction of the residual alveolar ridges in complete denture wearers: a mixed-longitudinal study covering 25 years. J Prosthet Dent. **1972** Feb; 27(2): 120–32. doi: 10.1016/0022-3913(72)90188-6.

Terheyden H. Augmentation Surgery. Biologic Principles | Surgical Techniques | Clinical Challenges. Berlin: Quintessence Publishing; **2022**. ISBN: 978-1-78698-113-4.

Testori T, Tavelli L, Scaini R, et al. How to avoid intraoperative and postoperative complications in maxillary sinus elevation. Periodontol 2000. **2023** Jun; 92(1): 299–328. doi: 10.1111/prd.12480.

Thoma DS, Naenni N, Figuero E, Hämmerle CHF, Schwarz F, Jung RE, Sanz-Sánchez I. Effects of soft tissue augmentation procedures on peri-implant health or disease: a systematic review and meta-analysis. Clin Oral Implants Res. **2018** Mar; 29 Suppl 15: 32–49. doi: 10.1111/clr.13114.

Thomason JM, Heydecke G, Feine JS, Ellis JS. How do patients perceive the benefit of reconstructive dentistry with regard to oral health-related quality of life and patient satisfaction? A systematic review. Clin Oral Implants Res. **2007** Jun; 18 Suppl 3: 168–188. doi: 10.1111/j.1600-0501.2007.01461.x.

Thomason JM, Kelly SA, Bendkowski A, Ellis JS. Two implant retained overdentures—a review of the literature supporting the McGill and York consensus statements. J Dent. **2012** Jan; 40(1): 22–34. doi: 10.1016/j.jdent.2011.08.017.

Thongpoung S, Masaki C, Nodai T, et al. A new mandibular deformation index predicts amount of bone deformation in edentulous patients treated with an implant-supported fixed prosthesis. J Prosthodont Res. **2022** Oct 7; 66(4): 582–588. doi: 10.2186/jpr.JPR_D_21_00145.

Tonellini G, Saez Vigo R, Novelli G. Double guided surgery in All-on-4 concept: When ostectomy is needed. Int J Dent. **2018** Feb 4; 2018: 2672549. doi: 10.1155/2018/2672549.

Tonetti MS, Greenwell H, Kornman KS. Staging and grading of periodontitis: Framework and proposal of a new classification and case definition. J Periodontol. **2018**; 89(Suppl 1): S159–S172. doi: 10.1002/JPER.18-0006.

Troeltzsch M, Troeltzsch M, Kauffmann P, et al. Clinical efficacy of grafting materials in alveolar ridge augmentation: a systematic review. J Craniomaxillofac Surg. **2016** Oct; 44(10): 1618–1629. doi: 10.1016/j.jcms.2016.07.028.

Tsigarida A, Chochlidakis K. A comparison between fixed and removable mandibular implant-supported full-arch prostheses: an overview of systematic reviews. Int J Prosthodont. **2021**; 34: s85-s92. doi: 10.11607/ijp.6911.

Tuna T, Kuhlmann L, Bishti S, Sirazitdinova E, Deserno T, Wolfart S. Removal of simulated biofilm at different implant crown designs with interproximal oral hygiene aids: An in vitro study. Clin Oral Implants Res. **2019** Jul; 30(7): 627–636. doi: 10.1111/clr.13448.

Tuna T, Setlaoui S, Bussmeier F, Wolfart S. Statisch navigierte Implantationsschablonen im zahnlosen Kiefer im digitalen Workflow. [Statically navigated implant surgical guides in the edentulous jaw in the digital workflow.] Implantologie. **2024;** 32(4): 397–411.

Turrentine FE, Wang H, Simpson VB, Jones RS. Surgical risk factors, morbidity, and mortality in elderly patients. J Am Coll Surg. **2006** Dec; 203(6): 865–877. doi: 10.1016/j.jamcollsurg.2006.08.026.

Van den Borre C, Rinaldi M, De Neef B, et al. Patient- and clinician-reported outcomes for the additively manufactured sub-periosteal jaw implant (AMSJI) in the maxilla: a prospective multicentre one-year follow-up study. Int J Oral Maxillofac Surg. **2022** Feb; 51(2): 243–250. doi: 10.1016/j.ijom.2021.05.015.

Vi S, Pham D, Du YYM, Arora H, Tadakamadla SK. Mini-implant-retained overdentures for the rehabilitation of completely edentulous maxillae: a systematic review and meta-analysis. Int J Environ Res Public Health. **2021** Apr 20; 18(8): 4377. doi: 10.3390/ijerph18084377.

Walton JN, Glick N, Macentee MI. A randomized clinical trial comparing patient satisfaction and prosthetic outcomes with mandibular overdentures retained by one or two implants. Int J Prosthodont. **2009** Jul–Aug; 22(4): 331–339.

Weigl P, Lauer HC. Advanced biomaterials used for a new telescopic retainer for removable dentures. J Biomed Mater Res. **2000**; 53(4): 337–347. doi: 10.1002/1097-4636(2000)53: 4<337::aid-jbm7>3.0.co;2-7.

Weigl P, Hahn L, Lauer HC. Advanced biomaterials used for a new telescopic retainer for removable dentures. J Biomed Mater Res. **2000**; 53(4): 320–336. doi: 10.1002/1097-4636(2000)53: 4<320::aid-jbm6>3.0.co;2-w.

WHO, Oral Health Factsheet, **2023** Mar; https://www.who.int/news-room/fact-sheets/detail/oral-health [accessed 2024 Oct 9]

Wirz J, Hoffmann A, eds. Galvanoprothetik. Neue Wege zum biologischen Zahnersatz. Berlin: Quintessence Publishing; **1999**. ISBN 978-3-87652-486-3.

Wirz J, Jäger K. Galvanoteleskope. Präzise, einfach und klinisch bewährt. [Galvano-telescopes. Precise, simple and clinically proven.] Quintessenz. **1998**; 49(3): 283–292.

Wismeijer D, van Waas MA, Vermeeren J. Overdentures supported by ITI implants: a 6.5-year evaluation of patient satisfaction and prosthetic aftercare. Int J Oral Maxillofac Implants. **1995** Nov-Dec;10(6):744–749.

Wismeijer D. The Breda implant overdenture study: an evaluation of clinical and radiological conditions, satisfaction and cost effectiveness in patients treated with mandibular overdentures on ITI implants. Dissertation. **1996**. ISBN 90-9009963-8.

Wismeijer D, van Waas MA, Vermeeren J, Mulder J, Kalk W. Patient satisfaction with implant-supported mandibular overdentures. A comparison of three treatment strategies with ITI-dental implants. Int J Oral Maxillofac Surg. **1997** Aug;26(4):263–267. doi: 10.1016/s0901-5027(97)80864-8.

Wismeijer D, van Waas MA, Mulder J, Vermeeren J, Kalk W. Clinical and radiological results of patients treated with three treatment modalities for overdentures on implants of the ITI Dental Implant System. A randomized controlled clinical trial. Clin Oral Implants Res. **1999** Aug;10(4):297–306. doi: 10.1034/j.1600-0501.1999.100406.x.

Wismeijer D, Joda T, Flugge T, et al. Group 5 ITI Consensus Report: Digital technologies. Clin Oral Implants Res. **2018** Oct; 29 Suppl 16: 436–442. doi: 10.1111/clr.13309.

Wolfart S. Implant prosthodontics: A patient-oriented strategy. Berlin: Quintessence Publishing; **2016**. ISBN: 978-1-85097-282-2.

Wolfart S. Implantatprothetik—ein patientenorientiertes Konzept. 2 ed. Berlin: Quintessence Publishing; **2023**. ISBN 978-3-86867-608-2.

Yao CJ, Cao C, Bornstein MM, Mattheos N. Patient-reported outcome measures of edentulous patients restored with implant-supported removable and fixed prostheses: A systematic review. Clin Oral Implants Res. **2018** Oct; 29 Suppl 16: 241–254. doi: 10.1111/clr.13286.

Zanetti EM, Pascoletti G, Calì M, Bignardi C, Franceschini G. Clinical assessment of dental implant stability during follow-up: what is actually measured, and perspectives. Biosensors (Basel). **2018** Jul 13; 8(3): 68. doi: 10.3390/bios8030068.

Zembic A, Wismeijer D. Patient-reported outcomes of maxillary implant-supported overdentures compared with conventional dentures. Clin Oral Implants Res. **2014** Apr; 25(4): 441–450. doi: 10.1111/clr.12169.

Zembic A, Tahmaseb A, Wismeijer D. Within-subject comparison of maxillary implant-supported overdentures with and without palatal coverage. Clin Implant Dent Relat Res. **2015** Jun; 17(3): 570–579. doi: 10.1111/cid.12125.

Zembic A, Tahmaseb A, Jung RE, Wiedemeier D, Wismeijer D. Patient-reported outcomes of maxillary edentulous patients wearing overdentures retained by two implants from insertion to 4 years. Int J Oral Maxillofac Implant. **2019** Mar–Apr; 34(2): 481–488. doi: 10.11607/jomi.6980.

Zhang XX, Shi JY, Gu YX, Lai HC. Long-term outcomes of early loading of straumann implant-supported fixed segmented bridgeworks in edentulous maxillae: a 10-year prospective study. Clin Implant Dent Relat Res. **2016** Dec; 18(6): 1227–1237. doi: 10.1111/cid.12420

Zitzmann NU, Marinello CP. Treatment plan for restoring the edentulous maxilla with implant-supported restorations: Removable overdenture versus fixed partial denture design. J Prosthet Dent **1999**; 82: 188–196. doi: 10.1016/s0022-3913(99)70155-1.

Zou D, Wu Y, Huang W, et al. A 3-year prospective clinical study of telescopic crown, bar, and Locator attachments for removable four implant-supported maxillary overdentures. Int J Prosthodont. **2013** Nov-Dez; 26(6): 566–573. doi: 10.11607/ijp.3485.

Zygogiannis K, Wismeijer D, Aartman IH, Osman RB. A systematic review on immediate loading of implants used to support overdentures opposed by conventional prostheses: factors that might influence clinical outcomes. Int J Oral Maxillofac Implant. **2016** Jan–Feb; 31(1): 63–72. doi: 10.11607/jomi.4028.